# Nutrition and Metabolism of The Surgical Patient, Part I

*Guest Editors*

STANLEY J. DUDRICK, MD, FACS
JUAN A. SANCHEZ, MD, MPA, FACS

# SURGICAL CLINICS OF NORTH AMERICA

www.surgical.theclinics.com

*Consulting Editor*
RONALD F. MARTIN, MD

June 2011 • Volume 91 • Number 3

SAUNDERS an imprint of ELSEVIER, Inc.

**W.B. SAUNDERS COMPANY**

*A Division of Elsevier Inc.*

1600 John F. Kennedy Blvd., Suite 1800, Philadelphia, PA 19103-2899

http://www.surgical.theclinics.com

**SURGICAL CLINICS OF NORTH AMERICA Volume 91, Number 3**
**June 2011 ISSN 0039–6109, ISBN-13: 978-1-4557-7993-2**

Editor: John Vassallo, j.vassallo@elsevier.com
Developmental Editor: Teia Stone

*Surgical Clinics of North America* (ISSN 0039–6109) is published bimonthly by Elsevier Inc., 360 Park Avenue South, New York, NY 10010-1710. Months of publication are February, April, June, August, October, and December. Business and Editorial Offices: 1600 John F. Kennedy Blvd., Suite 1800, Philadelphia, PA 19103-2899. Periodicals postage paid at New York, NY and additional mailing offices. Subscription prices are $311.00 per year for US individuals, $532.00 per year for US institutions, $152.00 per year for US students and residents, $381.00 per year for Canadian individuals, $661.00 per year for Canadian institutions, $429.00 for international individuals, $661.00 per year for international institutions and $210.00 per year for Canadian and foreign students/residents. To receive student/resident rate, orders must be accompanied by name of affiliated institution, date of term, and the *signature* of program/residency coordinator on institution letterhead. Orders will be billed at individual rate until proof of status is received. Foreign air speed delivery is included in all *Clinics* subscription prices. All prices are subject to change without notice. POSTMASTER: Send address changes to *Surgical Clinics*, Elsevier Health Sciences Division, Subscription Customer Service, 3251 Riverport Lane, Maryland Heights, MO 63043. **Customer Service (orders, claims, online, change of address): Telephone: 1-800-654-2452 (U.S. and Canada); 314-447-8871 (outside U.S. and Canada). Fax: 314-447-8029. E-mail: journalscustomerservice-usa@elsevier.com (for print support); journalsonline support-usa@elsevier.com (for online support).**

*Reprints.* For copies of 100 or more, of articles in this publication, please contact the Commercial Reprints Department, Elsevier Inc., 360 Park Avenue South, New York, New York 10010-1710. Tel. (212) 633-3812, Fax: (212) 462-1935, e-mail: reprints@elsevier.com.

The *Surgical Clinics of North America* is also published in Spanish by McGraw-Hill Interamericana Editores S.A., P.O. Box 5-237 06500 Mexico D.F. Mexico; and in Portuguese by Interlivros Edicoes Ltda., Rua Comandante Coelho 1085, CEP 21250, Rio de Janeiro, Brazil; and in Greek by Paschalidis Medical Publications, Athens Greece.

The *Surgical Clinics of North America* is covered in *MEDLINE/PubMed (Index Medicus), EMBASE/Excerpta Medica, Current Contents/Clinical Medicine, Current Contents/Life Sciences, Science Citation Index,* and *ISI/BIOMED.*

Printed and bound by CPI Group (UK) Ltd, Croydon, CR0 4YY

Transferred to Digital Print 2011

# Contributors

## CONSULTING EDITOR

**RONALD F. MARTIN, MD**
Staff Surgeon, Department of Surgery, Marshfield Clinic, Marshfield, Wisconsin; Clinical Associate Professor, University of Wisconsin School of Medicine and Public Health, Madison, Wisconsin; Colonel, Medical Corps, United States Army Reserve

## GUEST EDITORS

**STANLEY J. DUDRICK, MD, FACS**
Professor of Surgery, Department of Surgery, Yale University School of Medicine, New Haven, Connecticut; Chairman and Program Director Emeritus, Department of Surgery, Saint Mary's Hospital/Yale Affiliate, Waterbury, Connecticut

**JUAN A. SANCHEZ, MD, FACS**
Chairman and Program Director, Department of Surgery, Saint Mary's Hospital, Waterbury, Connecticut

## AUTHORS

**ROBERT H. BARTLETT, MD**
Professor Emeritus, Department of Surgery, University of Michigan, Ann Arbor, Michigan

**GEORGE L. BLACKBURN, MD, PhD**
S. Daniel Abraham Associate Professor of Nutrition, Associate Director, Division of Nutrition, Harvard Medical School, Center for the Study of Nutrition Medicine, Department of Surgery, Beth Israel Deaconess Medical Center, Boston, Massachusetts

**LUDWIK K. BRANSKI, MD**
Shriners Hospitals for Children and University of Texas Medical Branch, Galveston, Texas

**IMAD BTAICHE, PharmD**
Clinical Associate Professor, Department of Pharmacy, College of Pharmacy, University of Michigan, Ann Arbor, Michigan

**RONALD E. DECHERT, PhD**
Director, Metabolic Laboratory, University of Michigan; Department of Surgery, University of Michigan Hospitals, Ann Arbor, Michigan

**STANLEY J. DUDRICK, MD, FACS**
Professor of Surgery, Department of Surgery, Yale University School of Medicine, New Haven, Connecticut; Chairman and Program Director Emeritus, Department of Surgery, Saint Mary's Hospital/Yale Affiliate, Waterbury, Connecticut

**ERICA M. FALLON, MD**
Pediatric Surgery Research Fellow, The Vascular Biology Program, Department of Surgery, Children's Hospital Boston, Boston, Massachusetts

**JOSEF E. FISCHER, MD, FACS**
William V. McDermott Professor of Surgery, Harvard Medical School, Boston, Massachusetts

**RICHARD HERMAN, MD**
Clinical Lecturer, Section of Critical Care, Division of Pediatric Surgery, Mott Children's Hospital, University of Michigan, Ann Arbor, Michigan

**DAVID N. HERNDON, MD**
Professor, Department of Surgery and Pediatrics, Jesse H. Jones Distinguished Chair in Burn Surgery, University of Texas Medical Branch, Chief of Staff and Director of Research, Shriners Hospitals for Children Galveston, Galveston, Texas

**MARC G. JESCHKE, MD, PhD**
Ross Tilley Burn Centre, Sunnybrook Health Sciences Centre, and Department of Surgery, Division of Plastic Surgery, University of Toronto, Toronto, Canada

**ANDREW J. KERWIN, MD**
Associate Professor of Surgery, Division Chief, Acute Care Surgery, Department of Surgery, University of Florida College of Medicine Jacksonville; Trauma Medical Director, Shands Jacksonville, Jacksonville, Florida

**RIFAT LATIFI, MD, FACS**
Professor of Surgery, Trauma Division, Department of Surgery, University of Arizona, Tucson, Arizona; Director, Trauma Services, Hamad General Hospital, Hamad Medical Corporation, Doha, Qatar

**DAVID F. MERCER, MD, PhD**
Assistant Professor, Division of Transplantation, Department of Surgery, University of Nebraska Medical Center, Omaha, Nebraska

**DEEPIKA NEHRA, MD**
Pediatric Surgery Research Fellow, The Vascular Biology Program, Department of Surgery, Children's Hospital Boston, Boston, Massachusetts

**MICHAEL S. NUSSBAUM, MD**
Surgeon-in-Chief, Shands Jacksonville; Professor and Chair, Department of Surgery, University of Florida College of Medicine Jacksonville, Jacksonville, Florida

**JAMES PAUL O'NEILL, MD, MRCSI, MBA, MMSc, ORL-HNS**
Head and Neck Surgical Fellow, Department of Head and Neck Surgery, Memorial Sloan Kettering Cancer Center, New York, New York

**J. ALEXANDER PALESTY, MD, FACS**
Assistant Clinical Professor of Surgery, Department of Surgery, University of Connecticut School of Medicine, Farmington, Connecticut; Director of Surgical Oncology, Department of Surgery, Saint Mary's Hospital/Yale Affiliate, Waterbury, Connecticut

**JOSE MARIO PIMIENTO, MD**
Fellow in Surgical Oncology, Moffitt Cancer Center & Research Institute, Tampa, Florida

**MARK PUDER, MD, PhD**
The Vascular Biology Program, Department of Surgery, Associate in Surgery, Children's Hospital Boston; Associate Professor, Harvard Medical School, Boston, Massachusetts

**FEDJA A. ROCHLING, MB, BCh**
Assistant Professor, Division of Gastroenterology and Hepatology, Department of Medicine, University of Nebraska Medical Center, Omaha, Nebraska

**WILLIAM P. SCHECTER, MD**
Professor of Surgery, Department of Surgery, University of California San Francisco, San Francisco General Hospital, San Francisco, California

**ASHOK R. SHAHA, MD, FACS**
Professor of Surgery, Department of Head and Neck Surgery, Memorial Sloan Kettering Cancer Center, New York, New York

**DANIEL H. TEITELBAUM, MD**
Professor of Surgery, Division of Pediatric Surgery, Mott Children's Hospital, University of Michigan, Ann Arbor, Michigan

**JON S. THOMPSON, MD**
Division of General Surgery, Department of Surgery, University of Nebraska Medical Center, Omaha, Nebraska

**REBECCA WESEMAN, RD**
Medical Nutrition Education, University of Nebraska Medical Center, Omaha, Nebraska

**FELICIA N. WILLIAMS, MD**
Shriners Hospitals for Children and University of Texas Medical Branch, Galveston, Texas

# Contents

Metabolic changes after surgery, trauma, or serious illness have a complex pathophysiology. The early posttraumatic stress response is physiologic and associated with a state of hyperinflammation, increased oxygen consumption, and increased energy expenditure. These are part of a systemic reaction that encompasses a wide range of endocrinological, immunologic, and hematological effects. Surgery initiates changes in metabolism that can affect virtually all organs and tissues; the metabolic response results in hormone-mediated mobilization of endogenous substrates that leads to stress catabolism. Hypercatabolism has been associated with severe complications related to hyperglycemia, hypoproteinemia, and immunosuppression. Proper metabolic support is essential to restore homeostasis and ensure survival.

Management of enterocutaneous fistulas (ECFs) involves (1) recognition and stabilization, (2) anatomic definition and decision, and (3) definitive operation. Phase 1 encompasses correction of fluid and electrolyte imbalance, skin protection, and nutritional support. Abdominal imaging defines the anatomy of the fistula in phase 2. ECFs that do not heal spontaneously require segmental resection of the bowel segment communicating with the fistula and restoration of intestinal continuity in phase 3. The enteroatmospheric fistula (EAF) is a malevolent condition requiring prolonged wound care and nutritional support. Complex abdominal wall reconstruction immediately following fistula resection is necessary for all EAFs.

Short bowel syndrome is a challenging clinical problem that benefits from a multidisciplinary approach. Much progress has recently been made in all aspects of management. Medical intestinal rehabilitation should be the initial treatment focus, and several new potential pharmacologic agents are being investigated. Surgical rehabilitation using nontransplant procedures in selected patients may further improve intestinal function. Intestinal lengthening procedures are particularly promising. Intestinal transplantation has increasingly been used with improving success in patients with life-threatening complications of intestinal failure.

decades. The ability to feed patients who cannot eat has evolved from impossible to routine clinical practice in the last 4 decades. Nutrition in critically ill patients based on measurement of metabolism has evolved from a research activity to clinical practice in the last 3 decades. The authors have been involved in this evolution and this article discusses past, present, and likely future practices in nutrition in critically ill patients.

The hypermetabolic response to severe burn injury is characterized by hyperdynamic circulation and profound metabolic, physiologic, catabolic, and immune system derangements. Failure to satisfy overwhelming energy and protein requirements after, and during, severe burn injury results in multiorgan dysfunction, increased susceptibility to infection, and death. Attenuation of the hypermetabolic response by various pharmacologic modalities is emerging as an essential component of the management of patients with severe burn injury. This review focuses on the more recent advances in therapeutic strategies to attenuate the hypermetabolic response and its postburn-associated insulin resistance.

The importance of nutrition and the prognostic impact of malnutrition in patients with head and neck cancer are not fully appreciated in the surgical world where a pervasive attitude exists that weight loss during treatment is inevitable and nutritional expertise or intervention may be dismissed out of ignorance. In this article, the authors explore the nutritional requirements of these patients and the impact of a multidisciplinary therapeutic approach to head, neck, and skull base cancer care.

Despite the success of both parenteral and enteral nutrition in supporting patients who cannot eat, patients with either sepsis or cancer cannot be adequately supported. A proposed mechanism by which aerobic glycolysis leads to a shortage of energy production in the liver is discussed. According to this hypothesis, the proximity of sodium-potassium ATPase and glycogen, its fuel source, leads to the continuation of gluconeogenesis with continued proteolysis and muscle wasting. Myostatin and lipokine, newly discovered factors, may also play a role.

Cachexia has plagued clinicians for centuries. Although all cachexia is related to malnutrition, cachexia associated with malignant diseases differs from starvation cachexia in that it is more recalcitrant to nutritional therapy. All cachexia responds to judicious nutritional support; however, cancer cachexia worsens autonomously as the disease advances and cannot be arrested or reversed by any known form of nutrition, hormonal, or pharmacologic therapy. Cachexia must be treated cautiously to avoid overfeeding syndrome, which may result in serious or dangerous complications or death.

## THE CLINICS ARE NOW AVAILABLE ONLINE!

Access your subscription at:
**www.theclinics.com**

# Foreword

# Nutrition and Metabolism of The Surgical Patient, Part I

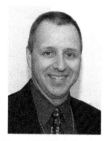

Ronald F. Martin, MD
*Consulting Editor*

*"Dis-moi ce que tu manges, je te dirai ce que tu es."* *[Tell me what you eat and I will tell you what you are].*

—*Anthelme Brillat-Savarin, 1826*

One would be hard pressed to find a medical topic that applies to all people so uniformly and is so widely misunderstood as nutrition. In fact, it is not just the "medical" aspects of nutrition but the everyday aspects of nutrition that are misunderstood as well. In some respects it is not surprising, since there are tremendous forces at play that shape our views and policies about food and nutrition in general. Cultural traditions, religious observances, local preferences, as well as a multitude of other social factors heavily influence the variety and amounts of foodstuffs we all consume. There are also economic (both large and small scale) and political pressures that play out much more than people sometimes realize. At this time of current financial distress on a worldwide basis, the relative prices and availability of food alone are adding to political and economic instability. It is ironic that two of the major medical problems facing us on a global scale are famine and obesity.

It is no surprise that the predominant concepts we all have about food and nutrition are more informed by our own history with food than by any scientific understanding of nutrition. Nearly two centuries ago the physiologist Brillat-Savarin asserted that he could tell us what we were if we told him what we ate. The quote above or one of its many derivatives has been used in so many contexts that most people have forgotten (or never knew) that the comment was included in a treatise on the physiology of gout.

This issue of the *Surgical Clinics of North America* is a slight departure from our usual process. Many years ago we decided to contain our topics to single issues. This issue will be the first of a two-part set. The reason for this temporary departure from policy is a confluence of opportunities. The most important reason is that we collectively perceived a gap in the readily available content sources for a comprehensive

Surg Clin N Am 91 (2011) xiii–xiv
doi:10.1016/j.suc.2011.04.012
0039-6109/11/$ – see front matter © 2011 Elsevier Inc. All rights reserved.

but concise collection of articles on the science of nutrition and we felt we had the capability to close that gap. We did, however, realize that if we were to attempt to limit the resources we had to a single issue, we would either lose depth or breadth of the topics to the point where we would not achieve our educational objectives.

Our priority is always dissemination of the highest quality content available. That said, all of our content comes from people with real lives and usually more demands put on their time than time to deliver on those requests. Dr Stan Dudrick, who guest edits these two issues with his colleague Dr Juan Sanchez, has played a major if not pivotal role in improving our understanding of nutrition. Dr Dudrick has spent nearly half a century developing an unparalleled understanding of nutrition and in particular how it affects the surgical patient. He has also touched the careers of hundreds if not thousands of surgeons as they trained and practiced. I can personally attest to his kindness and support of not only those people he has worked with directly but also to those who he has met briefly—he is a consummate surgical mentor. Thanks to Dr Dudrick, we have a unique access to an array of people who not only know the facts, as we understand them, about nutrition but many who were responsible for the development of this knowledge. Opportunities to collect such a group of contributors happen rarely; therefore, we decided to seize the chance to provide something truly spectacular for the readership by developing this two-part set.

I encourage the reader to devour this issue. Perhaps the knowledge corollary to Brillat-Savarin's posit might be, "show me what you read and I will tell you what you know." If so, the consumer of these articles will be considerably better informed about nutrition.

Ronald F. Martin, MD
Department of Surgery
Marshfield Clinic
1000 North Oak Avenue
Marshfield, WI 54449, USA

E-mail address:
martin.ronald@marshfieldclinic.org

# Preface

# Nutrition and Metabolism of The Surgical Patient, Part I

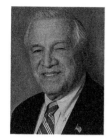 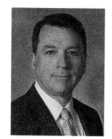

Stanley J. Dudrick, MD    Juan A. Sanchez, MD
*Guest Editors*

Two decades have passed since the publication of the *Surgical Clinics of North America* entitled, "Current Strategies in Surgical Nutrition" in June 1991, and almost five decades have elapsed since the initial investigative efforts were undertaken in the Harrison Department of Surgical Research at the University of Pennsylvania School of Medicine, which culminated in the demonstration of the first successful basic and clinical development of a practical, efficacious, and reasonably safe and affordable technique of total parenteral nutrition. This landmark contribution changed surgical and medical practice forever. No longer was it justifiable that malnourished or starving patients with serious or critical conditions, disorders, diseases, or injuries succumbed because they could not eat or receive their nutritional requirements adequately by tube feedings. Since 1967, it has been possible not only to expose in-patient starvation as the "skeleton in the hospital closet," but also mandatory that it be treated judiciously even by total intravenous feeding if necessary in order to minimize morbidity and mortality secondary to malnutrition and starvation, and to maximize the salvage and outcomes of critically ill patients.

The relevance of good nutritional status to the achievement of good clinical results was subsequently repeatedly demonstrated and established beyond a shadow of a doubt. Nutritional assessment also became more relevant and sophisticated, because the means were now available for clinicians to prevent, minimize, or correct the ravages of malnutrition and starvation under virtually all circumstances. Moreover, the successes associated with nutritional support by total parenteral nutrition served as the primary impetus for clinicians and scientists to learn more about individual nutrients, to improve nutrient constituents and formulations, and to design and develop new technology for nutrient delivery, monitoring, assessment, applications, and safety, etc.

Since the gastrointestinal tract has always been, is, and is highly likely to remain, the best means by which to be nourished, provided that it is in reasonably effective

Surg Clin N Am 91 (2011) xv–xvii
doi:10.1016/j.suc.2011.04.002
0039-6109/11/$ – see front matter © 2011 Elsevier Inc. All rights reserved.

working condition, attention was appropriately directed intensely and much more enthusiastically, imaginatively, and effectively, than ever before toward advancing novel substrates, formulations, techniques, and technology for optimal enteral feeding. Not only has the art of nutritional support grown and developed in leaps and bounds during the past twenty years, but the science of nutrition, which at times in the past has been suspect, marginal, or even disrespected by basic and clinical scientists, has made enormous strides and advances in the areas of clinical biochemistry, cellular and molecular biology, immunology, metabolism, gastrointestinal physiology, inflammation, organ functions, body composition and performance, genetics, nutrient substrate development, drug-nutrient interactions, delivery system engineering and technology, and countless other areas related to the many aspects of patient care in every specialty of the medical profession.

As predicted in the Preface of this publication twenty years ago, "Future innovative outgrowth and natural maturation of the medical technology and techniques are likely to occur in this field in the next decade and are most promising, almost incomprehensible and apparently unlimited." Clearly, this hopeful prediction has been amply realized, but the surface has barely been scratched relevant to what the future promises at this point in time. The more we learn, the more opportunities become apparent to discover even more, as the tree of knowledge develops and spreads its roots and branches in innumerable directions to challenge our own personal, professional, and clinical development. The future of this endeavor is still exciting to ponder with its myriad and titillating possibilities.

How fortunate we are to have attracted, and successfully imposed upon, the elite group of expert, experienced, talented scientists, clinicians, nutritionists, innovators, investigators, teachers, and cherished colleagues and friends to partner with us in the production of this two part edition in which we have attempted to summarize and update the current status of nutrition and metabolism. Originally, the plan was to produce one issue, but when the breadth of the field and the depth of the expertise were assessed, it was clear that even two issues would barely cover the essential areas of knowledge, experience, and philosophy required for a comprehensive presentation to our readers. We hope that the many selected references will help to augment the material and data in the articles, and that the readers will forgive the editors, authors, and publisher for any shortcomings that may be perceived as a result of our attempts to limit the number and length of the presentations for practical purposes. Above all, we have attempted to provide a summation and state-of-the-art handbook that might be useful to all who are interested in the complex areas of nutrition and metabolism and in providing the best metabolic and nutritional support of patients requiring and benefiting from our collective efforts on their behalf.

We are most beholden to our authors, who have shared their wealth of knowledge, experience, judgment, and wisdom, together with their invaluable efforts, skills, and time, in order to consummate this most worthwhile and commendable educational and training project in this vital field. We are extremely appreciative of the wonderful opportunity and encouragement offered to us by Ronald F. Martin, MD, Consulting Editor of the *Surgical Clinics of North America*, to serve as guest editors of this issue. His guidance, assistance, counsel, confidence, and patience have been most supportive and exemplary. We are also deeply indebted to Mr John Vassallo, Associate Publisher, Elsevier, who has been an indefatigable professional in his assistance at all points and in every area of importance in the production of this issue. We are especially grateful to our Executive Assistant, Mrs Joan Reeser, who ensured excellence, timeliness, consummate technical, editorial, and cognitive expertise, and eternal optimism and cheerfulness as we toiled through the maze of completing the countless tasks essential to the success of this venture. Finally, our thanks and love to Terry and Lise for their untold contributions, support, and sacrifices, willingly made so that we could undertake this demanding, yet satisfying, editorial responsibility.

Stanley J. Dudrick, MD
Chairman Emeritus and Program Director Emeritus
Department of Surgery
Saint Mary's Hospital
56 Franklin Street
Waterbury, CT 06706, USA

Juan A. Sanchez, MD
Chairman and Program Director
Department of Surgery
Saint Mary's Hospital
56 Franklin Street
Waterbury, CT 06706, USA

E-mail addresses:
sdudrick@stmh.org (S.J. Dudrick)
juan.sanchez@stmh.org (J.A. Sanchez)

# Metabolic Considerations in Management of Surgical Patients

George L. Blackburn, MD, PhD

**KEYWORDS**

- Stress response • Metabolic response
- Surgery • Injury • Trauma

Surgical procedures are followed by prompt changes in endocrine metabolic function and various host defense mechanisms.[1] These physiologic shifts must be quickly addressed (within 24–48 hours) to avoid the pathogenesis of postoperative morbidity. The stress response to surgery is characterized by increased secretion of pituitary hormones and activation of the sympathetic nervous system.[2] The overall metabolic effect of the hormonal changes is increased catabolism. This hormone-mediated mobilization of endogenous substrates provides energy sources, mechanisms to retain salt and water, and the means to maintain fluid volume and cardiovascular homeostasis. The net effect is an increased secretion of catabolic hormones.[3] Rather than pathogenic, however, the stress response to injury should be viewed as a finely tuned, integrated series of compensatory reactions that provide adequate quantities of fuel and amino acids for visceral protein synthesis.[4,5]

## METABOLIC RESPONSE TO INJURY
### History

In 1932, Sir David Cuthbertson[6] described the metabolic responses of four patients with lower limb injuries by documenting the time course of the changes. Ten years later, he was the first to describe distinct phases of the metabolic shifts that occur after major trauma by characterizing the ebb and flow of posttraumatic metabolic alterations.[7,8] The ebb phase is associated with a decline in body temperature and oxygen consumption, presumably aimed at reducing posttraumatic energy depletion. The clinical relevance of this phase is limited by its brevity. Conversely, the flow phase takes place after resuscitation from a state of shock.[9] It involves sustained

Disclosures: The author has nothing to disclose.
Center for the Study of Nutrition Medicine, Department of Surgery, Beth Israel Deaconess Medical Center, Harvard Medical School, Feldberg 880 East Campus, 330 Brookline Avenue, Boston, MA 02215, USA
E-mail address: gblackbu@bidmc.harvard.edu

Surg Clin N Am 91 (2011) 467–480
doi:10.1016/j.suc.2011.03.001
0039-6109/11/$ – see front matter © 2011 Elsevier Inc. All rights reserved.

hypermetabolism for at least 7 days and, in many severely injured patients, up to 3 weeks or longer.[10,11] This hypercatabolic condition leads to significantly increased oxygen consumption and energy expenditure—a state associated with severe complications related to hyperglycemia, hypoproteinemia, and immunosuppression.[4,9,12]

Dr Francis D. Moore was a pioneer in the field of metabolic responses to surgery. His studies culminated in two classic books, *The Metabolic Response to Surgery* co-authored with M.R. Ball[13] and *Metabolic Care of the Surgical Patient*.[14] These shifted the focus from improving the surgical craft to understanding the body's physiologic response to the trauma of surgery. Surgeons of the day did not understand how to optimize the physiologic status of their patients. A perfect anatomic operation could be followed by disastrous complications or death from a low level of circulating sodium chloride or magnesium, a high level of potassium chloride, or an undetected loss of plasma or water.

Dr Jonathan E. Rhoads at the Harrison Department of Surgical Research, University of Pennsylvania, focused on nutrition in surgical patients. He discovered that providing 100 g of glucose enables the body to draw on stores of fat for the remaining caloric supplement and promoted 100 g of protein as a stopgap measure. His work led to the later demonstration that an intravenous nutrient mixture could support normal growth in young animals and in children with severe bowel disease who received no food by mouth.[15]

Rhoads' younger colleague, Dr Stanley J. Dudrick,[16] invented total parenteral nutrition through the development of intravenous hyperalimentation and then advanced the clinical utility of surgical nutrition and its successful application in critically ill patients. In 1967, he demonstrated that a human infant could receive all nutrients entirely by intravenous feeding and still grow and develop normally. This seminal accomplishment, published in *JAMA*, laid the groundwork for many improvements in the technique and its further development and application. At a reception for the second Jonathan E. Rhoads Lectureship at the meeting of the American Society for Parenteral and Enteral Nutrition in 1979, this was the first time Dr Rhoads met Sir David Cuthbertson (**Fig. 1**).[17]

### Stress Catabolism

Surgical trauma initiates a complex series of metabolic host responses designed to maintain homeostasis and ensure survival.[18] Hormone-mediated mobilization of endogenous substrates (**Fig. 2**) leads to a functional redistribution of body cell mass after injury or surgery to provide nitrogen for protein synthesis. Catecholamines (epinephrine), corticosteroids, glucagon, and growth hormone mobilize stored protein and energy reserves in support of key pathways necessary for metabolic stabilization, host defense, and recovery. Free fatty acids, ketones, and glucose meet energy needs, whereas amino acids are used for the synthesis of acute phase proteins, gluconeogenesis, and thermogenesis essential for the homeostasis of injury metabolism.[4,9,12]

This initial period is characterized by increased oxygen consumption, insulin resistance, and protein catabolism. Modest hyperglycemia is common due to increased hepatic glucose production and peripheral insulin resistance in skeletal muscle.[19] Changes in lipid metabolism include increased lipolysis, fatty acid recycling, hypertriglyceridemia, and hepatic steatosis.[20] Postinjury metabolism is further characterized by increased skeletal and visceral muscle catabolism and negative nitrogen balance. This leads to depletion of lean body mass, a syndrome referred to as auto-cannibalism.[21] Glutamine released from muscle becomes the preferred energy substrate for enterocytes and immune cells and is used to synthesize the antioxidant glutathione.[22] Hepatic protein synthesis is prioritized to generate acute phase proteins

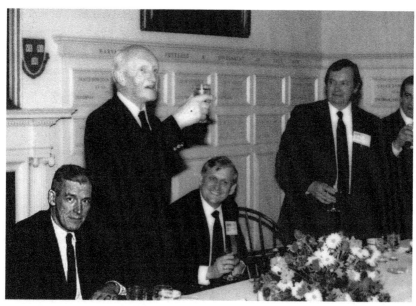

**Fig. 1.** (*Left to right*) Dr Jonathan E. Rhoads, Sir David Cuthbertson, and Drs George L. Blackburn, William Steffee, and Stanley Dudrick. Reception for the second Jonathan E. Rhoads Lectureship at the third meeting of the American Society for Parenteral and Enteral Nutrition at the Massachusetts Room, Harvard Club, Boston (1979). This was the first time Dr Rhoads met Sir David Cuthbertson. (*Courtesy of* George L. Blackburn, MD, PhD, Boston, MA.)

(eg, C-reactive protein) and immune cells (eg, leukocytes and neutrophils) at the expense of constitutive proteins, such as albumin.[23–25]

These metabolic changes are best understood as a redistribution of macronutrients from labile reserves (skeletal muscle and adipose tissue) to more active tissues (liver and bone marrow) for host defense, visceral protein synthesis, and heat production

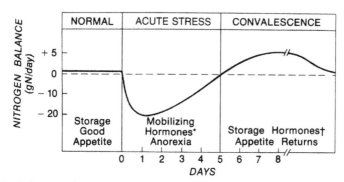

**Fig. 2.** Biphasic hormonal response to injury in the normal postoperative patient. Catecholamines*, cortocosteroids, glucagon, growth hormone, injury hormones, leukocytic mediators, storage hormones, insulin†. (*From* Blackburn GL, Harvey-Wilkes KB. Nutrition in surgical patients. In: Hardy JD, editor. Hardy's textbook of surgery. 1st edition. Philadelphia: J.B. Lippincott; 1983. p. 90–107; with permission.)

(Fig. 3). Micronutrients are also redistributed. The liver increases uptake of zinc, which is a cofactor in several enzymatic functions required during and after injury. Greater amounts of iron are also taken up by iron-binding proteins, such as transferrin, thus reducing the amount available for iron-dependent pathogenic microorganisms.[4]

## NEUROENDOCRINE RESPONSE TO INJURY
### Stress Hormones

Injury is associated with a pronounced neuroendocrine response characterized by increased secretion of various stress hormones, such as adrenaline and cortisol, but also by increased release of glucagon, growth hormone, aldosterone, and antidiuretic hormone.[26,27] The magnitude and duration of the hormonal response correlate well with the extent of the trauma.[28] Afferent impulses from the site of injury stimulate the secretion of hypothalamic-releasing hormones that further stimulate the pituitary gland.[29] Cortisol is secreted by hormonal stimulation of the adrenal cortex, whereas adrenaline in secreted by the adrenal medulla in response to activation of the sympathetic nervous system. Noradrenaline spills over into the plasma from the sympathetic nerve endings.

From a metabolic standpoint, cortisol is probably the most important hormone, with its widespread effects on glucose, amino acid, and fatty acid metabolism. No evidence to date shows that hormonal treatment can improve the outcome after major

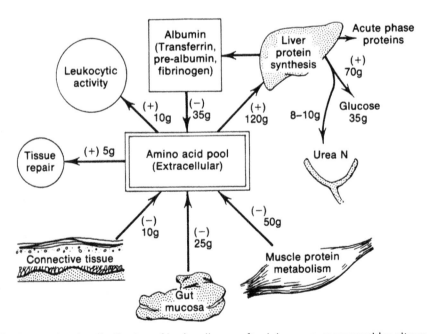

**Fig. 3.** Functional redistribution of body cell mass after injury or surgery provides nitrogen for protein synthesis. Arrows reflect the net release (−) in grams from connective tissue, gut mucosa, and muscle as well as uptake (+) of amino acids into tissues whose net metabolism is associated with survival. The conversion of protein into glucose and urea is a minor source of energy but an important part of the role of the liver to produce the heat necessary to maintain core temperature. (*From* Blackburn GL, Harvey-Wilkes KB. Nutrition in surgical patients. In: Hardy JD, editor. Hardy's textbook of surgery. 1st edition. Philadelphia: J.B. Lippincott; 1983. p. 90–107; with permission.)

trauma in humans,[29] although promising experimental trauma research has been performed suggesting some potential modulating effects on the response.[30]

### Cytokines—Host Defense

Considerable evidence indicates that infections occur more frequently, and with greater severity, in malnourished individuals. The immune system, however, encompasses a wide variety of host defenses and activities—phagocytosis, antibody synthesis, lymphokine production, complement-mediated cytolysis, interferon production, and sirtuin substrate actions.[31] These functions require the interaction of 3 types of leukocytes: thymus-derived (T), antibody synthesizing (B) lymphocytes, and accessory cells (eg, monocytes/macrophages, neutrophils, and endothelium).[9] Many cooperative interactions and activities depend on protein synthesis.

Nutritional depletion from anorexia, increased metabolic rate, malabsorption, or increased losses (fistulas and diarrhea) may compromise immunocompetence. Therefore, a variety of cytokines come into play when prompted by an inflammatory stimulus. The most widely studied proinflammatory cytokines with respect to metabolic regulation after injury, inflammation, and infection are tumor necrosis factor (TNF)-$\alpha$, interleukin (IL)-1, and IL-6. Other cytokines that may be involved in the metabolic response to injury and infection include IL-4, IL-7, IL-8, and interferon-$\gamma$ (IFN-$\gamma$). This list will probably grow longer as new cytokines and their functions continue to be identified. Known cytokines and additional ones, along with their functions, origin, target cells, and properties are provided in the Cytokines Online Pathfinder Encyclopaedia.[32]

The IL-6–type cytokines, TNF-$\alpha$, and IFN-$\gamma$,[33] are released in response to tissue injury or an inflammatory stimulus. They act locally and systemically to generate a variety of physiologic responses, in particular, the acute phase response. The IL-6 cytokines demonstrate pleiotropy and redundancy of actions.[34]

Different proinflammatory cytokines induce the activation of leukocytes. The leukocyte adhesion molecule, L-selectin, is important for the rolling of polymorphonuclear leukocytes (PMN), the first step of the cascade leading to adhesion, diapedesis, and subsequent organ dysfunction.[35] Mommsen and colleagues[35] recently found that the primary proinflammatory cytokine TNF-$\alpha$ regulates the L-selectin surface expression on PNM after surgical trauma, suggesting that a regulation of neutrophil adjustment on this level might be crucial in the development of posttraumatic complications. In this immune phase of the inflammatory response, the metabolic response to injury is characterized by hypercatabolism and hypermetabolism.[29,36–39]

### The Hormone-Cytokine Connection

Neuroendocrine stress reactions interact with the immunologic response to trauma.[40] The immunoinflammatory response is initiated immediately after injury and is mainly regulated by cytokines, which act as communication mediators between leukocytes, bridging the innate and adaptive immune responses.[41,42]

Evidence shows that hormones and cytokines interact at several levels in the regulation of the metabolic response to surgery. For example, TNF-$\alpha$, IL-1, and IL-6 stimulate the hypothalamus-pituitary-adrenal axis. In normal human subjects, TNF-$\alpha$ administration induces a stress hormone response with elevated plasma levels of corticotropin, cortisol, catecholamines, growth hormone, and glucagon.

Corticotropin-releasing factor, which is released from the hypothalamus during stress, is produced by leukocytes as well.[43] Immune cells are also considered a new, diffusely expressed adrenergic organ, with the ability to generate, release, and degrade catecholamines.[42] It seems that catecholamines use intracellular oxidative mechanisms to exert autoregulatory functions on immune cells.[44]

The physiologic counterpart of the adrenergic system, the cholinergic system, is also an integral part of human macrophage and lymphocyte regulation, and is termed the *cholinergic anti-inflammatory pathway*.[42]

## IMMUNOLOGIC ASSAYS

Experienced clinicians are unable to predict the extent to which trauma or injury will affect an individual's energy requirements.[45] Immunologic assays are valuable for assessing the functional and clinically significant severity of malnutrition. Simple measurements include an enumeration of total leukocytes (ie, total lymphocyte and neutrophil counts). Decreased lymphocyte counts (<1000 m$^3$) have been seen in hypoalbuminemic postsurgical patients and children with kwashiorkor but not in those with marasmus. Rapid protein depletion due to increased protein catabolism may have a different effect on immune response than the more gradual generalized depletion from anorexia and inadequate protein and carbohydrate intake. Other explanations for decreased leukocyte counts might include factors, such as blood loss, white blood cell migration to traumatized tissues, and cell sequestration in lymphoid tissues.[4]

The nonspecific immune defense systems—in particular, complement and immunoglobulin—are the primary mechanisms for containing bacterial contamination and preventing colonization, infection, and sepsis. Because complement and immunoglobulin synthesis have a high priority with respect to amino acid availability, they are not useful in the detection of mild or moderate nutritional deficiency in hospitalized patients. In cases of severe protein-calorie malnutrition, however, such as that seen in burn patients, decreased complement and immunoglobulin levels may become evident.

Delayed hypersensitivity skin testing, which evaluates cell-mediated immunity, is the most widely used assay for the analysis of immune function before elective surgery or before and during nutritional support (**Fig. 4**). A positive skin test requires functioning accessory cells, T and B lymphocytes, macrophage activation, lymphokine production, and monocyte chemotaxis. A wide variety of metabolic systems can interfere with this complex process. Anergy has been reported not only in immune deficient states but also in advanced age, uremia, bacterial and viral infections, and liver disease. Transient anergy often follows surgery or acute injury and is due to the appearance of a serum inhibitor or to T-lymphocyte reactions. One should, therefore, wait until the seventh or eighth postoperative day before evaluating the delayed hypersensitivity reaction.[4]

Radiation and chemotherapy, as well as cancer itself, may also act to depress the DH response to recall skin antigens. Thus, protein-calorie malnutrition is not the only cause of acquired anergy in the hospitalized patient. But regardless of the etiology, depression of cell-mediated immunity (as reflected by delayed hypersensitivity skin antigen testing) has been associated with increased sepsis and related mortality. This is so even though those organisms, against which cell-mediated immunity is not the primary host defense, are frequently the cause of the sepsis.

In most patients, the infectious agents are gram-negative rods or gram-positive cocci, ubiquitous organisms generally from a patient's own flora, rather than viruses, fungi, or intracellular parasites from the environment. In healthy, well-nourished individuals, indigenous flora are normally of low virulence. One possible mechanism for the increased incidence of sepsis associated with anergy is that the critical number of bacteria that ordinarily expected to be handled by the inflammatory response may be altered. DH testing does not identify the deficit; it is simply a marker that the immune system is not functioning adequately.

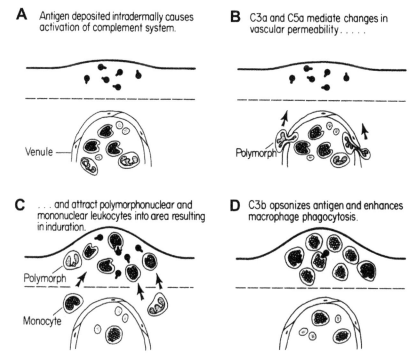

**A** Antigen deposited intradermally causes activation of complement system.

**B** C3a and C5a mediate changes in vascular permeability . . . . .

Venule

Polymorph

**C** . . . and attract polymorphonuclear and mononuclear leukocytes into area resulting in induration.

**D** C3b opsonizes antigen and enhances macrophage phagocytosis.

Polymorph

Monocyte

**Fig. 4.** Delayed hypersensitivity skin testing, which evaluates cell-mediated immunity, is the most widely used assay for the analysis of immune function before elective surgery or before and during nutritional support. (*From* Blackburn GL, Harvey-Wilkes KB. Nutrition in surgical patients. In: Hardy JD, editor. Hardy's textbook of surgery. 1st edition. Philadelphia: J.B. Lippincott; 1983. p. 90–107; with permission.)

Because of their high metabolic priority, immune functions of lymphocytes or accessory cells may be the first metabolic system to respond to nutritional support; thus, serial measurements of immune function may be of use to determine the appropriateness and effectiveness of nutritional therapy. Serial measurements are also valuable predictors of outcome (eg, mortality) in hospital therapy.

To measure the intactness of the delayed hypersensitivity response, 3 recall skin antigens—*Candida albicans,* mumps, and streptokinase-streptodornase—are commonly used. One-tenth milliliter of each solution is placed intradermally in the volar forearm, and the reaction is examined at 24 hours and 48 hours; a greater than or equal to 5-mm area of induration is considered positive. Immune competence is defined as a positive response to one or more of the antigens. Ninety-five percent accuracy of the test can be anticipated if it is meticulously performed. Although a negative response to recall skin antigen (in particular, mumps and *Candida*) may be due to a variety of causes, a positive serial response can provide important knowledge about the integrity of the host defense system and the effectiveness of nutrition support therapy—parenteral, enteral, or a combination of the two methods.[4]

## TRANSCRIPTION FACTORS

Transcription factors are proteins that under certain conditions bind to DNA and alter the rate of gene transcription and expression. They may enhance gene transcription, resulting in increased mRNA levels and, ultimately, upregulated protein expression. Alternatively, they may serve as repressors and inhibit gene transcription, thus decreasing production of a given protein. Examples of important transcription factors involved in the inflammatory response to injury and sepsis include nuclear factor κB (NF-κB), activating protein 1 (AP-1), signal transducer and activator of transcription factor (STAT)-3, and members of the CCAAT/enhancer-binding protein (C/EBP) family of transcription factors, in particular, C/EBPβ and C/EBPδ. Because of their key roles in gene regulation and as potential targets for treatment of inflammation, transcription factors have become subjects of intense scientific investigation. NF-κB is probably the most extensively studied inflammatory transcription factor, and is, therefore, discussed briefly.

A recent experiment in an animal model showed that the transplantation of mesenchymal stem cells modulated the inflammatory response to injury by neutralizing the activity of inflammatory cytokines. The study suggested that improvements in inflammatory responses in animal models after local transplantation of mesenchymal stem cells are explained, at least in part, by the NF-κB–dependent secretion of soluble TNF receptor 1 by mesenchymal stem cells.[46] Another experimental study found that activation of peroxisome proliferator-activated receptor -γ (PPARγ) seemed to play an important role in mediating salutary effects of 17β-estradiol on plasma cytokine levels and Kupffer cell cytokine production after trauma. PPARγ and Kupffer cell cytokine production are likely mediated via NF-κB and AP-1.

NF-κB is a redox sensitive transcription factor with regard to the production of proinflammatory molecules, including chemokines, cytokines, and adhesion molecules, that allow leukocytes to attach themselves to the endothelium and facilitate their extravasation to the interstitial spaces of tissues and organs.[47,48] The NF-κB family of proteins consists of several members, including p50, p52, c-Rel, p65 (Rel-A), and Rel-B. Each of these subunits can form homodimeric or heterodimeric complexes with other members of the family. Several other transcription factors also participate in gene regulation after trauma and during severe infection, including AP-1, STAT-1, hypoxia-inducible transcription factor, and C/EBPβ and C/EBPδ. In addition, new insights into the genetic response to inflammation may provide assays, potential biomarkers, or therapies, such as histone deacetylase inhibitors, that promote tissue repair while preventing inflammation from becoming chronic.[49–51]

## ENERGY EXPENDITURE AND PROTEIN REQUIREMENTS
### Energy Expenditure

The average nonstressed individual lying quietly in bed requires 23 kcal/kg per day to maintain body weight. Limited physical activity increases this requirement to 28 kcal/kg per day.[52,53] Ordinary, uncomplicated, open abdomen elective surgery does not lead to a significant increase in energy requirements. Increased metabolic response and protein catabolism result from the release of cytokines combined with more secretion of catabolic hormones.[54] This creates a heightened caloric requirement secondary to the catabolic response in severely injured or septic patients. Needs are increased approximately 25% in skeletal trauma, 50% in sepsis, and 75% to 100% in severe burns (**Fig. 5**).[55] Hypermetabolic patients are also subjected to an increased drain on protein stores. The following nitrogen losses are commonly seen in fasting patients: elective postsurgical patients, 7–9 g N per day; skeletal trauma or septic patients, 11–14 g N per day; severe burns, 12–18 g N per day.

Monitoring of nitrogen excretion is a simple, accurate assessment of the catabolic rate.[12] Assessment of body mass can be determined by the creatine index.[56] The

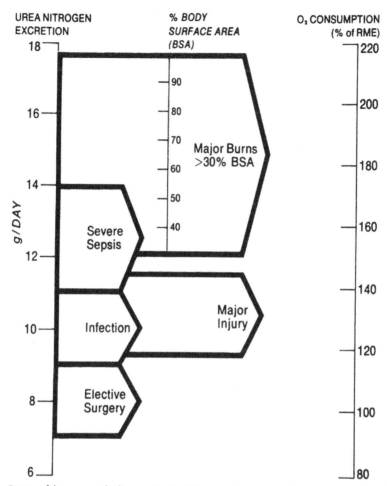

**Fig. 5.** Rates of hypermetabolism estimated from urinary urea nitrogen excretion. (*From* Blackburn GL, Bistrian BR, Maini BS, et al. Nutritional and metabolic assessment of the hospitalized patient. JPEN J Parenter Enteral Nutr 1977;1:11–22; with permission.)

addition of exogenous corticosteroids to the high circulating levels characteristic of stress can increase nitrogen losses even further.

Hypocaloric nutrition support offers another approach to meeting the energy needs of patients with evidence of accelerated gluconeogenesis and lipolysis that lead to hyperglycemia and elevated serum triglyceride levels.[57] In some cases, the traditional strategy of meeting or exceeding calorie requirements may compound the metabolic alterations of the stress response.[57] Increasing evidence suggests that critically ill patients have lower energy requirements than expected, but most guidelines[25,58] continue to recommend elevated caloric requirements in these patients, in particular those with sepsis.[59] This practice can lead to liver dysfunction.[59]

Most critically ill patients show an average resting energy expenditure of 23 kcal/ $kg^{-1}/d^{-1}$ before and during total parenteral nutrition, close to their total daily energy expenditure (without differences between septic and nonseptic patients).[60,61]

Although inconclusive, studies suggest that a nutrition support goal of 10 to 20 kcal/kg of ideal or adjusted weight and 1.5 to 2 g/kg ideal weight of protein may be beneficial during the acute stress response.[57]

### Protein Requirements

Protein catabolism is stimulated by increased cortisol concentrations. Predominantly, skeletal muscle is broken down, but some visceral muscle protein is also catabolized to release the constituent amino acids. The amino acids may be further catabolized for energy or used in the liver to form new protein, in particular acute-phase proteins. The liver also converts amino acids into other substrates (eg, glucose, fatty acids, or ketone bodies). Protein catabolism results in marked weight loss and muscle wasting in patients after major surgical and traumatic injury. The loss of protein can be measured and calculated indirectly by increased nitrogen excretion in the urine.

Both hormones and cytokines regulate protein metabolism after injury. The hormonal regulation may reflect a balance between catabolic hormones, such as glucocorticoids, and anabolic hormones, such as insulin and insulinlike growth factor 1. During trauma and infection, both types of hormones probably play a role in protein regulation. The role of the various mediators in protein metabolism after injury has been most extensively studied in skeletal muscle and liver, although evidence is emerging that the same substances regulate protein metabolism in other organs and tissues as well.[62]

Much interest has been shown in nutritional supplements for patients with critical illness and those undergoing major surgery. Certain nutrients may have a beneficial influence on the immune status of stressed patients. Glutamine, arginine, glycine, ω-3 polyunsaturated fatty acids, and nucleotides have been studied most extensively.[2] Glutamine and arginine are semiessential amino acids with a multiplicity of functions, including stimulation of immune activity. Studies of patients given enteral nutrition supplemented with arginine or glycine after major surgery have shown that patients benefited with a faster recovery of immunologic parameters, fewer infectious complications, and a shorter hospital stay.[3]

### SUMMARY

The stress response consists of the hormonal and metabolic changes that follow injury or trauma. It is part of the systemic reaction to injury,[62,63] which encompasses a wide range of endocrinological, immunologic, and hematological effects.[2,64] The endocrine response to surgery affects the hypothalamic-pituitary-adrenal axis. For example, surgery is one of the most potent activators of corticotropin and cortisol secretion; increased plasma concentrations of both hormones can be measured within minutes of the start of surgery.[2]

The metabolic sequelae of the endocrine response center around increased secretion of catabolic hormones. Surgery affects metabolism of carbohydrates, protein, fat, and water and electrolytes.[2] Most critically ill patients have evidence of an increased metabolic response and protein catabolism that results from the release of cytokines combined with increased secretion of catabolic hormones.[54,59] With prolonged stress and catabolism, substrate levels (in particular amino acids) fall, resulting in decreased synthesis of plasma proteins, especially those concerned with host defense. For clinical purposes, a 5-day rule is an important marker, indicating the time that supplemental nutrition support should begin to sustain the metabolic response to injury without development of malnutrition and risk of impaired host defense and wound healing.[2,4,65]

Early observations by Cuthbertson confirmed that severe injury initiated systemic catabolic responses and eventually enabled him to assign a causal association between this response and the increased presence of the stress hormones, catecholamines, and glucocorticoids. Today we know that the stress response encompasses a wide range of endocrinological, immunologic, and hematological effects. A variety of approaches have been used to attenuate the stress response and improve outcomes.[66] Reducing the trauma associated with surgical illness has decreased morbidity and mortality and has made significant contributions to improved outcomes in surgical patients. Further advances in these approaches will continue to enhance surgical care in the future.[65,67–69]

## REFERENCES

1. Kehlet H. Surgical stress response: does endoscopic surgery confer an advantage? World J Surg 1999;23:801–7.
2. Desborough JP, Hall GM. Endocrine response to surgery. In: Kaufman L, editor. Anaethesia review. Edinburgh (United Kingdom): Churchill Livingston; 1993. p. 131–48.
3. Desborough JP. The stress response to trauma and surgery. Br J Anaesth 2000; 85:109–17.
4. Blackburn GL, Harvey-Wilkes KB. Nutrition in surgical patients. In: Hardy JD, editor. Hardy's textbook of surgery. 1st edition. Philadelphia: J.B. Lippincott Co; 1983. p. 90–107.
5. Blackburn GL, Bothe A Jr, Lahey MA. Organization and administration of a nutrition support service. Surg Clin North Am 1981;61:709–19.
6. Cuthbertson D. Observations on the disturbance of metabolism produced by injury to the limbs. Q J Med 1932;1:233–46.
7. Cuthbertson DP. Post-shock metabolic response. Lancet 1942;1:433–6.
8. Cuthbertson DP. The metabolic response to injury and other related explorations in the field of protein metabolism: an autobiographical account. Scott Med J 1982;27:158–71.
9. Stahel PF, Flierl MA, Moore EE. "Metabolic staging" after major trauma - a guide for clinical decision making? Scand J Trauma Resusc Emerg Med 2010;18:34.
10. Biffl WL, Moore EE, Haenel JB. Nutrition support of the trauma patient. Nutrition 2002;18:960–5.
11. Hasenboehler E, Williams A, Leinhase I, et al. Metabolic changes after polytrauma: an imperative for early nutritional support. World J Emerg Surg 2006;1:29.
12. Blackburn GL, Maini BS, Pierce EC Jr. Nutrition in the critically ill patient. Anesthesiology 1977;47:181–94.
13. Moore FD, Ball MR. The metabolic response to surgery. Springfield (IL): Charles C. Thomas; 1949.
14. Moore FD. Metabolic care of the surgical patient. Philadelphia: W.B. Saunders; 1959.
15. Death of Dr. Jonathan Rhoads, A Preeminent Penn Paragon weekly publication of faculty and staff of University of Pennsylvania, vol. 48. Philadelphia (PA): University of Pennsylvania; 2002. Number 17.
16. Stanley J. Dudrick, MD, FACS, is recipient of the 2005 Jacobson Innovation Award. Press Release. Available at: http://www.facs.org/news/jacobson.html. Accessed February 4, 2011.
17. Blackburn GL. Introduction of the Jonathan B. Rhoads Lectureship: Sir David P. Cuthbertson 1979 Awardee. JPEN J Parenter Enteral Nutr 1979;3:107.

18. Kinross JM, Alkhamesi N, Barton RH, et al. Global metabolic phenotyping in an experimental laparotomy model of surgical trauma. J Proteome Res 2011;10(1): 277–87.

19. Mizock BA. Alterations in fuel metabolism in critical illness: hyperglycaemia. Best Pract Res Clin Endocrinol Metab 2001;15:533–51.

20. Mizock BA. Metabolic derangements in sepsis and septic shock. Crit Care Clin 2000;16:319–36, vii.

21. Cerra FB, Siegel JH, Coleman B, et al. Septic autocannibalism. A failure of exogenous nutritional support. Ann Surg 1980;192:570–80.

22. Bongers T, Griffiths RD, McArdle A. Exogenous glutamine: the clinical evidence. Crit Care Med 2007;35(Suppl 9):S545–52.

23. Shaw JHF, Wolfe RR. An integrated analysis of glucose, fat, and protein metabolism in severely traumatized patients. Studies in the basal state and the response to total parenteral nutrition. Ann Surg 1989;209:63–72.

24. Cerra FB, Benitez MR, Blackburn GL, et al. Applied nutrition in ICU patients. A consensus statement of the American College of Chest Physicians. Chest 1997;111:769–78.

25. McClave SA, Martindale RG, Vanek VW, et al. Guidelines for the Provision and Assessment of Nutrition Support Therapy in the Adult Critically Ill Patient: Society of Critical Care Medicine (SCCM) and American Society for Parenteral and Enteral Nutrition (A.S.P.E.N.). JPEN J Parenter Enteral Nutr 2009;33:277–316.

26. Weissman C. The metabolic response to stress: an overview and update. Anesthesiology 1990;73:308–27.

27. Buckingham JC. Hypothalamo-pituitary responses to trauma. Br Med Bull 1985; 41:203–11.

28. Ni Choileain N, Redmond HP. Cell response to surgery. Arch Surg 2006;141: 1132–42.

29. Brøchner AC, Toft P. Pathophysiology of the systemic inflammatory response after major accidental trauma. Scand J Trauma Resusc Emerg Med 2009;17:43.

30. Hsieh CH, Nickel EA, Chen J, et al. Mechanism of the salutary effects of estrogen on kupffer cell phagocytic capacity following trauma-hemorrhage: pivotal role of Akt activation. J Immunol 2009;182:4406–14.

31. Gallí M, Van Gool F, Leo O. Sirtuins and inflammation: Friends or foes? Biochem Pharmacol 2011;81(5):569–76.

32. Ibelgaufts H. COPE: Cytokines Online Pathfinder Encyclopaedia. Available at: http://www.copewithcytokines.de/cope.cgi. Accessed January 7, 2011.

33. Svoboda P, Kantorová I, Ochmann J. Dynamics of interleukin 1, 2, and 6 and tumor necrosis factor alpha in multiple trauma patients. J Trauma 1994;36: 336–40.

34. Jawa RS, Anillo S, Huntoon K, et al. Analytic review: interleukin-6 in surgery, trauma, and critical care: part I: basic science. J Intensive Care Med 2011;26: 3–12.

35. Mommsen P, Barkhausen T, Hildebrand F, et al. Regulation of L-selectin expression by trauma-relevant cytokines. Pathol Res Pract 2011;207(3):142–7.

36. Moore FD. Bodily changes in surgical convalescence. I. The normal sequence observations and interpretations. Ann Surg 1953;137:289–315.

37. Hill AG, Hill GL. Metabolic response to severe injury. Br J Surg 1998;85:884–90.

38. Douglas RG, Shaw JH. Metabolic response to sepsis and trauma. Br J Surg 1989; 76:115–22.

39. Stoner HB. Interpretation of the metabolic effects of trauma and sepsis. J Clin Pathol 1987;40:1108–17.

40. Waymack JP, Fernandes G, Yurt RW, et al. Effect of blood transfusions on immune function. Part VI. Effect on immunologic response to tumor. Surgery 1990;108: 172-7.
41. Stahel PF, Smith WR, Moore EE. Role of biological modifiers regulating the immune response after trauma. Injury 2007;38:1409-22.
42. Aller MA, Arias JI, Alonso-Poza A, et al. A review of metabolic staging in severely injured patients. Scand J Trauma Resusc Emerg Med 2010;18:27.
43. Stephanou A, Jessop DS, Knight RA, et al. Corticotrophin-releasing factor-like immunoreactivity and mRNA in human leukocytes. Brain Behav Immun 1990;4: 67-73.
44. Flierl MA, Rittirsch D, Huber-Lang M, et al. Catecholamines-crafty weapons in the inflammatory arsenal of immune/inflammatory cells or opening pandora's box? Mol Med 2008;14:195-204.
45. Fung EB. Estimating energy expenditure in critcally ill adults and children. AACN Clin Issues 2000;11:480-97.
46. Yagi H, Soto-Gutierrez A, Navarro-Alvarez N, et al. Reactive bone marrow stromal cells attenuate systemic inflammation via sTNFR1. Mol Ther 2010;18:1857-64.
47. Rushing GD, Britt LD. Reperfusion injury after hemorrhage: a collective review. Ann Surg 2008;247:929-37.
48. Hanada T, Yoshimura A. Regulation of cytokine signaling and inflammation. Cytokine Growth Factor Rev 2002;13:413-21.
49. Li Y, Liu B, Dillon ST, et al. Identification of a novel potential biomarker in a model of hemorrhagic shock and valproic acid treatment. J Surg Res 2010;159:474-81.
50. Li Y, Liu B, Fukudome EY, et al. Surviving lethal septic shock without fluid resuscitation in a rodent model. Surgery 2010;148:246-54.
51. Li Y, Yuan Z, Liu B, et al. Prevention of hypoxia-induced neuronal apoptosis through histone deacetylase inhibition. J Trauma 2008;64:863-70.
52. Klein S, Kinney J, Jeejeebhoy K, et al. Nutrition support in clinical practice: review of published data and recommendations for future research directions. National Institutes of Health, American Society for Parenteral and Enteral Nutrition, and American Society for Clinical Nutrition. JPEN J Parenter Enteral Nutr 1997;21: 133-56.
53. Stroud M, Duncan H, Nightingale J, et al. Guidelines for enteral feeding in adult hospital patients. Gut 2003;52(Suppl 7):vii1-12.
54. Chrousos GP. The hypothalamic-pituitary-adrenal axis and immune-mediated inflammation. N Engl J Med 1995;332:1351-62.
55. Blackburn GL, Bistrian BR, Maini BS, et al. Nutritional and metabolic assessment of the hospitalized patient. JPEN J Parenter Enteral Nutr 1977;1:11-22.
56. Bistrian BR. A simple technique to estimate severity of stress. Surg Gynecol Obstet 1979;148:675-8.
57. Boitano M. Hypocaloric feeding of the critically ill. Nutr Clin Pract 2006;21:617-22.
58. Kreymann KG, Berger MM, Deutz NE, et al. ESPEN Guidelines on Enteral Nutrition: intensive care. Clin Nutr 2006;25:210-23.
59. Grau T, Bonet A. Caloric intake and liver dysfunction in critically ill patients. Curr Opin Clin Nutr Metab Care 2009;12:175-9.
60. Zauner C, Schuster BI, Schneeweiss B. Similar metabolic responses to standardized total parenteral nutrition of septic and nonseptic critically ill patients. Am J Clin Nutr 2001;74:265-70.
61. Reid CL. Poor agreement between continuous measurements of energy expenditure and routinely used prediction equations in intensive care unit patients. Clin Nutr 2007;26:649-57.

62. Hasselgren PO, Hubbard WJ, Chaudry IH. Metabolic and inflammatory responses to trauma and infection. In: Fischer JE, editor. 5th edition, Mastery of Surgery, vol. 1. Philidelphia: Lippincott Williams & Wilkins; 2007. p. 2–22.

63. McCowen KC, Malhotra A, Bistrian BR. Stress-induced hyperglycemia. Crit Care Clin 2001;17:107–24.

64. Kavanagh BP, McCowen KC. Clinical practice. Glycemic control in the ICU. N Engl J Med 2010;363:2540–6.

65. Wilmore DW. From Cuthbertson to fast-track surgery: 70 years of progress in reducing stress in surgical patients. Ann Surg 2002;236:643–8.

66. Ziegler TR. Parenteral nutrition in the critically ill patient. N Engl J Med 2009;361: 1088–97.

67. Blackburn GL, Wollner S, Bistrian BR. Nutrition support in the intensive care unit: an evolving science. Arch Surg 2010;145:533–8.

68. Blackburn GL. Interaction of the science of nutrition and the science of medicine. JPEN J Parenter Enteral Nutr 1979;3:131–6.

69. Khaodhiar L, Blackburn GL. Enteral nutrition support. In: Fischer JE, editor. 5th edition. Mastery of surgery, vol. 1. Philadelphia: Lippincott Williams & Wilkins; 2007. p. 45–56.

# Management of Enterocutaneous Fistulas

William P. Schecter, MD

**KEYWORDS**

- Enterocutaneous fistula • Enteroatmospheric fistula
- Open abdomen • Abdominal wall reconstruction

The sudden appearance of intestinal contents draining from an abdominal incision is an emotionally devastating experience for both patient and surgeon. An organized management plan and optimistic attitude based on a thorough understanding of the pathophysiology do much to reassure the fistula patient and other members of the surgical team. The spectrum of enterocutaneous fistulas (ECFs) ranges from an easily managed, low-output colocutaneous fistula to a high-output enteroatmospheric fistula (EAF) in the midst of an open abdomen requiring many months of intensive care, nutritional support, and complex reconstructive surgery. A comprehensive review of ECF must begin with its history.

## HISTORY

Alexis St Martin, a Canadian trapper, developed a chronic gastrocutaneous fistula after a musket shot injury to the abdomen in 1822. It remained open until his death 58 years later.[1] However, in general, the mortality of ECFs was high and remained high even after Bohrer and Miller[2] advocated conservative management in acute cases and "maintenance of chemical balance" in 1931. Thirty-four years later, Chapman and colleagues[3] identified 4 key principles of fistula care: fluid resuscitation, drainage of local abscesses, control of fistula effluent, and skin protection. The major breakthrough occurred in 1969 when Dudrick and colleagues[4] introduced total parenteral nutrition, reversing the catabolic state and permitting many fistulas to heal spontaneously. Further advances in knowledge and technology now permit precise diagnosis, interventional drainage of associated intra-abdominal abscesses,[5] and soft tissue coverage of persistent fistulas.[6] In addition, fistula management in specialized intestinal failure units is associated with a significant reduction in mortality.[7–9]

This article relies heavily on the following previously published article: Schecter WP, Hirshberg A, Chang DS, et al. Enteric fistulas: principles of management. Journal of the American College of Surgeons. 2009 Oct;209(4):484–91; with permission.

Department of Surgery, University of California, San Francisco, San Francisco General Hospital, 1001 Potrero Avenue, Ward 3A17, San Francisco, CA 94110, USA
*E-mail address:* bschect@sfghsurg.ucsf.edu

Surg Clin N Am 91 (2011) 481–491
doi:10.1016/j.suc.2011.02.004
0039-6109/11/$ – see front matter © 2011 Elsevier Inc. All rights reserved.

Improvements in resuscitation and the widespread use of damage-control laparotomy[10] have resulted in an epidemic of enteric fistulas in the midst of an open abdomen in intensive care units throughout the country.[11] These EAFs (or exposed fistulas), first described in the early 1980s,[12,13] are particularly challenging[14] because the absence of overlying soft tissue virtually precludes spontaneous closure.

## CLASSIFICATION OF ECF

An ECF is an abnormal communication between the bowel lumen and skin, often associated with sepsis, fluid and electrolyte abnormalities, and malnutrition.[15] ECFs are classified based on their anatomy, cause, or physiology (**Box 1**).[16] The anatomic classification describes the segment of gut from which the fistula originates. The etiologic classification is based on the underlying disease process. Most ECFs occur after an operative or interventional procedure. Approximately 20% of all ECFs are associated with Crohn disease, especially after bowel resection.[17] The physiologic classification is based on the volume of fistula output.

EAFs are classified based on the surrounding wound.[18] A deep EAF drains intestinal content directly into the peritoneal cavity, causing peritonitis. A superficial EAF occurs in the midst of a granulating wound covering a fused intestinal block. The peritoneal cavity is obliterated by the wound healing process. Therefore, a superficial EAF is primarily a stoma control problem, as opposed to a deep EAF, which is characterized by ongoing peritonitis and catabolism.[11]

---

**Box 1**
**ECF classification**

Anatomic classification

    Gastrocutaneous

    Enterocutaneous

    Colocutaneous

Etiologic classification

    Iatrogenic

        Operation

        Percutaneous drainage

    Trauma

    Foreign body

    Crohn disease

    Infectious disease

        Tuberculosis

        Actinomycosis

    Malignancy

Physiologic classification

    Low output (<200 mL/d)

    Moderate output (200–500 mL/d)

    High output (>500 mL/d)

About one-third of ECFs close after conservative treatment with wound care, control of infection, and nutritional support.[14] The familiar acronym "FRIENDS" (**Box 2**) is useful to help students recall the various causes of a persistent ECF. The barriers to spontaneous closure include distal obstruction, a short or epithelialized tract, malignancy, and underlying infection.[19] The EAF is especially hostile because the absence of overlying skin or soft tissue precludes spontaneous closure.[20]

## MANAGEMENT OF ECF

There are 3 phases of ECF management: (1) recognition and stabilization, (2) anatomic definition and decision, and (3) definitive operation.

### Phase 1: Recognition and Stabilization

Attention is directed to 4 clinical problems as soon as a fistula is identified: fluid and electrolyte repletion, skin care, sepsis, and nutritional support.[11] Aggressive fluid resuscitation and correction of electrolyte abnormalities is the first concern. Effluent from high-output fistulas should be replaced with normal saline and potassium (KCl at 10 mEq/L). Duodenal and pancreatic fistulas may require replacement of bicarbonate losses. In problem cases, electrolyte replacement is guided by the electrolyte content of the fistula effluent and serum.

Control of the fistula output is essential to protect the surrounding skin from the caustic effects of the intestinal contents. The best drainage systems are designed by a committed nurse or stoma therapist adapting to the unique and evolving characteristics of each wound.[21–23]

Vacuum-assisted wound management has been widely used for ECF care[24] in the past decade, significantly reducing the number of required dressing changes. Some investigators argue that vacuum-assisted wound management accelerates fistula closure by stimulating wound healing.[25,26] However, there is some evidence that this method may increase the risk of fistula formation if a fistula is not already present, and may delay closure of an existing fistula.[27,28] At present, there are no controlled trials comparing vacuum-assisted wound management with traditional wound drainage systems to resolve this controversy.

Somatostatin and octreotide can pharmacologically reduce the volume of fistula output. Although somatostatin rapidly reduces the fistula drainage, its clinical usefulness is limited by a short half-life (1–3 minutes). Its synthetic analogue, octreotide, has a half-life of 2 hours and results in a reduction of fistula output (40%–90%) after 48 hours[29] and a reduction in time to fistula closure (from 50 to 5–10 days).[30] Despite

---

**Box 2**
**Causes of persistent ECF**

F: foreign body

R: radiation enteritis

I: inflammation bowel disease

E: epithelialized fistula tract

N: neoplasm

D: distal obstruction

S: sepsis

the improvement in time to fistula closure, there is no evidence that octreotide improves the overall rate of fistula closure.[31] If a patient has a condition precluding spontaneous fistula closure, octreotide will only increase cost without affecting outcome, (see **Box 2**). In addition, octreotide inhibits growth hormone, thereby potentially inhibiting immune function.[32–34] However, there are no clinical studies confirming or excluding this possibility.

Infection associated with ECF can present as a contained intra-abdominal abscess or peritonitis. Most intra-abdominal abscesses can be drained percutaneously with radiographic or ultrasound image guidance. Peritonitis requires laparotomy with either exteriorization of the leak or proximal diversion of intestinal effluent. Very rarely, a leak can be closed primarily or resected with primary anastomosis.

Nutritional support to correct the catabolic consequences of ECF is essential. Baseline nutrient requirements consist of 20 kcal/kg/d of carbohydrate and fat and 0.8 g/kg/d of protein. However, caloric and protein requirements can increase to 30 kcal/kg/d and 1.5 to 2.5 g/kg/d, respectively, in patients with high-output fistulas.[35]

Fish oil or ω-3 fatty acid supplementation of enteral diets improves gut immune function.[36] These supplements have been associated with lower infection rates after injury,[37] during intensive care,[38] and following abdominal surgery.[39] However, other studies have failed to show a salutary effect.[40–42] There are no randomized trials investigating the use of these supplements in patients with ECF.

As a general rule, enteral feedings are preferred whenever possible because they preserve the intestinal mucosal barrier, gut hormonal and immunologic function, and avoid the problem of central line sepsis. However, enteral feedings are often not feasible because of feeding intolerance, inability to access the gastrointestinal (GI) tract, or high fistula output. Most patients with moderate-output and high-output ECFs will require total parenteral nutrition, which improves the rate of spontaneous closure.[29,43] Nutritional support should be advanced slowly for several days to optimal feeding goals in severely malnourished patients to reduce the risk of refeeding syndrome.[44] Correction of fluid, electrolyte, and vitamin deficiencies should precede aggressive feeding.

### Phase 2: Anatomic Definition and Decision

The next step after patient stabilization is anatomic delineation of the ECF. The abdominal computed tomography (CT) scan with appropriate intraluminal and intravenous contrast has largely replaced conventional radiography because it identifies not only the fistula tract, but also associated intra-abdominal abscesses and related disorders. If the information from the CT scan is insufficient for planning purposes, additional GI contrast radiograms may be helpful.

Reconstructive surgery should be delayed if the fistula output is decreasing, or if there is evidence of wound (or tract) healing.[26] Sufficient time should be allotted for the ECF to heal with conservative treatment. Spontaneous fistula closure rates vary from 15% to 71%.[3,12,21,26,45–53] Visschers and colleagues[20] reported a spontaneous closure in only 16% of their 135 patients, but the mean time from fistula onset to surgery was only 53 days. Adjuvant use of an anal fistula plug or fibrin glue in the fistula tract may promote healing in selected cases.[54]

As a general principle, the patient should be infection free and nutritionally replete with supple soft tissues in the region of the wound before definitive reconstruction. ECFs are associated with obliterative peritonitis[55] causing dense vascular adhesions. This intense inflammatory response persists for a minimum of 6 weeks after the onset of the ECF and can persist as long as a year in EAFs associated with an open abdomen. Ill-advised early operation in this hostile environment is associated with a high risk of potentially fatal complications.

### Phase 3: Definitive Operation

Resection of an ECF is a long, complex operation requiring patience, precision, and planning. The GI tract must be dissected from the ligament of Treitz to the rectum, if necessary, to mobilize all adhesions and to eliminate potential points of obstruction. The incision should be planned to ensure well-vascularized soft tissue coverage of the entire bowel. All serosal defects and enterotomies that occur during the dissection must be meticulously repaired. The goal of surgery is resection of the bowel segment giving rise to the fistula, and reestablishment of intestinal continuity. Singh and colleagues[56] recommend long intestinal tube stenting of the entire small bowel after fistula resection based on their 30-year experience with this technique. Of their 282 patients with high-output fistulas, 99 (35%) required surgery. Six patients (6%) died after surgery. All patients were stented, and no complications of stenting occurred. Ninety-three patients (93.9%) had a successful surgical repair, and there were no episodes of bowel obstruction or fistula recurrence within 6 months of surgery. Although I have limited personal experience with this technique, their results are impressive.

Intestinal failure caused by extensive bowel resection is a risk of complex fistula reconstructive surgery. Small bowel transplantation is an alternative to lifelong total parenteral nutrition in carefully selected patients with this devastating complication.[57]

### THE CHALLENGE OF EAF

The most important step in the management of EAF is prevention. If present, the greater omentum should be placed over exposed bowel in all patients with an open abdomen. Negative-pressure sponges and gauze dressings should never be placed in direct contact with bowel, especially if suture lines are exposed. In the absence of omentum, other biologic dressings, such as cadaver skin, should be used to protect the bowel, prevent desiccation, and reduce the risk of fistula formation. Routine wound care of the open abdomen should not be delegated to inexperienced members of the surgical team. Access to an open wound with exposed bowel should be limited to 1 or 2 highly experienced clinicians: an ounce of prevention is worth a pound of cure.[58]

### MANAGEMENT OF DEEP EAF

A deep EAF in an open abdomen results in spillage of intestinal contents, causing ongoing peritonitis and hemodynamic instability. Resuscitation and urgent laparotomy to achieve source control are essential. However, source control is often easier said than done. Massive edema of the gut and abdominal wall, combined with foreshortening and edema of the mesentery, frequently precludes exteriorization or proximal diversion of the leak. Furthermore, the appearance of dense vascular adhesions within 10 to 14 days of bowel exposure (the open abdomen equivalent of obliterative peritonitis) converts the intestinal tract into an impenetrable fused visceral block, precluding safe dissection.[59]

If exteriorization or proximal diversion of the bowel is not possible, the key to management is isolation of the intestinal contents from the peritoneal cavity until the abdominal wound granulates around the fistula, thereby converting it to a superficial EAF. Definitive closure of the fistula is only rational and possible many months later.

Simple tube drainage of fistulas is an appealing but ineffective method of source control. The tube only enlarges the hole, potentially eroding into adjacent bowel, and fails to control the drainage completely. One innovative management technique is the floating stoma.[60] A plastic sheet cut to appropriate size is used as a temporary abdominoplasty. A stoma hole is cut in the plastic sheet, and the margin of the opening in the bowel is then sutured to the perimeter of the hole in the plastic sheet, thus diverting the intestinal contents from the peritoneal cavity until a carpet of granulation tissue covers the exterior surface of the free peritoneal cavity. A colostomy appliance is applied to the plastic sheet over the improvised stoma to collect the effluent.

More commonly, vacuum-assisted wound management is used for source control by continuous suction of the intestinal fluid. This method also minimizes manipulation of the wound associated with the exposed bowel, simplifies nursing care, and keeps the patient's skin dry. In the case of a complex fistula with multiple holes, tubes sometimes have a role. They can be placed into each hole and brought out through conforming openings created in the sponge. The adhesive sponge thus serves as a platform to suspend the tubes, preventing contact of the tubes with adjacent bowel, and sucking up residual fluid draining around the tubes. The adhesive plastic dressing placed over the sponge must be carefully fashioned around the tubes to achieve an airtight closure.[18]

If vacuum-assisted wound management is chosen, it is essential to avoid direct contact between the bowel and the sponge. Plastic sheets, petroleum gauze, or even cadaver split-thickness skin grafts can be used as a biologic dressing.[61] Placement of any foreign body that adheres to the bowel increases the risk of fistula formation. The role of negative pressure in fistula formation is unknown. Reports of fistula formation after vacuum-assisted wound management[27] led Fischer[28] to urge caution in its use, particularly in the presence of a fresh intestinal anastomosis. However, in certain cases of deep EAF, vacuum-assisted wound management may be the only available practical option for source control.

A deep EAF in the midst of an open abdomen is the catabolic equivalent of a major full-thickness burn. Enteral nutrition alone is rarely, if ever, able to supply the calories and protein required because of gut dysfunction caused by peritonitis, bowel edema, and massive loss of fluid and protein. Combined enteral and parenteral nutritional support, together with source control, is critical to prevent catabolic collapse.

## MANAGEMENT OF SUPERFICIAL EAF

A superficial EAF occurs in the midst of a carpet of granulation tissue covering a fused block of viscera with an obliterated peritoneal cavity. These patients rarely exhibit uncontrolled sepsis because the intestinal contents do not ordinarily come in contact with, or accumulate in, the peritoneal cavity. However, they do present major wound and stoma management problems. The key principle is protection of the bowel adjacent to the fistulas to prevent development of additional leaks. Occasionally, small bud fistulas can be closed and covered with autogenous or cadaver split-thickness skin grafts.[62] On rare occasions, it is possible to close very small holes with acellular human dermal matrix[63] or autogenous split-thickness skin grafts.[62] Fibrin glue can be helpful in affixing the grafts to the bowel. The probability of success is low, but the cost of failure with use of these local procedures is minimal.

In most cases, the carpet of granulation tissue around the superficial EAF must be covered with autogenous split-thickness skin grafts. A negative-pressure wound dressing placed over the grafts is an effective dressing. After the grafts heal, there are many options for stoma management. The basic principle is use of stoma bases and creams to protect the grafts and skin from the stomal drainage. Committed, skilled nurses and stoma therapists are essential and valuable members of the team.

## ABDOMINAL WALL RECONSTRUCTION

All patients with an EAF have an open abdomen by definition that will ultimately require reconstruction. A sufficient period of time (at least 6–12 months) must pass to allow the wound to mature and the surrounding tissues to soften before definitive surgery. Patience on the part of both the patient and the surgeon is essential. Ill-advised early operation greatly increases the risk of failure. If the viscera is covered by a skin graft, surgery should be delayed until the graft can be pinched off the underlying bowel between the index finger and the thumb.[64] This pinch test indicates that a plane exists between the graft and the underlying bowel, permitting safe dissection of the graft from the bowel.

The goals of the procedure are resection of the segment of bowel communicating with the fistula, restoration of intestinal continuity, and coverage of the bowel with well-vascularized soft tissue. Careful planning of the abdominal wall reconstruction includes an assessment of the deficient abdominal wall components and the tissues available for reconstruction. Many patients benefit from consultation with an experienced reconstructive surgeon. Use of either autogenous or biologic materials for abdominal wall reconstruction is preferable because of the heavy contamination caused by the fistula. Although human[65] and porcine[66] acellular dermal matrix and porcine submucosa[67] may be necessary for visceral coverage in some cases, increasing experience suggests that these materials are not durable and ultimately become expensive hernia sacs. Nevertheless, the primary goal of the procedure is cure of the fistula; ventral herniorrhaphy is a secondary goal. If any of these materials are necessary to protect the bowel, they should be used as needed.

Autogenous tissue can usually be used for reconstruction. The components separation technique[68] is the mainstay for abdominal closure if the rectus abdominis muscle is present. The rectus abdominis myofascial units on both sides of the defect are advanced, capable of bridging gaps up to 10 cm in the upper abdomen, 20 cm in the midabdomen, and 6 to 8 cm in the lower abdomen.[68]

However, the rectus abdominis muscle is frequently unavailable. In this situation, a variety of available skin, as well as pedicle and free muscle and myocutaneous flaps, are potential choices for coverage. If skin flaps are not a viable option, random other tissue flaps and/or placement of tissue expanders before definitive surgery should be considered.

The muscle flaps useful in abdominal wall reconstruction can be based on the tensor fascia lata,[69] the rectus femoris,[70] and the latissimus dorsi.[71] Chang and colleagues[72] recently described an island pedicled anterolateral thigh flap for closure of an intractable Crohn small bowel fistula. The reconstructive options are limited only by the available tissue components and the skill and imagination of the reconstructive surgeon. The best results are obtained by treatment in centers capable of providing dedicated comprehensive care.[8,9,13]

## SUMMARY

ECF is a life-threatening condition requiring longitudinal care for many months. A spectrum of vexing clinical problems ranging from hypovolemic shock to malnutrition to complex abdominal wall reconstruction challenge the skill of even highly experienced surgeons. High-output fistulas and EAFs are best managed in centers providing comprehensive care of intestinal failure.

## REFERENCES

1. Beaumont W. Experiments and observations on the gastric juices and physiology of digestion. Edinburgh (UK): MacLaughlin & Stewart, Southbridge; and Simpkin, Marshall, & Co London; 1838.
2. Bohrer JV, Milici A. Duodeno-cutaneous fistulae. Ann Surg 1931;93(6):1174–90.

3. Chapman R, Foran R, Dunphy JE. Management of intestinal fistulas. Am J Surg 1964;108:157–64.
4. Dudrick SJ, Wilmore DW, Vars HM, et al. Can intravenous feeding as the sole means of nutrition support growth in the child and restore weight loss in an adult? An affirmative answer. Ann Surg 1969;169(6):974–84.
5. Gerzof SG, Robbins AH, Birkett DH, et al. Percutaneous catheter drainage of abdominal abscesses guided by ultrasound and computed tomography. AJR Am J Roentgenol 1979;133(1):1–8.
6. Mathes SJ, Bostwick J 3rd. A rectus abdominis myocutaneous flap to reconstruct abdominal wall defects. Br J Plast Surg 1977;30(4):282–3.
7. Irving M, White R, Tresadern J. Three years' experience with an intestinal failure unit. Ann R Coll Surg Engl 1985;67(1):2–5.
8. Gyorki DE, Brooks CE, Gett R, et al. Enterocutaneous fistula: a single-centre experience. ANZ J Surg 2010;80(3):178–81.
9. Datta V, Engledow A, Chan S, et al. The management of enterocutaneous fistula in a regional unit in the United Kingdom: a prospective study. Dis Colon Rectum 2010;53(2):192–9.
10. Burch JM, Ortiz VB, Richardson RJ, et al. Abbreviated laparotomy and planned reoperation for critically injured patients. Ann Surg 1992;215(5):476–83 [discussion: 483–4].
11. Schecter WP, Hirshberg A, Chang DS, et al. Enteric fistulas: principles of management. J Am Coll Surg 2009;209(4):484–91.
12. Levy E, Frileux P, Cugnenc PH, et al. Exposed fistula of the small intestine, a complication of peritonitis or laparotomy. Apropos of 120 cases. Ann Chir 1986;40(3):184–95 [in French].
13. Schein M, Decker GA. Gastrointestinal fistulas associated with large abdominal wall defects: experience with 43 patients. Br J Surg 1990;77(1):97–100.
14. Schein M. What's new in postoperative enterocutaneous fistulas? World J Surg 2008;32(3):336–8.
15. Edmunds LH Jr, Williams GM, Welch CE. External fistulas arising from the gastrointestinal tract. Ann Surg 1960;152:445–71.
16. Berry SM, Fischer JE. Classification and pathophysiology of enterocutaneous fistulas. Surg Clin North Am 1996;76(5):1009–18.
17. Keighley M, Heyen F, Winslet MC. Entero-cutaneous fistulas and Crohn's disease. Acta Gastroenterol Belg 1987;50(5):580–600.
18. Al-Khoury G, Kaufman D, Hirshberg A. Improved control of exposed fistula in the open abdomen. J Am Coll Surg 2008;206(2):397–8.
19. Reber HA, Roberts C, Way LW, et al. Management of external gastrointestinal fistulas. Ann Surg 1978;188(4):460–7.
20. Visschers RG, Olde Damink SW, Winkens B, et al. Treatment strategies in 135 consecutive patients with enterocutaneous fistulas. World J Surg 2008;32(3):445–53.
21. Martinez JL, Luque-de-Leon E, Mier J, et al. Systematic management of postoperative enterocutaneous fistulas: factors related to outcomes. World J Surg 2008; 32(3):436–43 [discussion: 444].
22. Franklin C. The suction pouch for management of simple or complex enterocutaneous fistulae. J Wound Ostomy Continence Nurs 2010;37(4):387–92.
23. Hardwicke J, Wright TC, Hargest R, et al. The use of the Flexi-Seal Faecal Management System in laparostomy wounds involving enterocutaneous fistula. Ann R Coll Surg Engl 2010;92(4):W12–4.
24. Cro C, George KJ, Donnelly J, et al. Vacuum assisted closure system in the management of enterocutaneous fistulae. Postgrad Med J 2002;78(920): 364–5.

25. Banwell P, Withey S, Holten I. The use of negative pressure to promote healing. Br J Plast Surg 1998;51(1):79.
26. Wainstein DE, Fernandez E, Gonzalez D, et al. Treatment of high-output enterocutaneous fistulas with a vacuum-compaction device. A ten-year experience. World J Surg 2008;32(3):430–5.
27. Rao M, Burke D, Finan PJ, et al. The use of vacuum-assisted closure of abdominal wounds: a word of caution. Colorectal Dis 2007;9(3):266–8.
28. Fischer JE. A cautionary note: the use of vacuum-assisted closure systems in the treatment of gastrointestinal cutaneous fistula may be associated with higher mortality from subsequent fistula development. Am J Surg 2008; 196(1):1–2.
29. Nubiola P, Badia JM, Martinez-Rodenas F, et al. Treatment of 27 postoperative enterocutaneous fistulas with the long half-life somatostatin analogue SMS 201-995. Ann Surg 1989;210(1):56–8.
30. Dorta G. Role of octreotide and somatostatin in the treatment of intestinal fistulae. Digestion 1999;60(Suppl 2):53–6.
31. Alivizatos V, Felekis D, Zorbalas A. Evaluation of the effectiveness of octreotide in the conservative treatment of postoperative enterocutaneous fistulas. Hepatogastroenterology 2002;49(46):1010–2.
32. Lattuada D, Casnici C, Crotta K, et al. Inhibitory effect of pasireotide and octreotide on lymphocyte activation. J Neuroimmunol 2007;182(1/2):153–9.
33. Wiedermann CJ, Reinisch N, Braunsteiner H. Stimulation of monocyte chemotaxis by human growth hormone and its deactivation by somatostatin. Blood 1993; 82(3):954–60.
34. Dudrick SJ, Maharaj AR, McKelvey AA. Artificial nutritional support in patients with gastrointestinal fistulas. World J Surg 1999;23(6):570–6.
35. Makhdoom ZA, Komar MJ, Still CD. Nutrition and enterocutaneous fistulas. J Clin Gastroenterol 2000;31(3):195–204.
36. Kudsk KA. Immunonutrition in surgery and critical care. Annu Rev Nutr 2006;26: 463–79.
37. Kudsk KA, Minard G, Croce MA, et al. A randomized trial of isonitrogenous enteral diets after severe trauma. An immune-enhancing diet reduces septic complications. Ann Surg 1996;224(4):531–40 [discussion: 540–3].
38. Bower RH, Cerra FB, Bershadsky B, et al. Early enteral administration of a formula (Impact) supplemented with arginine, nucleotides, and fish oil in intensive care unit patients: results of a multicenter, prospective, randomized, clinical trial. Crit Care Med 1995;23(3):436–49.
39. Schilling J, Vranjes N, Fierz W, et al. Clinical outcome and immunology of postoperative arginine, omega-3 fatty acids, and nucleotide-enriched enteral feeding: a randomized prospective comparison with standard enteral and low calorie/low fat I.V. solutions. Nutrition 1996;12(6):423–9.
40. Saffle JR, Wiebke G, Jennings K, et al. Randomized trial of immune-enhancing enteral nutrition in burn patients. J Trauma 1997;42(5):793–800 [discussion: 800–2].
41. Heyland DK, Novak F, Drover JW, et al. Should immunonutrition become routine in critically ill patients? A systematic review of the evidence. JAMA 2001;286(8): 944–53.
42. Marik PE, Zaloga GP. Immunonutrition in critically ill patients: a systematic review and analysis of the literature. Intensive Care Med 2008;34(11):1980–90.
43. Lloyd DA, Gabe SM, Windsor AC. Nutrition and management of enterocutaneous fistula. Br J Surg 2006;93(9):1045–55.

44. Stanga Z, Brunner A, Leuenberger M, et al. Nutrition in clinical practice-the refeeding syndrome: illustrative cases and guidelines for prevention and treatment. Eur J Clin Nutr 2008;62(6):687–94.
45. Halversen RC, Hogle HH, Richards RC. Gastric and small bowel fistulas. Am J Surg 1969;118(6):968–72.
46. Campos AC, Andrade DF, Campos GM, et al. A multivariate model to determine prognostic factors in gastrointestinal fistulas. J Am Coll Surg 1999;188(5):483–90.
47. Fazio VW, Coutsoftides T, Steiger E. Factors influencing the outcome of treatment of small bowel cutaneous fistula. World J Surg 1983;7(4):481–8.
48. Fischer JE. The pathophysiology of enterocutaneous fistulas. World J Surg 1983; 7(4):446–50.
49. Aguirre A, Fischer JE, Welch CE. The role of surgery and hyperalimentation in therapy of gastrointestinal-cutaneous fistulae. Ann Surg 1974;180(4): 393–401.
50. McIntyre PB, Ritchie JK, Hawley PR, et al. Management of enterocutaneous fistulas: a review of 132 cases. Br J Surg 1984;71(4):293–6.
51. Prickett D, Montgomery R, Cheadle WG. External fistulas arising from the digestive tract. South Med J 1991;84(6):736–9.
52. Sitges-Serra A, Jaurrieta E, Sitges-Creus A. Management of postoperative enterocutaneous fistulas: the roles of parenteral nutrition and surgery. Br J Surg 1982; 69(3):147–50.
53. Draus JM Jr, Huss SA, Harty NJ, et al. Enterocutaneous fistula: are treatments improving? Surgery 2006;140(4):570–6 [discussion: 576–8].
54. Satya R, Satya RJ. Successful treatment of an enterocutaneous fistula with an anal fistula plug after an abdominal stab wound. J Vasc Interv Radiol 2010; 21(3):414–5.
55. Hill GL. Operative strategy in the treatment of enterocutaneous fistulas. World J Surg 1983;7(4):495–501.
56. Singh B, Haffejee AA, Allopi L, et al. Surgery for high-output small bowel enterocutaneous fistula: a 30-year experience. Int Surg 2009;94(3):262–8.
57. Vianna RM, Mangus RS, Tector AJ. Current status of small bowel and multivisceral transplantation. Adv Surg 2008;42:129–50.
58. Schecter WP, Ivatury RR, Rotondo MF, et al. Open abdomen after trauma and abdominal sepsis: a strategy for management. J Am Coll Surg 2006;203(3): 390–6.
59. Scott BG, Feanny MA, Hirshberg A. Early definitive closure of the open abdomen: a quiet revolution. Scand J Surg 2005;94(1):9–14.
60. Subramaniam MH, Liscum KR, Hirshberg A. The floating stoma: a new technique for controlling exposed fistulae in abdominal trauma. J Trauma 2002;53(2): 386–8.
61. Jamshidi R, Schecter WP. Biological dressings for the management of enteric fistulas in the open abdomen: a preliminary report. Arch Surg 2007;142(8):793–6.
62. Sarfeh IJ, Jakowatz JG. Surgical treatment of enteric 'bud' fistulas in contaminated wounds. A riskless extraperitoneal method using split-thickness skin grafts. Arch Surg 1992;127(9):1027–30 [discussion: 1030–1].
63. Girard S, Sideman M, Spain DA. A novel approach to the problem of intestinal fistulization arising in patients managed with open peritoneal cavities. Am J Surg 2002;184(2):166–7.
64. Jernigan TW, Fabian TC, Croce MA, et al. Staged management of giant abdominal wall defects: acute and long-term results. Ann Surg 2003;238(3):349–55 [discussion: 355–7].

65. Maurice SM, Skeete DA. Use of human acellular dermal matrix for abdominal wall reconstructions. Am J Surg 2009;197(1):35–42.
66. Hsu PW, Salgado CJ, Kent K, et al. Evaluation of porcine dermal collagen (Permacol) used in abdominal wall reconstruction. J Plast Reconstr Aesthet Surg 2009; 62(11):1484–9.
67. Johnson EK, Paquette EL. Use of surgisis for abdominal wall reconstruction/ closure in battlefield casualties during Operation Iraqi Freedom. Mil Med 2007; 172(10):1119–24.
68. Shestak KC, Edington HJ, Johnson RR. The separation of anatomic components technique for the reconstruction of massive midline abdominal wall defects: anatomy, surgical technique, applications, and limitations revisited. Plast Reconstr Surg 2000;105(2):731–8 [quiz: 739].
69. Williams JK, Carlson GW, deChalain T, et al. Role of tensor fasciae latae in abdominal wall reconstruction. Plast Reconstr Surg 1998;101(3):713–8.
70. Koshima I, Moriguchi T, Inagawa K, et al. Dynamic reconstruction of the abdominal wall using a reinnervated free rectus femoris muscle transfer. Ann Plast Surg 1999;43(2):199–203.
71. de Weerd L, Kjaeve J, Aghajani E, et al. The sandwich design: a new method to close a high-output enterocutaneous fistula and an associated abdominal wall defect. Ann Plast Surg 2007;58(5):580–3.
72. Chang SH, Hsu TC, Su HC, et al. Treatment of intractable enterocutaneous fistula with an island pedicled anterolateral thigh flap in Crohn's disease–case report. J Plast Reconstr Aesthet Surg 2010;63(6):1055–7.

# Current Management of the Short Bowel Syndrome

Jon S. Thompson, MD[a],*, Rebecca Weseman, RD[b],
Fedja A. Rochling, MB, BCh[c], David F. Mercer, MD, PhD[d]

**KEYWORDS**

- Short bowel syndrome • Intestinal failure
- Intestinal transplantation

Intestinal failure from loss of intestine, or short bowel syndrome (SBS), is associated with the inability to maintain protein, energy, fluid, electrolytes, or micronutrient balances while on a conventionally accepted normal diet.[1] SBS generally occurs when less than 200 cm of functional intestine remains in adults.[2] **Table 1** lists the causes of SBS in adults at the University of Nebraska Medical Center from 1990 to 2005. Postoperative SBS has emerged as the most common condition. The severity of the clinical features depends on several factors, including primarily the extent of resection, but also the site of resection, underlying intestinal disease, presence or absence of the ileocecal valve, functional status of the remaining digestive organs, and adaptive capacity of the intestinal remnant (**Fig. 1**). Long-term outcome is primarily determined by patient age and underlying disease.[3,4] However, several deaths are caused by complications directly related to the management of SBS. Approximately two-thirds of patients who develop SBS survive after the initial hospitalization, and a similar proportion of patients are alive 1 year later.[5,6]

The pathophysiologic changes that occur in SBS relate primarily to the loss of intestinal absorptive surface and more rapid intestinal transit.[2] Gastric hypersecretion, inactivation of pancreatic enzymes, and loss of bile salts also contribute. Malabsorption of nutrients results in malnutrition and weight loss, diarrhea and steatorrhea, vitamin deficiency, and electrolyte imbalance. More specific complications include

The authors have nothing to disclose.
[a] Division of General Surgery, Department of Surgery, University Nebraska Medical Center, 983280 Nebraska Medical Center, Omaha, NE 68198-3280, USA
[b] Medical Nutrition Education, University Nebraska Medical Center, 983285 Nebraska Medical Center, Omaha, NE 68198-3285, USA
[c] Division of Gastroenterology and Hepatology, Department of Medicine, University Nebraska Medical Center, 982000 Nebraska Medical Center, Omaha, NE 68198-2000, USA
[d] Division of Transplantation, Department of Surgery, University Nebraska Medical Center, 983285 Nebraska Medical Center, Omaha, NE 68198-3285, USA
* Corresponding author.
*E-mail address:* jthompso@unmc.edu

**Table 1**
**Causes of short bowel syndrome in adults**

|  | Number | % |
|---|---|---|
| Postoperative resection | 84 | 28 |
| Malignancy/irradiation | 63 | 21 |
| Mesenteric vascular disease | 63 | 21 |
| Crohn's disease | 49 | 16 |
| Trauma | 22 | 8 |
| Other benign conditions | 19 | 6 |
| Total | 300 |  |

an increased incidence of nephrolithiasis from hyperoxaluria, cholelithiasis secondary to altered bile salt and bilirubin metabolism, and gastric hypersecretion. Bacterial overgrowth can also occur secondary to stasis from mechanical bowel obstruction or primary motor abnormalities. Liver disease is an important factor in mortality, especially in patients dependent primarily on parenteral nutrition (PN).[7]

Functional and structural adaptation of the remaining intestine occurs after massive intestinal resection.[8] This process results in improved absorption of nutrients, begins within the first few months after resection, and can continue for 1 to 2 years. Thus, permanent intestinal failure is determined 2 years after resection. The degree of adaptation depends partly on the extent and site of resection, the provision of enteral nutrients, and the response to gastrointestinal hormones and other regulatory polypeptides.[2,8]

Management of SBS progresses through several phases. Early management usually involves stabilization of a critically ill surgical patient who recently underwent intestinal resection, often together with other procedures. Controlling sepsis, maintaining fluid and electrolyte balance, and initiation of nutritional support are important areas in initial management of these patients. As the patient recovers, the primary goals of management are to maintain adequate nutritional status, maximize the absorptive capacity of the remaining intestine, and prevent the development of complications related to both the underlying pathophysiology and the nutritional therapy itself.[2] Surgical approaches have become increasingly important and include preserving the intestinal remnant, maximizing or improving the function of the intestinal remnant, and augmenting intestinal length.[4] Intestinal transplantation is also being performed more frequently in selected patients.

Comprehensive care of patients with intestinal failure requires a multidisciplinary approach (**Fig. 2**). Efforts should be coordinated by a physician leader with expertise

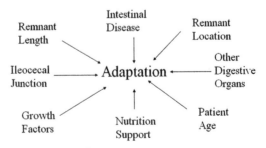

**Fig. 1.** Factors affecting outcome of SBS.

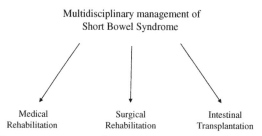

**Fig. 2.** Multidisciplinary management of SBS.

in gastrointestinal disease. Gastrointestinal surgical expertise in both adult and pediatric patients is required, and the presence of a transplant surgeon broadens the therapeutic options. A nutritionist is essential, and a nurse coordinator is indispensable in daily management, as are psychologists and social workers to address psychosocial issues. Administrative support to coordinate the process and database is also required. This multidisciplinary effort should optimize patient outcome.[9,10]

## MEDICAL REHABILITATION

The overall goal of medical rehabilitation is to return patients to as normal a lifestyle as possible with as little dependence on PN as can be achieved. Optimal management should improve patient survival. Intestinal rehabilitation is the process of enhancing intestinal absorption and function through the use of modified diet, enteral nutrition, oral rehydration solution, antimotility and antisecretory agents, antibiotics, and growth factors.

### *Maintain Nutritional Status*

The most important therapeutic objective in the management of SBS is to maintain the patient's nutritional status, primarily through PN support in the early postoperative period. This therapy includes provision of not only energy substrates and protein but also fluid, electrolytes, minerals, vitamins, and micronutrients. Most patients require 25 to 30 kcal/kg per day and 1.0 to 1.5 g of protein per kilogram per day with appropriate additives. Fluid and electrolyte losses from the gastrointestinal tract may be great during the early postoperative period. Specific attention to the individual patient's requirements for optimal fluid replacement is necessary to prevent dehydration.[2]

Enteral nutrition support should be started as early as feasible after operation when the ileus has resolved. This step is important for maximizing intestinal adaptation and preventing complications related to PN. Many patients will be able to absorb the necessary nutrients entirely through the enteral route as their condition improves and intestinal adaptation occurs. Intestinal remnant length has important prognostic implications for nutrition support. Patients with more than 180 cm of small intestine remaining generally require no PN; those with more than 90 cm of small intestine and particularly with colon will generally require PN for less than 1 year; and those with less than 60 cm of small intestine will likely require permanent PN depending on the remaining length of colon.[6,11] Patients with remaining colon in continuity have greater fluid and nutrient absorption as the colon adapts as a digestive organ.[12,13]

During the transition from parenteral to enteral nutrition support, the primary objectives are maintenance of a stable body weight and prevention of large fluctuations in fluid balance.[14] Ongoing metabolic monitoring is necessary for early detection and correction of potential metabolic abnormalities and micronutrient deficiencies. PN should be gradually decreased only after enteral intake is clearly increasing in amount and tolerability, because whether parenteral nutrients suppress appetite is unclear. Sustained increases in gastrointestinal fluid losses may be a sign that further advancements in enteral feeding will not be tolerated and should prompt review of a patient's overall management strategy, with consideration of reducing or halting the pace of enteral advancement. Within the confines of maintaining overall nutritional state, consideration should be given to reducing parenteral lipids to minimize cholestasis and progressive liver dysfunction associated with soy-based lipids. Over time, as parenteral requirements diminish, intermittent PN can be cycled, reducing hours of therapy during the day and perhaps eventually eliminating days of PN support.

### Maximize Enteral Nutrient Absorption

Dietary management for individual patients with SBS is determined by a variety of factors, including the intestinal remnant length and location, presence of any underlying intestinal disease, and status of the remaining digestive organs.[2] Whether the patient has a stoma will also be an important consideration, because diarrhea and perianal complications may markedly diminish oral intake. However, patients with stomas may be more likely to take a greater percentage of their calories enterally. Patients with SBS may develop hyperphagia to overcome their inefficient absorption.[15] Continuous enteral feeding may permit greater absorption of nutrients than intermittent enteral feeding in patients with remnants less than 90 cm.[16]

Dietary recommendations for patients with SBS are determined primarily by remnant length and whether the colon is in continuity (**Table 2**).[2,9,17] Hyposmolar diets are started initially to minimize gastrointestinal fluid losses. More complex diets can be ingested later. Because jejunal mucosa is relatively permeable, isotonic feedings are particularly important with jejunal remnants shorter than 100 cm. Ingestion of a glucose–electrolyte oral rehydration solution with a sodium concentration of at least 90 mmol/L will optimize water and sodium absorption in the proximal jejunum and minimize secretion into the lumen.[18] Initially, a high-carbohydrate, high-protein diet is appropriate to maximize absorption.

Providing nutrients in their simplest form so that digestion does not become a limiting factor in the absorptive process is one strategic approach. Simple sugars

| Table 2<br>Dietary recommendations for short bowel syndrome | | |
|---|---|---|
| | **Colon in Continuity** | **No Colon in Continuity** |
| Fluids | Hypotonic and/or ORS | ORS |
| Carbohydrate | 50%–60% of caloric intake<br>Complex carbohydrates<br>Limit simple sugars<br>Low lactose | 40%–50% of caloric intake<br>Complex carbohydrates<br>Limit simple sugars |
| Fat | 20%–30% of caloric intake<br>Adequate essential fats<br>MCT/LCT | 30%–40% of caloric intake<br>Adequate essential fats<br>LCT |
| Protein | 20%–30% of caloric intake | 20%–30% of caloric intake |
| Fiber | 5–10 g/d soluble fiber for net secretors | 5–10 g/d soluble fiber for net secretors |
| Oxalate | Restriction | No restriction |

Abbreviations: LCT, long-chain triglycerides; MCT, medium-chain triglycerides; ORS, oral rehydration solution.

and di- and tripeptides are rapidly absorbed from the intestinal tract. Partially hydro-lyzed diets seem to be just as effective. Fat absorption requires more digestion unless the fat is supplied in the form of medium-chain triglycerides (MCT). Stool fat increases markedly, however, in patients with remnants less than 60 cm. Because the ability to absorb these nutrients improves with time, the diet should be continually modified. Other problems, such as lactase deficiency, may also be present and require appro-priate management. The addition of dietary fiber is useful in patients who are net fluid secretors. Pectin may improve absorption through prolonging transit time and serving as a source of short-chain fatty acids. The role of specific nutrients such as glutamine and growth factors such as growth hormone and glucagon-like peptide 2 (GLP-2) in improving nutrient absorption is discussed later.

Another important aspect of dietary management is to provide a diet that will accel-erate and maximize the intestinal adaptive response. Enteral nutrients are important in this phase. Provision of fat, particularly long-chain triglycerides and dietary fiber, may be particularly important in this regard.[19] Glutamine is the preferred enterocyte fuel and may be trophic to the gut.[20] Although these nutrients may act directly to stimulate intestinal adaptation, the meal may also stimulate intestinal adaptation through endo-crine or paracrine effects. Growth factors and hormones may also stimulate intestinal adaptation.[21–25]

Minimizing gastrointestinal secretion and controlling diarrhea are also important goals for maximizing absorption (**Table 3**). Several agents are useful for improving absorption through their antisecretory and antimotility effects, including narcotics, such as codeine and diphenoxylate, and the peripherally acting narcotic, loperamide.[2] These agents tend to have diminished effects over time, necessitating progressive dosage increases or periodic drug holidays to restore sensitivity.

Cholestyramine may also be beneficial when the diarrhea is related to the cathartic effect of unabsorbed bile salts in the colon. Because bile acid malabsorption is difficult to detect clinically and cholestyramine is generally well tolerated, it is a reasonable empiric early intervention, especially in patients with limited ileal resections. Because of interactions limiting absorption of other drugs, however, establishing a compatible and durable dosing schedule for patients can be challenging. Care must be taken over

| Table 3 Medical treatment of short bowel syndrome | |
|---|---|
| **Treatment Goal** | **Medications** |
| Slow transit and decrease diarrhea | Loperamide Diphenoxylate Narcotics Cholestyramine Pancreatic enzymes |
| Reduce gastrointestinal secretion | $H_2$ receptor antagonists Proton pump inhibitors Octreotide[a] Clonidine[a] |
| Treat bacterial overgrowth | Antibiotics Probiotics Prokinetics |
| Pharmacologic treatment | Glutamine Growth hormone |

[a] Off-label use.

time to ensure that patients do not develop fat-soluble vitamin deficiencies as a result of chronic cholestyramine use.

Both the $H_2$ receptor antagonists and proton pump inhibitors (PPIs) have been shown to be effective in controlling gastric hypersecretion.[26] However, prolonged therapy with PPIs may be associated with bowel symptoms and bacterial overgrowth.[27] Somatostatin and its long-acting analog octreotide can improve diarrhea through increasing small-intestinal transit time, reducing salt and water excretion, and reducing gastric hypersecretion. Because of tachyphylaxis, however, they typically become less effective over the long term and may have deleterious effects, including steatorrhea, inhibition of intestinal adaptation, and increased incidence of cholelithiasis.[28,29] Therefore, although it might be helpful, octreotide should not be used routinely for the first-line management of chronic diarrhea. Recent studies suggest that the $\alpha_2$-adrenergic receptor agonist clonidine may also reduce fluid loss in these patients.[30] Treatment of bacterial overgrowth will also improve absorption. The intestinal microflora is altered in patients with SBS, and prebiotics and probiotics may become helpful in management.[31,32]

Pharmacologic therapy for SBS is a rapidly expanding area of investigation. A variety of growth factors and hormones have been identified that can promote intestinal growth or enhance absorptive function.[33] Although several agents with these effects have been studied experimentally, only a few are being used clinically. Growth hormone has trophic and proabsorptive effects on the gut and other metabolic effects. Glutamine helps maintain the structural integrity of the gut.[20] Epidermal growth factor (EGF) and GLP-2 are being studied in clinical trials. Several issues related to timing, dosage, duration of therapy, and route of delivery for these agents remain unresolved. These agents have most frequently been used to augment nutritional management in stable patients after initial intestinal adaptation.

Almost 15 years ago, Byrne and Wilmore initiated a treatment protocol that included a high-carbohydrate, low-fat diet; glutamine; and high-dose growth hormone in patients with stable SBS. In an initial unblinded, uncontrolled study, fluid and electrolyte absorption and nutrient absorption improved together with weight gain in patients with SBS.[21] Subsequent studies by these investigators showed that 60% of patients were weaned off PN and another one-third had reduced PN requirements.[22] This 4-week intensive regimen led to apparent benefit at 1-year follow-up. However, which of these therapies was actually responsible for improved absorption was unclear. Subsequently, a randomized, placebo-controlled, double-blinded clinical trial showed that regimens involving growth hormone, glutamine, and diet and those involving growth hormone and diet permitted more PN weaning than the regimen of glutamine and diet, but only growth hormone, glutamine, and diet maintained the effect at 3 months.[23] However, growth hormone alone has not shown a consistent beneficial effect in other randomized, blinded, placebo-controlled crossover studies.[34–36] Both growth hormone and glutamine are available for clinical use, but growth hormone is generally not used routinely because of cost, side effects, and questionable efficacy.[37]

Currently, GLP-2 seems to be another agent that has promise for promoting intestinal absorption and adaptation. GLP-2 is produced by enteroendocrine L-cells in the distal small intestine and colon and stimulates mucosal growth and absorption. In an open-label study, Jeppesen et al.[24] reported improved absorption in eight patients with SBS without colon who received exogenous GLP-2. A longer-acting analog, teduglutide, is now available.[25] Initial studies with this agent suggest a transient improvement in intestinal absorption of fluid, but not energy, during therapy but loss of effect later. Modest changes in villus height and crypt depth were also seen in the remnant. Patients have shown good compliance and safety with treatment for up to 2 years.[38] However, teduglutide remains investigational and is undergoing further study in patients with SBS.

EGF is proabsorptive and stimulates intestinal adaptation in experimental studies.[39] A recent clinical trial of enteral recombinant EGF in pediatric patients with SBS found increased carbohydrate absorption and tolerance to enteral feeds.[40] However, ongoing administration was required for sustained improvement, and this agent remains investigational.

### Prevent Complications

Metabolic complications are common in patients with SBS (**Box 1**).[41] Hyperglycemia and hypoglycemia are ever-present potential complications of patients receiving large amounts of calories parenterally. Patients are also always at risk for dehydration and renal dysfunction. Hypocalcemia is a common problem related to poor absorption and binding by intraluminal fat. Maintaining adequate levels of calcium, magnesium, and vitamin D supplementation is important to minimize bone disease. Increasingly, clinicians are recognizing that patients with SBS can require extremely large doses of vitamin D to rebuild and maintain body stores. Although typically doses of vitamin D range from 1000 to 2000 units per day, patients with SBS can require as much as 50,000 units or more per day for a period to repair deficits.

Both metabolic acidosis and alkalosis can occur. A unique problem that can occur is D-lactic acidosis. The mechanism results from colonic bacterial fermentation of unabsorbed nutrients, particularly simple sugars, into the D-enantiomer of lactic acid rather than the more typical L-enantiomer. This condition leads to progressive metabolic acidosis and altered mental status, slurred speech, and ataxia. The authors have had success in correcting recalcitrant cases of D-lactic acidosis through treating bacterial overgrowth and providing supplemental calcium and enteral thiamine to drive bacteria toward production of the L-enantiomer.

Specific nutrient deficiencies that must be prevented and monitored closely[2] include iron and vitamin deficiencies and micronutrients, such as selenium, zinc, and copper. Because fat is poorly absorbed, fatty acid deficiency can also occur. Serum free fatty acid levels and triene:tetraene ratios should be monitored periodically to determine the need for supplementation and response to treatment. In general, the

---

**Box 1**
**Complications in short bowel syndrome**

*Therapy-related*

Diarrhea and steatorrhea

Metabolic abnormalities

Nutritional deficiencies

Infectious complications

Liver disease

*Physiologic*

Cholelithiasis

Nephrolithiasis

Gastric hypersecretion

Bacterial overgrowth

enteral intake must exceed the malabsorptive losses to ensure that these requirements are being met.

Catheter-related sepsis is an important problem that often necessitates rehospitalization and replacement of catheters.[41,42] Meticulous attention to technique and conscientious patient education are important to prevent this complication. The use of antibiotic-impregnated central lines and caps may have a role in preventing line sepsis, as may the use of antibiotic locks. The value of the latter must be balanced against the risk of inducing antibiotic resistance in this infection-prone population. However, the use of indwelling catheter ethanol locks has recently been shown to reduce line infection rates.[43]

During a window in PN provision, a volume of (typically) 70% ethanol, equal to the volume of the line, is instilled into the central line and remains as a "lock" until being removed before restarting PN. Over time, catheter-related central vein thrombosis is another potential complication in patients who require PN permanently. This complication may become an important factor in patient survival and a major indication for consideration of intestinal transplantation.

PN-induced liver disease is another potential long-term problem. This complication seems to be a multifactorial process that may be reversible at earlier stages but that can lead to severe steatosis (more typical in adults), cholestasis (more typical in children), progressive fibrosis, and eventually cirrhosis.[7,44] This complication occurs more frequently in children and accounts for one-third of deaths in patients on long-term PN. It can be minimized through following the principles of good PN management in patients, such as maximizing enteral calories, avoiding PN overfeeding, and preventing specific nutrient deficiencies.[44]

Intravenous lipid emulsions seem to have a significant role in liver disease associated with SBS, perhaps through elevated levels of A phytosterols in the predominantly soy-derived lipids available in the market. Elevated levels of certain phytosterols have been shown to be associated with paralysis of bilirubin transport mechanisms in the hepatocyte membrane, perhaps contributing to progressive hyperbilirubinemia and inflammation. Treating bacterial growth and preventing recurrent sepsis are also important. The role of ursodeoxycholic acid administration is uncertain but may be beneficial.

Small intestine bacterial overgrowth (SIBO) may result from impaired motility or stasis caused by obstructive lesions and can lead to villous blunting, inflammation, deconjugation of vitamin $B_{12}$, and competition for enteral nutrients.[45,46] Depending on the bacterial species present, secretory diarrhea may also occur. Typically presenting as increased flatulence, bloating or meteorism, crampy abdominal pain, changes in stool habits, foul-smelling bowel movements, or progressive intolerance of previously tolerated enteral feeds, SIBO requires a high degree of suspicion for diagnosis. The most common diagnostic tests include hydrogen breath testing and duodenal aspiration with quantitative bacterial culture. Bacterial growth at greater than 100,000 colonies per milliliter may be considered pathologic, and are treated based on sensitivities. In general, poorly absorbed antibiotics are preferable, but over time almost any regimen will induce bacterial resistance, and thus cycling of antibiotics is often required. Additionally, the use of probiotics, either alone or in a rotation with antibiotics, can be another potential therapy. SIBO may result from a mechanical obstruction or a blind loop, which can be relieved by operation.

Cholelithiasis has been shown to occur in one-third of patients with SBS.[47,48] Long-term PN is associated with both altered hepatic bile metabolism and gallbladder stasis. Biliary sludge forms within a few weeks of initiating PN in the absence of enteral intake, but rapidly disappears when enteral nutrition is resumed. Patients receiving PN are at risk for both cholelithiasis and hepatocellular dysfunction and thus require careful clinical monitoring. Intestinal mucosal disease and resection, particularly of the ileum, cause bile acid malabsorption, leading to lithogenic bile and the formation of cholesterol stones. The risk for cholelithiasis is significantly increased if less than 120 cm of intestine remains after resection, the terminal ileum has been resected, and PN is required.[44] The incidence of cholelithiasis can be minimized through providing nutrients enterally whenever possible. Patients totally dependent on PN may be treated with intermittent CCK injections to prevent stasis and formation of sludge. Small amounts of oral lipids also stimulate gallbladder emptying. Cholelithiasis is more likely to be complicated in patients with SBS and may require more extensive surgical treatment. Prophylactic cholecystectomy should be considered in patients with SBS when laparotomy is being performed for other reasons.[49]

Nephrolithiasis, primarily calcium oxalate stones, also occurs with some frequency, especially in patients with SBS and colonic continuity. Ingested oxalate is normally bound to calcium in the intestinal lumen and is not absorbed.[47] Decreased availability of calcium secondary to reduced intake or binding by intraluminal fat leaves free oxalate in the lumen. Free oxalate is absorbed in the colon and forms calcium oxalate in the urine. Thus, nephrolithiasis is unusual in patients with intestinal resection and jejunostomy, but occurs in one-fourth of patients with an intact colon within 2 years of resection. Nephrolithiasis can be prevented through maintaining a diet low in oxalate, minimizing intraluminal fat, supplementing calcium orally, and maintaining a high urinary volume. Cholestyramine, which binds oxalic acid in the colon, might also be useful as an adjunct to treatment.

Gastric hypersecretion is a potential problem in patients with SBS.[2] Massive intestinal resection can cause gastric hypersecretion as a result of parietal cell hyperplasia and hypergastrinemia. This transient phenomenon usually lasts several months, and presumably involves loss of an inhibitor from the resected intestine. Hyperacidity exacerbates malabsorption and diarrhea, and one-fourth of patients undergoing massive resection develop peptic ulcer disease.[50] Thus, reducing gastric acid secretion should both improve absorption and prevent peptic ulcer disease. Control of acid secretion by $H_2$ receptor antagonists or PPIs should be initiated in the perioperative period after resection and maintained until the increased acid production resolves, perhaps up to 1 year after resection. A few patients eventually require surgical intervention, but gastric resection should be avoided whenever possible.

## SURGICAL REHABILITATION
### Preserve Intestinal Remnant Length

Abdominal reoperation is required over time in approximately one-half of patients with SBS, with intestinal problems being the most frequent indication.[50] An important goal in any reoperation in patients with SBS is to preserve the intestinal remnant length. Resection can often be avoided by using intestinal tapering to improve the function of dilated segments, strictureplasty for benign strictures, and serosal patching for certain strictures and chronic perforations.[51] Intestinal resection should be limited in extent when it cannot be avoided. Depending on previous operations, patients will occasionally have isolated or bypassed intestinal segments that can be recruited into continuity at reoperation; this should always be given careful consideration. It is always important to document the length of intestine remaining during any operation on a patient with SBS to help guide subsequent management.

Whether to establish intestinal continuity in patients who have a colonic remnant is an important clinical issue. Restoring continuity has both advantages and disadvantages.[52] Quality of life is usually improved for patients when the stoma is avoided. Furthermore, stomas increase the risk of catheter sepsis.[53] The colon may improve chances of enteral autonomy through increasing the absorptive surface area, producing energy in the form of short-chain fatty acid, and prolonging overall transit time, particularly if the ileocecal valve is intact. However, the response of the colon to luminal contents is somewhat unpredictable, and bile acids in the colon may in fact cause a secretory diarrhea.

Perianal problems can be disabling and can lead to a decrease in the patient's voluntary oral intake. Patients with an intact colon are at increased risk for the formation of calcium oxalate stones.[47] The authors found that only 20% of patients who initially had a stoma ultimately had continuity restored later with a satisfactory outcome.[52] This decision should be considered on an individual basis, depending on the length of the intestinal remnant, the status of the ileocecal valve and colon, and the patient's overall condition. Generally, at least 90 cm of small intestine is required to prevent severe diarrhea and perianal complications. However, restoring continuity generally should be encouraged.

### Surgical Therapy for the Short Bowel Syndrome

The surgical approach to patients with SBS depends on several factors.[4] The nature of nutritional support is obviously the primary determinant as to whether surgery should be considered. In the authors' experience, at least one-half of patients with SBS can sustain themselves on enteral nutrition alone.[4] Surgery should be considered cautiously and generally performed in these patients only if they show worsening malabsorption, are at risk for requiring PN, or have other symptoms related to malabsorption. Almost one-half of the patients who are stable on long-term PN are candidates for surgery, with weaning the patient off PN as the primary goal.

Patients who develop significant persistent, recalcitrant, or recurrent complications while dependent on PN have more compelling reasons to undergo surgery. These patients should consider undergoing intestinal transplantation, because many will die prematurely.

Patient age and underlying disease are also important factors. Younger patients are much more likely to adapt to enteral nutrition but are also more likely to be candidates for operative treatment. Adult patients with mesenteric vascular disease undergo surgery less frequently in the authors' experience. When the decision is made to offer surgical therapy, the choice of procedure is influenced by intestinal remnant length, intestinal function, and the diameter of the intestinal remnant (**Table 4**). This determination allows identification of several patient groups who might be treated with specific surgical procedures.

Adult patients with intestinal remnants longer than 120 cm are more likely to be sustained on enteral nutrition alone, particularly if colon is also present. If intestinal diameter is normal, the main goal is to preserve remnant length or recruit additional bowel as permitted. When adults develop intestinal dilation, it is typically secondary to obstruction, either as a result of recurrent intra-abdominal adhesions or stricture at the site of a previous anastomosis. Chronically dilated bowel will typically be poorly functional and predisposed to malabsorption and bacterial overgrowth.

Although conservative management is the preferred initial management, definitive therapy will often require relief of intestinal obstruction through lysis of adhesions, strictureplasty, or short-segment bowel resections as deemed necessary.[54] Dilation of the intestinal remnant occurs more frequently in children and seems to have a different basis that is more adaptive in nature than pathologic.[55] Obstruction, if suspected radiographically, should be treated surgically as required. In patients with appropriate length of the bowel segment, the authors generally

**Table 4**
**Surgical therapy for short bowel syndrome**

| Intestinal Anatomy | Clinical Status | Surgical Therapy |
|---|---|---|
| Adequate length with normal diameter (remnant >120 cm) | Enteral nutrition only | Optimize intestinal function Recruit additional length |
| Adequate length with dilated bowel | Bacterial overgrowth | Treat obstruction Intestinal tapering |
| Marginal length with normal diameter (remnant 60–120 cm) | Rapid transit Need for PN | Recruit additional length Procedures to slow transit |
| Marginal length with dilated bowel | Bacterial overgrowth Need for PN | Intestinal lengthening |
| Short length with normal diameter (remnant <60 cm) | Need for PN | Optimize intestinal function |
| Short length with dilated bowel | Bacterial overgrowth Need for PN | Intestinal lengthening |
| Short length | Complications of PN | Intestinal transplantation |

*Abbreviation:* PN, parenteral nutrition.

perform longitudinal tapering enteroplasties to restore a uniform lumen diameter. When tapering enteroplasties are used, they may be either resective or imbricating, and the authors have not found significant differences between the approaches.[55] In general, the authors do not advocate performing lengthening procedures on obstructed bowel in an effort to "create length," but rather recommend relieving the obstruction and allowing the bowel to recover more natural, unimpeded function. Although they have found lengthening procedures to be invaluable in managing children with adaptive dilation, long-term data on function and outcome are insufficient to advocate aggressive stapling of the bowel when length appears otherwise adequate to maintain nutrition.

A challenging group of patients are those who have a marginal remnant (60–120 cm in adults) and signs of rapid transit. Slowing the rapid intestinal transit may permit these patients to be supported by enteral means alone. Several approaches to this problem are possible.[56] Reversing a 10- to 15-cm intestinal segment in situ has been used most frequently to slow transit in SBS. Longer segments are more likely to be associated with chronic obstruction, whereas shorter segments have less influence on intestinal transit and function. More than 40 patients have been reported in the literature, and although documentation is usually not extensive, clinical improvement has often been reported.[56] Outcome is difficult to evaluate because segments are sometime reversed during ostomy closure[57,58] and some concerns have been raised about long-term function after the procedure.[57]

Creation of various artificial valves to replace the ileocecal valve has been attempted. The authors have generally performed the valve procedure through creating a sphincter similar to that used in the continent ileostomy procedure but of shorter length (2 cm). They have had a favorable result in one adult and one child with this valve.[4] However, outcomes have not been uniformly successful in the few other cases reported. Both isoperistaltic and antiperistaltic colon interposition have also been attempted. Although transit time may be prolonged because of the intrinsic differences in motility between the colon and small intestine, actual benefit has been difficult to show in a few anecdotal reports. Intestinal pacing also has been attempted based on laboratory studies, suggesting that it may be possible to pace the small intestine in a retrograde fashion with electrodes. However, attempts to accomplish this clinically have been unsuccessful. The overall success rat of procedures to improve transit is approximately 50%.[54]

Patients with short remnant length (<60 cm in adults) and dilated intestinal segments represent a more difficult problem. In this scenario, the goal is to preserve functional length, restore luminal diameter, and improve the overall absorption of the surface area of residual intestine. Preserving functional length can mean removing short dysmotile segments that seem to cause more harm than good. To restore luminal diameter, the authors and others have found the so-called intestinal lengthening procedures to be the optimal treatment.[55] Although easiest to describe as lengthening, these procedures actually represent an attempt to optimize the surface area: volume ratio of the intestine to improve contact time between luminal contents and absorption surface. The procedures may have some actual benefit in increasing mucosal mass, although this is difficult to prove conclusively. When the underlying cause for dilation is most likely obstruction based on preoperative imaging and clinical scenario, the authors advocate prompt intervention to relieve obstruction, but not necessarily a concurrent enteroplasty if the dilation appears to be acute rather than chronic. When dilatation is progressive in the absence of obstruction, and so-called adaptive dilation and attempts at medical management are unsuccessful, surgical intervention is indicated. Two techniques are currently available for application and are described later.

The initial lengthening approach reported was longitudinal lengthening via the Bianchi procedure (**Fig. 3**).[55] This procedure involves dissection along the mesenteric edge of the bowel to allocate terminal blood vessels anatomically to either side of the bowel wall. Longitudinal transection of the bowel is then performed, usually with a stapling device, which creates two parallel limbs, each of a smaller diameter. These

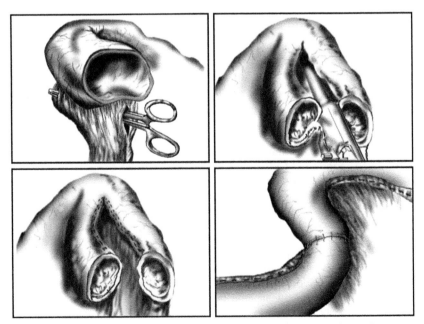

**Fig. 3.** Longitudinal enteroplasty (Bianchi procedure). (*Reproduced from* Thompson JS. Surgical rehabilitation of intestine in short bowel syndrome. Surgery 2004;135:465–70; with permission.)

limbs can then be anastomosed to lengthen the intestinal remnant, through which intestine nutrients flow. More than 100 cases have been reported, mostly in children.[55] Segments have been lengthened up to 90 cm, and overall improved nutrition was seen in approximately 80% of patients. Complications have been reported in 20% of procedures, which, unsurprisingly, include ischemia and anastomotic leaks. Recurrent dilation can occur, but follow-up for up to 10 years suggests that this procedure has long-term benefit in 50% of patients.[59] However, 10% ultimately underwent intestinal transplantation.

More recently, an alternative method of lengthening, serial transverse enteroplasty (STEP), was introduced (**Fig. 4**).[60] This procedure involves repeated applications of a linear stapling device from opposite directions in a zigzag fashion, which partially divides the bowel from either the mesenteric and antimesenteric sides or transversely. The length of the transverse division is determined by the intestinal diameter. Success involves complete release of adhesions from duodenum to colon, and then a combination of tapering or STEP enteroplasties to restore a uniform bowel lumen appropriate for the size of the patient. The authors typically require a diameter of at least 4 cm before performing a STEP enteroplasty to maintain a resulting lumen diameter of approximately 2 cm. Motility can be somewhat slow to return, and the authors have observed that the full benefit of a STEP taper procedure generally is not realized until 8 to 12 weeks after surgery. Recurrent dilation can certainly occur and is managed in a similar fashion.

Clinical improvement in SBS has occurred in 80% of patients who underwent STEP, and 5% have undergone subsequent intestinal transplantation. More than 70 cases of

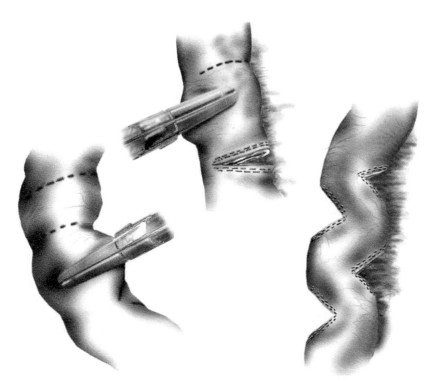

**Fig. 4.** STEP procedure. (*Reproduced from* Thompson JS. Surgical rehabilitation of intestine in short bowel syndrome. Surgery 2004;135:465–70; with permission.)

STEP have been published in the literature.[55] Follow-up is not as long as for the Bianchi procedure, which has been in use longer.

The authors' experience with the STEP technique has been favorable, and it is now their preferred procedure.[59,61] They found that 58% of 64 patients undergoing either the Bianchi procedure or STEP were able to discontinue PN. This finding correlated with the functional length gained eventually and total functional length after the procedure. Overall clinical outcome is similar for the STEP and Bianchi procedures in the authors' experience. STEP avoids the difficult dissection along the mesenteric border and the end-to-end anastomosis of the Bianchi procedure. Although bowel may have to be more dilated for this technique, it is more feasible in challenging areas, such as near the ligament of Treitz. No prohibitions exist to performing either repeat STEP procedures or tapering enteroplasties at later surgeries.

## INTESTINAL TRANSPLANTATION

Patients with SBS who develop life-threatening complications related to PN are candidates for intestinal transplantation, and when complications include portal hypertension or progressive liver failure, they become candidates for combined liver/small intestine transplantation.[62] The generally accepted indications for intestinal transplantation are recurrent life-threatening central venous line infection (especially fungal infections), progressive loss of central venous access, and development of progressive liver disease. Intestinal transplants have also been used for certain tumors (neuroendocrine, desmoids) in the area of the superior mesenteric vasculature, for which complete resection involves removing an extensive length of the bowel as a consequence of resecting its blood supply with the tumor. Attempts to expand indications to include conditions such as splanchnic venous thrombosis alone and poor tolerance of or unwillingness to use total parenteral nutrition have not become universally accepted, because the current survival rates for these latter conditions are higher than those for transplantation in selected patients who can achieve 50% enteral independence and have a good potential for further rehabilitation. Isolated liver transplantation may be advocated for patients with irreversible liver failure.[63] The significant mortality rate among patients developing PN-associated liver failure justifies the approach of organ replacement therapy.

Currently, almost 2000 intestinal transplants have been performed in the United States, approximately 75% of which have been performed in patients younger than 18 years.[62] Currently, 1-year graft survival rates are as high as 89% in adults aged 18 to 34 years, and fall to as low as 64% in children younger than 1 year. Graft survival at 5 years falls off, with published rates from as low as 31% in children younger than 1 year to as high as 69% in children aged 6 to 10 years. Patient survival rates are similar at 1 and 5 years after transplant.[62,64,65] Chronic rejection and infectious complications remain important determinants of survival. In general, induction immunosuppression is performed with an antithymocyte or anti–interleukin-2 receptor therapy, followed by therapy with tacrolimus or steroids, or adjunctive immunosuppressants such as mycophenolate mofetil. Improvements in survival over the past 2 decades have largely been related to improved pediatric critical care and careful management of immunosuppression to reduce incidence of opportunistic infections and posttransplant lymphoproliferative disorder.[65] Overall, it is increasingly being recognized that the treatment of intestinal failure involves both rehabilitation and transplantation, and that these approaches are complementary and not competitive or contradictory.

More information about long-term nutritional outcome and quality of life is emerging.[62,66,67] Approximately one-third of patients undergoing intestinal transplantation require PN at discharge. However, at 1 year, 90% are independent of PN.[62] This procedure has improved quality of life in almost all domains, but particularly in digestive function, vocational status, medical compliance, optimism, and energy.[66] However, these claims should be interpreted cautiously because more recent studies suggest that quality of life remains lower in these patients than in nontransplant controls.[67]

Among all the surgical approaches to SBS, intestinal transplantation has the greatest theoretical potential for treating patients with SBS, both in terms of the number of patients who would benefit and the functional improvement derived. With greater experience and improved results, this therapy is expected to be able to extend to other patients with SBS. Suitable donor organs remain scarce, particularly for pediatric patients. The ethics and technical aspects of using living related donors for intestinal transplantation continue to be considered. Transplantation is clearly an appropriate option for individuals with anticipated survival of less than 12 months related to PN-associated complications. A more aggressive approach to the use of intestinal transplantation, particularly solitary transplantation, is justified in patients with signs of early liver dysfunction and other severe complications of nutritional therapy. Patients with high-risk complications of intestinal failure should be referred early to a center specializing in intestinal transplantation so that they may be carefully monitored and, if indicated, listed for transplant before complications develop that preclude the operation or increase its risks.

## SUMMARY

SBS is a challenging clinical problem that benefits from a multidisciplinary approach. Much progress has recently been made in all aspects of management. Medical intestinal rehabilitation should be the initial treatment focus, and several new potential pharmacologic agents are being investigated. Surgical rehabilitation using nontransplant procedures in selected patients may further improve intestinal function. Intestinal lengthening procedures are particularly promising. Intestinal transplantation increasingly has been used with improving success in patients with life-threatening complications of intestinal failure.

## REFERENCES

1. O'Keefe SJ, Buchman AL, Fishbein TM, et al. Short bowel syndrome and intestinal failure: consensus, definitions, and overview. Clin Gastroenterol Hepatol 2006;4:6–10.
2. Buchman AL, Scolapio J, Fryer J. American Gastroenterological Association Medical Position Statement: short bowel syndrome and intestinal transplantation. Gastroenterology 2003;124:1105–10.
3. Howard L, Ament M, Fleming CR, et al. Current use and clinical outcome of home parenteral and enteral nutrition therapies in the United States. Gastroenterology 1995;109:355–65.
4. Thompson JS, Langnas AN, Pinch LW, et al. Surgical approach to the short bowel syndrome. Ann Surg 1995;222:600–7.
5. Thompson JS. Comparison of massive versus repeated resections leading to the short bowel syndrome. J Gastrointest Surg 2000;4:101–4.
6. Messing B, Crenn P, Beau P, et al. Long-term survival and parenteral nutrition dependence in adult patients with short bowel syndrome. Gastroenterology 1999;117:1043–50.

7. Cavicchi M, Beau P, Crenn P, et al. Prevalence of liver disease as a contributing factor in patients receiving home parenteral nutrition for permanent intestinal failure. Ann Intern Med 2000;132:525–32.

8. Drozdowski L, Thomson AB. Intestinal mucosal adaptation. World J Gastroenterol 2006;12:4614–27.

9. Dibaise J, Young RJ, Vanderhoof JA, et al. Intestinal rehabilitation and the short bowel syndrome. Am J Gastroenterol 2004;99:1823–32.

10. Rhoda KM, Parekh NR, Lennon E, et al. The multidisciplinary approach to the care of patients with intestinal failure at a tertiary care facility. Nutr Clin Pract 2010;25:183–91.

11. Carbonnel F, Cosnes J, Chevret BL, et al. The role of anatomic factors in nutritional autonomy after extensive bowel resection. JPEN J Parenter Enteral Nutr 1996;20:275–80.

12. Nordgaard I, Hensen BS, Mortensen PB. Colon as a digestive organ in patients with short bowel. Lancet 1994;343:373–6.

13. Jeppesen PB, Mortensen PB. The influence of a preserved colon on the absorption of medium chain fat in patients with small bowel resection. Gut 1998;43:478–83.

14. Dibaise J, Matarese LE, Messing B, et al. Strategies for parenteral nutrition weaning in adult patients with short bowel syndrome. J Clin Gastroenterol 2006;40:594–8.

15. Crenn P, Morin MC, Joly F, et al. Net digestive absorption and adaptive hyperphagia in adult short bowel patients. Gut 2004;3:1279–86.

16. Levy E, Frileux P, Sandrucci S, et al. Continuous enteral nutrition during the early adaptive stage of the short bowel syndrome. Br J Surg 1988;75:549–53.

17. Shatnawei A, Parekh NR, Rhoda KM, et al. Intestinal failure management at the Cleveland Clinic. Arch Surg 2010;145:521–7.

18. Atia AN, Buchman AL. Oral rehydration solutions in non-cholera diarrhea: a review. Am J Gastroenterol 2009;104:2596–604.

19. Jeppesen PB, Hoy CE, Mortensen PB. Deficiencies of essential fatty acids, vitamin and E and changes in plasma lipoproteins in patients with reduced fat absorption or intestinal failure. Eur J Clin Nutr 2000;54:632–42.

20. Van der Hulst RR, Van Kreel BK, Von Meyenfeldt MF, et al. Glutamine and the preservation of gut integrity. Lancet 1993;341:1363–5.

21. Byrne TA, Persinger RL, Young LS, et al. A new treatment for patients with short-bowel syndrome: growth hormone, glutamine, and a modified diet. Ann Surg 1995;222:243–55.

22. Byrne TA, Morrissey TB, Nattakom TV, et al. Growth hormone, glutamine, and a modified diet enhance nutrient absorption in patients with severe short bowel syndrome. JPEN J Parenter Enteral Nutr 1995;19:296–302.

23. Byrne TA, Wilmore DW, Iyer K, et al. Growth hormone, glutamine and an optimal diet reduces parenteral nutrition in patients with short bowel syndrome. Ann Surg 2005;242:655–61.

24. Jeppesen PB, Hartmann B, Thulesen J, et al. Glucagon-like peptide 2 improves nutrient absorption and nutritional status in short-bowel patients with no colon. Gastroenterology 2001;120:806–15.

25. Jeppesen PB, Sanquinetti EL, Buchman A, et al. Teduglutide (ALX-0600), a dipeptidyl peptidase-IV resistant glucagon like peptide-2 (GLP-2) analog, improves intestinal function in short bowel syndrome patients. Gut 2005;54:1224–31.

26. Jeppeson PB, Stann M, Tjellessen L. Effect of intravenous ranitidine and omeprazole on intestinal absorption of water, sodium and macronutrients in patients with intestinal resection. Gut 1998;43:763–9.

27. Compare D, Pica L, Rocco A, et al. Effects of long-term PPI treatment on producing bowel symptoms and bacterial overgrowth. Eur J Clin Invest 2010;10:1365.
28. O'Keefe SJ, Haymond MW, Bennet WM, et al. Long-acting somatostatin analogue therapy and protein metabolism in patients with jejunostomies. Gastroenterology 1994;107:379–88.
29. Catnach SM, Anderson JV, Fairclough PD, et al. Effect of octreotide on gallstone prevalence and gallbladder motility in acromegaly. Gut 1993;34:270–3.
30. McDaniel K, Taylor B, Huey W, et al. Use of clonidine to decrease intestinal fluid losses in patients with high-output short bowel syndrome. JPEN J Parenter Enteral Nutr 2004;28:265–8.
31. Joly FL, Mayeuv C, Bruneau A, et al. Drastic changes in fecal and mucosa associated microbiota in adult patients with short bowel syndrome. Biochimie 2010; 92:753–61.
32. Stoidis CN, Misiakos EP, Patapis P, et al. Potential benefits of pro and prebiotics on intestinal mucosal immunity and intestinal barrier in short bowel syndrome. Nutr Res Rev 2010;21:1–9.
33. Jeppesen PB. The use of hormonal growth factors in the treatment of patients with short bowel syndrome. Drugs 2006;66:581–9.
34. Seguy D, Kvahedi K, Kapel N, et al. Low-dose growth hormone in adult home parenteral nutrition dependent short bowel syndrome patients: a positive study. Gastroenterology 2003;124:293–302.
35. Scolapio JS, Camilleri M, Fleming CR, et al. Effect of growth hormone, glutamine, and diet on adaption in short bowel syndrome: a randomized controlled trial. Gastroenterology 1997;115:1074–81.
36. Szkudlarek J, Jeppesen PB, Mortensen PB. Effect of high dose growth hormone with glutamine and no change in diet on intestinal absorption in short bowel patient: a randomized, double blind, crossover, placebo controlled study. Gut 2000;47:199–205.
37. Wales PW, Nasr A, deSilva N, et al. Human growth hormone and glutamine for patients with short bowel syndrome. Cochrane Database Syst Rev 2010;6:CD006321.
38. Jeppesen PB, Lund P, Gottschalck IB, et al. Short bowel patients treated for 2 years with GLP 2: compliance, safety and effects on quality of life. Gastroenterol Res Pract 2009;2009:425759.
39. Thompson JS. EGF and the short bowel syndrome. JPEN J Parenter Enteral Nutr 1999;23:S113–6.
40. Sigalet DL, Martin GR, Butzner JD, et al. A pilot study of the use of epidermal growth factor in pediatric short bowel syndrome. J Pediatr Surg 2005;40:763–8.
41. Howard L, Ashley C. Management of complications in patients receiving home parenteral nutrition. Gastroenterology 2003;124:1651–61.
42. O'Keefe SJ, Burnes JU, Thompson RL. Recurrent sepsis in home parenteral nutrition patients: an analysis of risk factors. JPEN J Parenter Enteral Nutr 1994;18: 256–63.
43. Opilla MT, Kirby DF, Edmund MB. Use of ethanol lock therapy to reduce the incidence of catheter related blood stream infections in home parenteral nutrition patients. JPEN J Parenter Enteral Nutr 2007;31:302–5.
44. Kelly DA. Preventing parenteral nutrition liver disease. Early Hum Dev 2010;86: 683–7.
45. DiBaise JK, Young RJ, Vanderhoof JA. Enteric microbial flora, bacterial overgrowth and short bowel syndrome. Clin Gastroenterol Hepatol 2006;4:11–20.
46. Quigley EM, Abu-Shanab A. Small intestinal bacterial overgrowth. Infect Dis Clin North Am 2010;24:943–59.

47. Nightingale JM, Lennard-Jones JE, Gertner DJ, et al. Colonic preservation reduces need for parenteral therapy, increases incidence of renal stones, but does not change high prevalence of gallstones in patients with a short bowel. Gut 1992;33:1493–7.

48. Dray X, Joly F, Reijasse D, et al. Incidence, risk factors and complications of cholelithiasis in patients with home parenteral nutrition. J Am Coll Surg 2007; 204:13–21.

49. Thompson JS. The role of prophylactic cholecystectomy in the short bowel syndrome. Arch Surg 1996;131:556–660.

50. Thompson JS. Reoperation in patients with the short bowel syndrome. Am J Surg 1992;164:453–7.

51. Thompson JS. Surgical rehabilitation of intestine in short bowel syndrome. Surgery 2004;35:465–70.

52. Nguyen BT, Blatchford GJ, Thompson JS, et al. Should intestinal continuity be restored after massive intestinal resection? Am J Surg 1989;158:577–80.

53. Siepler JK, Nishikawa RA, Diamantidi ST, et al. Exit site infections are more common in patients with ostomies. JPEN J Parenter Enteral Nutr 2007;31:55.

54. Thompson JS, Langnas AN. Surgical approaches to improving intestinal function in Short Bowel Syndrome. Arch Surg 1999;134:706–71.

55. Thompson JS, Sudan DA. Intestinal lengthening in the short bowel syndrome. In: Cameron J, editor, Advances in Surgery, volume 42. St Louis (MO): Mosby; 2008. p. 49–61.

56. Thompson JS. Surgical approach to the short bowel syndrome: procedures to slow intestinal transit. Eur J Pediatr Surg 1999;9:263–6.

57. Thompson JS, Sudan DA, Gilroy R. Predicting outcome of procedures to slow intestinal transit. Transplant Proc 2006;38:1838–9.

58. Panis Y, Messing B, Rivet P, et al. Segmental reversal of the small bowel as an alternative to intestinal transplantation in patients with short bowel syndrome. Ann Surg 1997;225:401–7.

59. Sudan D, Thompson JS, Botha J, et al. Comparisons of intestinal lengthening procedures for patients with short bowel syndrome. Ann Surg 2007;246:593–604.

60. Kim H, Fauza D, Garza J, et al. Serial transverse enteroplasty (STEP): a novel bowel lengthening procedure. J Pediatr Surg 2003;38:425–9.

61. Yannam G, Sudan D, Grant W, et al. Intestinal lengthening in adults with short bowel syndrome. J Gastrointest Surg 2010;14:1931–6.

62. Mazariegos GV, Steffick DE, Horslen S, et al. Intestinal transplantation in the United States 1999-2008. Am J Transplant 2010;10:1020–34.

63. Botha JF, Grant WJ, Torres C, et al. Isolated liver transplantation in infants with end stage liver disease due to short bowel syndrome. Liver Transpl 2006;12:1062–6.

64. Grant D, Abu-Elmagd K, Reyes J, et al. 2003 report of the intestine transplant registry: a new era has dawned. Ann Surg 2005;241:607–13.

65. Abu-Elmagd K, Costa G, Bond GJ, et al. Five hundred intestinal and multivisceral transplantations at a single center. Ann Surg 2009;250:567–81.

66. O'Keefe SID, Emerling M, Kovitsky D, et al. Nutrition and quality of life following small intestinal transplantation. Am J Gastroenterol 2007;102:1093–100.

67. Sudan D. Long term outcomes and quality of life after intestinal transplantation. Curr Opin Organ Transplant 2010;15:357–60.

# Nutrition Support in the Pediatric Surgical Patient

Richard Herman, MD[a], Imad Btaiche, PharmD[b],
Daniel H. Teitelbaum, MD[c],*

**KEYWORDS**

• Pediatric nutrition • Surgical nutrition • Pediatric growth

Maintaining adequate nutrition of pediatric surgical patients is critical not only to aid in healing but also to continue normal growth and development. The use of central venous catheters and the development of parenteral nutrition (PN) has dramatically increased the survival of previously fatal pediatric surgical conditions. The past 50 years have led to dramatic developments in both specialized enteral and parenteral products for infants and children.

## NORMAL PEDIATRIC GROWTH

Growth and development are unique features to pediatric patients that greatly affect the goals and objectives of nutritional support. Term newborn infants grow at a rate of 25 to 30 g per day over the first 6 months of life, leading to a doubling of the birth weight by 5 months of age and tripling by 12 months.[1] Body weight increases 20-fold by the end of the first decade, and body length increases by 50% by the end of the first year of life and increases 3-fold by the end of the first decade of life. Preterm infants' growth pattern is distinct from that of term infants. Most nutrients are accumulated by a fetus in the third trimester of pregnancy. Thus, fat accounts for only 1% to 2% of body weight in a 1-kg infant compared with 16% in a term (3.5-kg) infant. During the first 7 to 10 days of life, term infants lose approximately 7% to 10% of their body weight, whereas not only do preterm infants lose more of their weight, approximately 15%, but also they regain it at a slower rate, only 10 to 20 g per day, because they have yet to enter the accelerated weight gain of the third trimester.[2]

The authors have nothing to disclose.
[a] Section of Critical Care, Division of Pediatric Surgery, Mott Children's Hospital, University of Michigan, 1500 East Medical Center Drive, F3970, Ann Arbor, MI 48109-0245, USA
[b] College of Pharmacy, University of Michigan, UH UHB 2D301, 1500 East Medical Center Drive, Ann Arbor, MI 48109-5008, USA
[c] Division of Pediatric Surgery, Mott Children's Hospital, University of Michigan, 1500 East Medical Center Drive, F3970, Ann Arbor, MI 48109-0245, USA
* Corresponding author.
*E-mail address:* dttlbm@med.umich.edu

Surg Clin N Am 91 (2011) 511–541
doi:10.1016/j.suc.2011.02.008
0039-6109/11/$ – see front matter © 2011 Elsevier Inc. All rights reserved.

## NUTRITIONAL ASSESSMENT
### Initial Objective Assessment

Nutritional assessment is a critical aspect of the initial evaluation of all surgical patients.[3] Work by Cooper and colleagues[4] showed that 18% to 40% of pediatric surgical patients have malnutrition. This rate of malnutrition has also been shown in other pediatric patients.[5] Nutritional assessment can be divided into subjective and objective components. Two basic tools are available, the Mini Nutrition Assessment[6] and Subjective Global Assessment. Modification of the Subjective Global Assessment has been made for pediatrics, but it is not as well validated as for adults.[7] The objective portion of the assessment begins with the basic anthropometric measurements of height, weight, and head circumference. Measurements are placed on a standardized growth curve, such as that of the National Center for Health Statistics, from which the expected weight for height indexes can be calculated. Because length and head circumference are less affected than weight by excess fat or postoperative fluid fluctuations, length is an excellent indicator of long-term body growth. Acute changes in nutritional status have a more immediate effect on body weight, whereas chronic undernutrition results in a lag in both height and weight. These changes in growth are probably best expressed using a z score for weight-to-length ratio as well as weight, length, and head circumference for age. Once patients are over 2 years of age, weight-to-length ratio can best be reflected by a child's body mass index (BMI), and expression of BMI as a z score can often add a useful perspective. Special growth charts are also available for monitoring the growth of children with special health care needs (eg, Down syndrome, Prader-Willi syndrome, myelomeningocele, achondroplasia, and cerebral palsy). Use of these charts can give an important perspective as to where a child's growth should lie.[8]

### Biochemical Measurements of Nutritional Status

Because there are no established norms for prealbumin or retinol binding protein in infants and young children, these traditional methods used to measure nutrition in adults cannot be translated to pediatric patients.[9] Additionally, because these visceral proteins lack specificity under stress and inflammatory conditions and are affected by non-nutritional factors, further caution must be used in assigning values to pediatric surgical patients. Therefore, their levels should be interpreted in the context of nutritional history, underlying diseases, and medication therapy. Other parameters that can be useful for measuring nutritional status include bone age and dental status, because malnutrition is a common cause of delayed bone maturation.[10]

## NUTRITIONAL REQUIREMENTS
### Energy Requirements

The energy needs of infants and children are unique; requirements are listed in **Table 1**. In children, energy is required for maintenance of body metabolism and growth. A gross estimate of calorie expenditure can be obtained by using the Dietary Reference Intakes for energy requirements, based on a child's age, weight, height, and physical activity, based on the Food and Nutrition Board, Institute of Medicine, National Academy of Sciences, *Dietary Reference Intakes: Recommended Intakes for Individuals* in 2006.[11] Although careful clinical examination is important in making a determination of a child's nutritional status, Baker and colleagues[12] showed that the depleted state could not be reliably detected on the basis of weight-to-height ratio, triceps skin fold, mid- to upper-arm circumference, hand strength, albumin concentration, total protein level, or creatinine-to-height ratio. Measurement or estimation of metabolic rate and energy needs is the best method of following the nutritional status.[13–15] One of the most

| Table 1 |  |
|---|---|
| **Daily energy requirements (total kcal/kg) for pediatric patients** | |
| Preterm neonate | 90–120 |
| <6 Months | 85–105 |
| 6–12 Months | 80–100 |
| 1–7 Years | 75–90 |
| 7–12 Years | 50–75 |
| >12–18 Years | 30–50 |

*Data from* Mirtallo J, Canada T, Johnson D. Task force for the revision of safe practices for parenteral nutrition. Safe practices for parenteral nutrition. JPEN J Parenter Enteral Nutr 2004;28:S39–70.

accurate methods of measuring energy expenditure is indirect calorimetry.[16] In indirect calorimetry, $CO_2$ production and $O_2$ consumption are measured using a metabolic cart. The sample is best measured in intubated infants yielding a resting energy expenditure (REE). The energy expenditure or metabolic rate, as measured in cubic centimeters of oxygen per minute, can be converted to calories per hour or per day, if the substrates are known. All measurements are only approximations of caloric needs for which a surgeon must further adjust according to the clinical course of a patient. Such measurements give an excellent way to monitor patients, in particular those children who are in an ICU setting.[17] Unfortunately, indirect calorimetry may be difficult in young infants with uncuffed endotracheal tubes, in which an air leak may lead to significant inaccuracies in results. In contrast to adults, the rise in REE postsurgery in infants and children is much less. Mitchell and colleagues[15] found that the REE of postoperative cardiac patients fell to values below those of normal healthy children who had not undergone surgery. This finding was confirmed by Letton and colleagues,[18] who examined energy expenditure in young infants in the postoperative period. These studies suggested that reliance on recommended daily allowance values may result in overfeeding postoperatively.

## Water

The water content of infants is higher than that of adults (75% vs 65% of body weight) and is proportional to muscle mass. Fluids provide the principal source of water; however, some water is derived by the oxidation of food and body tissues. Requirements for water are related to caloric consumption; therefore, infants must consume much larger amounts of water per unit of body weight than adults. In general, calorie requirements (kcal/kg/d) are matched to the amount of fluid needs (mL/kg/d). The daily consumption of fluid by healthy infants is equivalent to 10% to 15% of their body weight in contrast to only 2% to 4% by adults. In addition, the normal water content in food for infants and children is much higher than that of adults. Only 0.5% to 3% of fluid intake is retained by infants and children. Estimation of daily maintenance fluid requirements in infants and children is shown in (**Table 2**).[19]

## Protein

The requirement for protein in infants is based on the combined needs of growth and maintenance (**Table 3**). Two percent of an infant's body weight, compared with 3% of an adult's body weight, consists of nitrogen. The average intake of protein should comprise approximately 15% of total calories administered. In addition to the 8 essential amino acids in adults, 4 additional amino acids (cysteine, tyrosine, arginine, and histidine) are considered essential in infants. New tissue cannot be formed unless all of the essential amino acids are present in the diet simultaneously; the absence

**Table 2**
**Daily fluid requirements for pediatric patients**

| Body Weight | Amount |
|---|---|
| <1500 g | 130–150 mL/kg |
| 1500–2000 g | 110–130 mL/kg |
| 2–10 kg | 100 mL/kg |
| >10–20 kg | 1000 mL for 10 kg + 50 mL/kg for each kg >10 |
| >20 kg | 1500 mL for 20 kg + 20 mL/kg for each kg >20 |

*Data from* Mirtallo J, Canada T, Johnson D. Task force for the revision of safe practices for parenteral nutrition. Safe practices for parenteral nutrition. JPEN J Parenter Enteral Nutr 2004;28:S39–70.

of only one essential amino acid results in a negative nitrogen and protein balance. Further, the use of taurine supplementation has been shown to decrease the severity of PN-associated cholestasis.[20] It has also been suggested that proline is essential in preterm infants, although this has yet to be confirmed.[21]

Protein requirements are typically based on age and adjusted based on nutritional status, stress level, severity and type of injury, kidney and liver functions, and other clinical conditions. Delivery of greater amounts of protein to neonates may lead to elevated blood urea nitrogen levels. Protein requirements in premature infants are higher than in term infants and range from 3 to 3.5 g/kg per day.[9,22] Such delivery is critical to provide optimal growth and neurodevelopment in infants. In very-low-birth-weight infants, this requirement may approach 3.85 g/kg per day.[23] In particular, taurine is essential for normal neural and retinal development.[24]

### Carbohydrates

Carbohydrates provide a major and most immediate source of energy through parenteral and enteral routes. Newborn infants have limited glycogen reserves (34 g), most of which reside in the liver. Thus, short periods of fasting can lead to a hypoglycemic state. The primary enteral carbohydrate delivered to neonates and young infants is lactose, and small bowel lactase levels remain sufficiently high in most infants until they are at least 2 or 3 years of age. Nonlactose formulas that are soy based and contain sucrose or corn syrup may provide adequate amounts of carbohydrates (discussed later). Preterm infants may be unable to digest certain carbohydrates, in particular lactose, because lactase activity in the intestines is inadequate. Thus, for premature infants, formulas that have a 50:50 mixture of lactose and glucose polymers are ideal.

### Fat

Lipids have the advantage of being an excellent source of energy and essential fatty acids. Linoleic acid is essential, and deficiencies may occur in as little as 2 to

**Table 3**
**Daily protein requirements (g/kg) for pediatric patients[a]**

| | |
|---|---|
| Preterm neonates | 3–4 |
| Infants (1–12 months) | 2–3 |
| Children (>10 kg or 1–10 y) | 1–2 |
| Adolescents (11–17 y) | 0.8–1.5 |

[a] Assumes normal age-related organ function.
*Data from* Mirtallo J, Canada T, Johnson D. Task force for the revision of safe practices for parenteral nutrition. Safe practices for parenteral nutrition. JPEN J Parenter Enteral Nutr 2004;28:S39–70.

3 days in neonates.[25,26] A deficiency of fatty acids in infants may result when less than 1% of the caloric intake is linoleic acid; in general, 2% to 4% of dietary energy should come from essential fatty acids. Manifestations of fatty acid deficiency include scaly skin, hair loss, visual or behavioral disorders, diarrhea, thrombocytopenia, and impaired wound healing.[27] The two major polyunsaturated fatty acids are linoleic acid, which is an $\omega$-6 fatty acid, and $\alpha$-linolenic acid, which is an $\omega$-3 fatty acid. $\omega$-6 fatty acids are usually derived from plants and $\omega$-3 fatty acids are usually derived from fish oils. Both of these polyunsaturated fats are essential for the development of cell membranes and the central nervous system, as well as for the synthesis of arachidonic acid and related prostaglandins. Thromboxanes derived from $\omega$-6 fatty acids are potential mediators of platelet aggregation, whereas thromboxanes derived from $\omega$-3 fatty acids, such as docosahexaenoic acid, are potent anticoagulants and have important uses for neonatal central nervous system development and modulation of inflammatory conditions. Further, $\omega$-6 fatty acids, which form arachidonic acid, also contribute to the formation of prostaglandin (PG) $E_2$, a known immunosuppressant, whereas $\omega$-3 fatty acids contribute to the formation of $PGE_1$ and $PGE_3$, which do not have an immunosuppressive effect. If full delivery of lipids is not done, essential fatty acid deficiency should be monitored at least once a month.

## Minerals, Trace Elements, and Vitamins

### Vitamins
The normal daily requirement of vitamins has been recently revised by the Food and Drug Administration.[28] Vitamins are essential components or cofactors of various metabolic reactions. Most commercial infant formulas contain adequate amounts of vitamins to meet known daily requirements. Infants who receive other types of formula or human milk may require additional vitamin supplementation (**Table 4**).

### Trace elements
Trace elements comprise less than 0.01% of the total body weight in humans.[29] **Table 5** lists functions and **Table 6** lists the recommended doses of trace elements. Deficiencies in zinc can arise from various sources that are common in pediatric surgical patients; such sources include short bowel syndrome, thermal burns, peritoneal dialysis, inflammatory bowel disease, and other causes of diarrhea. Clinical manifestations of zinc deficiency include growth retardation, alopecia, skin lesions (acrodermatitis enteropathica), impaired lymphocyte function, and impaired wound healing; zinc deficiency can lead to diarrhea.[30] Supplementation in infants should be a minimum of 400 mg/kg per day. Copper deficiency has been reported in patients receiving PN formulas that are not supplemented with copper.[31] Manifestations of copper deficiency include a microcytic, hypochromic anemia; neutropenia; hypothermia; mental status changes; and, in children, growth retardation and skeletal demineralization. Removal of copper from infants and children may lead to an aplastic anemic condition, which can be fatal.[32] Selenium levels dramatically decline after as few as 6 weeks of PN.[33] Without the addition of selenium, deficiencies are generally manifested by cardiomyopathy as well as by peripheral myositis with associated muscle tenderness.

## ENTERAL NUTRITION

Enteral nutrition (EN) includes oral nutritional supplementation and tube feedings. EN should be the primary source of nutrients if the gastrointestinal tract is functional. Even when full feedings are not tolerated enterally, the provision of small volumes of trophic feedings may prevent further deterioration of intestinal function.

**Table 4**
Vitamins/minerals

| Mineral/Vitamin | Essential Function in Pediatrics | Conditions if Excess | Deficiency Effects in Pediatric Patients | Supplementation Required |
|---|---|---|---|---|
| Vitamin A | Retinoic acid for vision Coordination of cell cycle | Anorexia in infants (6000 μg) | Pulmonary disease in infants | Added in formula |
| Vitamin D | Bone formation and mineral homeostasis | Hypercalcemia | Deficient immune function, asthma and allergies, poor bone growth | In formula, excess not needed |
| Vitamin E | Antioxidant effects, prevents neuropathy & biliary atresia, helps prevent lung injury and retinopathy | Weakness, nausea, dizziness, bleeding, diarrhea | Nerve damage, (ataxia, neuropathy, myopathy) | |
| Vitamin K | Prevents coagulopathy | Jaundice, anemia, flushing | Bleeding | If excess diarrhea |
| Water-soluble Vitamins | Carbohydrate, protein, fat metabolism, oxidation and reduction reactions | Excess vitamin C can lead to nephrolithiasis and interference with vitamin $B_{12}$ absorption | Chelosis, lethargy | |

Data from Refs.[66-75]

**Table 5**
Trace elements: metalloenzymes maximize enzymatic reactions, deficiency and supplementation needed for those on longer-term PN

| Element | Functions | Deficiency Causes | Deficiency Effects | Pediatric Manifestations |
|---|---|---|---|---|
| Zinc | Formation of metalloenzymes, RNA, membrane stabilization, maintenance immunity | Short bowel syndrome, thermal burns, dialysis, diarrhea | Alopecia, skin lesions, impaired wound healing | Growth retardation |
| Copper | Metalloenzyme function (stored and excreted in liver) | Nonsupplemented parenteral nutrition | Microcytic hypochromic anemia, neutropenia, hypothermia, mental status changes | Growth retardation, skeletal demineralization, fatal aplastic anemia |
| Selenium | Involved with enzymes reducing free radicals | Parenteral nutrition | Cardiomyopathy, peripheral myositis, muscle tenderness | |
| Manganese | | Excess in total parenteral nutrition | Growth retardation in animals | Excess deposit in liver and brain (remove from total parenteral nutrition in infants with liver disease) |
| Chromium | Potentiator of insulin | | Poor glucose tolerance | |
| Molybdenum | Oxidative metabolism of purines and sulfur | | Increase uric acid levels | |

Data from Refs. [77–86]

**Table 6**
Daily parenteral trace element requirements and supplementation in parenteral nutrition according to American Society for Parenteral and Enteral Nutrition guidelines

| Age Group | Zinc | Copper | Manganese | Chromium | Selenium |
|---|---|---|---|---|---|
| Adults (mg/d) | 2.5–5 | 0.3–0.5 | 0.06–0.1 | 0.01–0.015 | 0.02–0.06 |
| Adolescents >40 kg (mg/d) | 2–5 | 0.2–0.5 | 0.04–0.1 | 0.005– 0.015 | 0.04–0.06 |
| Preterm infants <3 kg (μg/kg/d) | 400 | 20 | 1 | 0.05–0.3 | 1.5–2 |
| Term infants 3–10 kg (μg/kg/d) | 50–250 | 20 | 1 | 0.2 | 2 |
| Children 10–40 kg (μg/kg/d) | 50–125 | 5–20 | 1 | 0.14–0.2 | 1–2 |
| Supplementation (μg/kg/d) | 400 | — | — | — | — |

*Data from* Mirtallo J, Canada T, Johnson D. Task force for the revision of safe practices for parenteral nutrition. Safe practices for parenteral nutrition. JPEN J Parenter Enteral Nutr 2004;28:S39–70.

## Indications

Infants in a state of good health before surgery or trauma can sustain 5 to 7 days without significant energy intake without serious systemic consequences provided that adequate nutritional support is initiated thereafter. Premature infants less than 32 to 34 weeks' gestation do not generally have a maturely coordinated suck and swallow; therefore, feeding must be provided enterally either by bolus every 2 to 3 hours or by continuous feedings. Oral feedings should be attempted when feasible, because delay in initiating oral nutrient swallowing results in long-term oral aversion. Additionally, the younger an infant's gestational age, the greater the percentage who are discharged with growth restriction. Almost 100% of infants born at 24 weeks' gestational age are discharged with a diagnosis of growth restriction. Therefore, aggressive feeding even within the first 24 hours of life is generally considered advisable. Children who have specific underlying diseases associated with malabsorption may benefit from specialized formulas. There are many high-calorie formulas available to address variable needs (**Tables 7** [infant] and **8** [pediatric]).

## Delivery Modalities

Children receiving gastric feedings tolerate a higher osmolarity and volume than those being fed into the small bowel. Furthermore, gastric acid may benefit digestion, has a bactericidal effect, and is associated with less-frequent gastrointestinal complications.[1] For patients requiring feedings for more than 8 weeks, a more permanent feeding access (eg, gastrostomy tube) should be considered. Several complications have been described, including improper placement (ie, placement too close to the pylorus), inadvertent placement through an adjacent loop of bowel, necrosis of the tract of the gastrostomy tube, and technical failures that require laparotomy.[34]

Use of jejunal tubes is plagued with problems, including involuntary dislodgement of transpylorically placed tubes and catheter obstruction due to inspissations of feedings or instillation of medications. Short-term complications of surgically placed jejunostomy tube include intra-abdominal abscess and volvulus with bowel infarction. Long-term complications include intestinal obstruction and peritonitis. When using tubes passed distal to the pylorus, continuous drip feedings are recommended to prevent the development of diarrhea and other symptoms of dumping.

## Enteral Formulas

The choice of formula depends on the age of the patient and the condition of the gastrointestinal tract. In general, term infants should be maintained on human milk (discussed later) or standard 20 kcal/30 mL formula (see **Table 7; Table 8**). Cow's milk–based formulas for term infants contain nutrients that closely approximate the nutritional profile of human milk. Some formulas have added arachidonic acid and docosahexaenoic acid, the two fatty acids that are found in human milk that are believed essential for brain and eye development; however, no strong evidence-based literature supports the need for this. A lactose-based formula is generally the first choice because it is the most physiologically similar to human milk and is the least expensive. Soy formulas are indicated to manage galactosemia and primary or secondary lactase deficiency. A protein hydrolysate or elemental formula is recommended in infants who have milk-protein intolerance, because one-third of infants who have an allergen-induced reaction to cow's milk are also intolerant of soy. Further, soy formulas are not recommended for premature infants because of their high aluminum content that may contribute to osteopenia.

Calories from EN can be added by increasing the volume delivered, increasing the concentration of the formula, or supplementing the feedings. Formula concentrations may be increased to 30 kcal/30 mL; however, highly concentrated formulas may be difficult for some infants to digest and have a higher renal solute load, and it may take time for them to build up tolerance. Higher concentrations have also been associated with a necrotizing enterocolitis (NEC)-type process.[35] Formula supplementation can be done by the addition of up to 2 g of a glucose polymer or 1 g of fats as medium-chain triglycerides (MCTs) or vegetable oil. Caution must be taken when supplementing calories in this fashion because it may compromise the ability of an infant to consume sufficient amounts of protein or minerals if the amount of formula is limited.

Standard premature infant formulas are milk-based formulas, which provide 22 to 24 cal/30 mL and are optimized for required vitamins, minerals, and trace element needs. A portion of fat is provided as MCTs to compensate for the limited bile salt pool in young infants. MCTs, however, cannot be used to prevent essential fatty acid deficiency (all of which are long-chain triglycerides). Premature infants are at increased risk for NEC. This risk is not increased with gastrointestinal priming feeds; however, excessive advancements in the rates of these feedings have been shown to put neonates at increased risk. Whether feedings are given via bolus or continuous methods does not seem to influence hospital outcomes or days to reach full feeding.[36,37]

### Administration of Enteral Nutrition

For preterm infants, a feeding protocol is typically followed to maintain consistency of practice and reduce the incidence of NEC, and these guidelines are now well established.[3,38] For term infants, intermittent enteral feeding can be initiated at 2 to 5 mL/kg every 3 to 4 hours. Feeding is advanced in increments of 2 to 5 mL/kg every 2 feedings to goal rate as tolerated. Guidelines have been revamped for safe delivery of EN and are given in **Table 9** for term and premature infants. Feeding residuals are checked before each intermittent feeding, and EN is held if the residual volume is greater than twice the administered volume.

### Human Milk

Human milk has a variety of advantages over commercial formulas. The American Academy of Pediatrics advocates nursing until 1 year of age, yet the majority of mothers in the United States stop nursing by the infant's second month of life.[39] Breastfeeding provides both nutrition as well as passive immunologic protection to the neonate. Breast milk contains 87% water and provides 0.64 to 0.67 kcal/mL. The fat content of breast milk is high, at 3.4 g/dL, whereas the protein content of

**Table 7**
Infant formulas

| Formula | kcal/ mL | Protein (g/L) | Protein (%kcal) | Protein Source | CHO Source | CHO (%kcal) | Fat Source | Fat (%kcal) | Indications |
|---|---|---|---|---|---|---|---|---|---|
| Similac Special Care (Abbott Nutrition) | 0.81 | 24 | 12 | Nonfat milk, whey | Lactose, corn syrup solids | 41 | MCT oil, soy oil, coconut oil | 47 | Prematurity |
| NeoSure (Abbott Nutrition) | 0.73 | 21 | 11 | Nonfat milk, whey | Lactose, corn syrup solids | 42 | MCT oil, soy oil, coconut oil | 48 | Prematurity, discharge formula |
| Enfamil (Mead Johnson) | 0.67 | 14 | 8.5 | Whey, nonfat milk | Lactose | 43.5 | Palm olein, soy oil, coconut oil, sun oil | 48 | Standard |
| Similac (Abbott Nutrition) | 0.67 | 14 | 8 | Nonfat milk, whey | Lactose | 43 | Soy oil, coconut oil, safflower oil | 49 | Standard |
| | 0.81 | 17 | 8 | Nonfat milk, whey | Lactose | 43 | Soy oil, coconut oil, safflower oil | 49 | |
| ProSobee (Mead Johnson) | 0.67 | 17 | 10 | Soy isolate, methionine | Corn syrup solids | 42 | Palm olein, soy oil, coconut oil, sun oil | 48 | Lactose intolerance, galactosemia |
| Isomil (Abbott Nutrition) | 0.67 | 17 | 10 | Soy isolate, methionine | Corn syrup, sucrose | 41 | Soy oil, coconut oil, safflower oil | 49 | Lactose malabsorption, galactosemia |
| Nutramigen (Mead Johnson) | 0.67 | 19 | 11 | Casein hydrolysate, cystine, tyrosine, tryptophan | Corn syrup solids, modified cornstarch | 41 | Palm olein, soy oil, coconut oil, sun oil | 48 | Protein intolerance |

| Pregestimil (Mead Johnson) | 0.67 | 19 | 11 | Casein hydrolysate, cystine, tyrosine, tryptophan | Corn syrup solids, modified cornstarch, dextrose | 41 | MCT oil, corn oil, soy oil, safflower oil | 48 | Protein intolerance, cystic fibrosis, neonatal cholestasis, short bowel syndrome |
|---|---|---|---|---|---|---|---|---|---|
| Alimentum (Abbott Nutrition) | 0.67 | 19 | 11 | Casein hydrolysate, cystine, tyrosine, tryptophan | Sucrose, modified tapioca, starch | 41 | MCT oil, safflower oil, soy oil | 48 | Protein intolerance, neonatal cholestasis |
| Neocate (Nutricia North America) | 0.67 | 21 | 12 | Free amino acids | Corn syrup solids | 47 | MCT oil, safflower oil, corn oil, soy oil, sun oil | 41 | Food allergy, protein intolerance, short bowel syndrome |
| Enfaport Lipil (Mead Johnson) | 1 | 35 | 14 | Calcium caseinate, sodium caseinate | Corn syrup solids | 41 | MCT oil (84%), soy oil | 45 | Chylothorax, LCHAD deficiency |

*Abbreviations:* CHO, carbohydrate; LCHAD, long-chain 3-hydroxyacyl-CoA dehydrogenase.

Composition of infant and pediatric formulas is summarized in **Tables 7** and **8**, respectively. Enfamil (Mead Johnson) and Similac (Abbott Nutrition) both have milk-based proteins and contain lactose as the carbohydrate source. There are only limited reasons to use soy formulas. The soy-based products include ProSobee (Mead Johnson) and Isomil (Abbott Nutrition). Both contain corn syrup solids as a carbohydrate source. Isomil also contains sucrose. Soy formulas are indicated to manage galactosemia and primary or secondary lactase deficiency. Soy formulas should not be used in patients with a documented allergy or intolerance to milk protein because one-third of infants who have an allergen-induced reaction to cow's milk are also intolerant of soy. Therefore, a protein hydrolysate or elemental formula is recommended in infants who have a milk-protein intolerance. Protein hydrolysates include Nutramigen (Mead Johnson), Alimentum (Abbott Nutrition), and Pregestimil (Mead Johnson). Alimentum and Pregestimil also provide 50% to 55% of fat as MCTs. If infants have continued symptoms of protein-intolerance when ingesting a protein-hydrolysate, then an amino acid–based formula may be provided. For the infant population, Neocate (Nutricia North America) is the only amino acid–based formula available. Children older than 12 months of age who continue to be intolerant of milk protein may respond well to Peptamen Junior· (Nestle Nutrition), which is a whey protein hydrolysate. If an amino acid–based formula is needed in children older than 12 months of age, options include, L-emental (Hormel Health Labs/Nutrition Medical), and EleCare (Abbott Nutrition). EleCare has long-chain triglycerides. Sixty-eight percent of the fat in L-emental is derived from MCT.

**Table 8**
**Pediatric formulas**

| Formula | kcal/mL | Protein (g/L) | Protein (%kcal) | Protein Source | CHO Source | CHO (%kcal) | Fat Source | Fat (%kcal) | Indications |
|---|---|---|---|---|---|---|---|---|---|
| PediaSure (Abbott Nutrition) | 1.0 | 30 | 12 | Milk protein concentrate, whey protein, soy isolate | Corn maltodextrin, sucrose | 53 | Safflower oil, soy oil, MCT oil | 35 | Standard, oral feeds, tube feeds |
| Boost (Mead Johnson) | 1 | 42 | 17 | Milk | Corn syrup, sucrose | 68 | Canola oil, corn oil, sunflower oil | 15 | Standard, oral feeds, tube feeds |
| Peptamen Junior (Nestle Nutrition) | 1.0 | 30 | 12 | Hydrolyzed whey | Maltodextrin | 55 | MCT, soy oil, canloa oil | 33 | Short bowel syndrome, cholestasis, pancreatitis |
| L-Emental (Hormel Health labs/Nutrition Medical) | 0.8 | 40 | 16 | L-amino acids | Maltodextrin, modified starch | 82 | Safflower oil | 2 | Short bowel syndrome, inflammatory bowel disease, pancreatitis |
| EleCare (Abbott Nutrition) | 0.67 | 21 | 15 | L-amino acids | Corn syrup solids | 43 | MCT, safflower oil, soy oil | 42 | Malabsorption, food allergies |
| Suplena (Abbott Nutrition) | 1.8 | 45 | 10 | Sodium caseinate, milk protein isolate | Corn maltodextrin, sucrose | 51 | Safflower oil, soy oil, canola oil | 48 | Renal failure |

*Abbreviation:* CHO, carbohydrate.

| Table 9 |
|---|
| **Enteral nutrition administration to preterm infants** |

| Birth Weight (g) | ≤1000 | >1000–<1250 | 1250–1500 | >1500–2000 | >2000–2500 |
|---|---|---|---|---|---|
| Volume of First Feeding | 10–20 mL/kg/d | 10–20 mL/kg/d | 20 mL/kg/d | 20 mL/kg/d | 5 mL every 3 hours |
| Volume Rate of Feeding Advances | 10–20 mL/kg/d | 10–20 mL/kg/d | 20 mL/kg/d | 20 mL/kg/d | 5 mL may advance, as tolerated every other feed as tolerated |

*Data from* Btaiche I, Khalidi N, Kovacevich D. The parenteral and enteral nutrition manual. 9th edition. Ann Arbor (MI): The University of Michigan Hospitals and Health Centers. Ann Arbor: University of Michigan; 2010.

human milk (0.9%) is lower than that of bovine milk or commercial formulas but seems much better absorbed. Ingestion of human milk allows for the acquisition of passive immunity via the transfer of both immunoglobulins and lymphocytes from the mother.[40] The immunologic advantages of breast milk include the transmission of both humoral and cellular factors to the neonate.[40] Despite similar amounts of trace elements, human milk allows for a more efficient absorption of these elements compared with commercial formulas. Although human milk has many advantages, high demands for calcium, phosphorus, electrolytes, vitamins, and trace elements cannot be achieved with human milk alone. Because of this, human milk fortifiers (one pack per ounce) should be added to breast milk that is fed to preterm infants. Supplementation should continue until a child achieves the weight of a term infant. When human milk fortifier is added to human milk, the hang time of the final reconstituted formula is 2 hours.

### Complications of Enteral Feeding

The gastrointestinal tract generally tolerates feedings well once the postoperative ileus has resolved. Not uncommonly, critically ill children sustain a loss of a significant portion of the absorptive function, often due to a lactase deficiency. Symptoms are generally manifested by cramping, diarrhea, or emesis. Symptoms often improve with the initiation of a lactose-free diet. In critically ill children, frequent interruptions of enteral feeding for procedures, feeding intolerances, fluid restriction, or gastrointestinal dysmotility result in suboptimal EN delivery.[41,42] The gastrointestinal tract generally tolerates increased volume more readily than increased osmolarity. Rapid-bolus nasogastric feedings may lead to a high incidence of reflux, which can be associated with aspiration, a major known risk of enteral feedings. Complications can be decreased with the use of a slow, continuous infusion or preferably with jejunal feedings, a now controversial method.[43] Use of small bowel feeding has been shown to improve energy and nutrition delivery in children.[44] In stable patients, continuous infusion through a nasogastric tube is associated with no higher incidence of aspiration than is infusion through a nasoduodenal tube, even in those with delayed gastric emptying.[45] When a patient's clinical condition allows, raising the backrest or the head of the bed to 30° to 45° during continuous feeding also decreases the risk of aspiration.[46] Other complications include contamination of the enteral feeds, so care must be taken during preparation and at the bedside. Expiration times should be observed. Assessment of adequate absorption can be performed most readily by the testing of the stool for the absorption of carbohydrates, by measuring stool pH, and by detecting for reducing substances. The presence of a stool pH less than or equal to 5.5, or a reducing substance of greater than 0.5 %, indicates the passage of unabsorbed carbohydrates into the stool and, once detected, should lead to a decrease in the formula concentration of carbohydrate.

## PARENTERAL NUTRITION
### Indications for PN

PN is ideal for maintaining nutrition in infants and children who are unable to tolerate enteral feedings. Clinical conditions in children likely requiring PN include gastrointestinal disorders (short bowel syndrome, malabsorption, intractable diarrhea, bowel obstruction, protracted vomiting, inflammatory bowel disease, and enterocutaneous fistulas), congenital anomalies (gastroschisis, bowel atresia, volvulus, and meconium ileus), radiation therapy to the gastrointestinal tract, chemotherapy resulting in gastrointestinal dysfunction, and severe respiratory distress syndrome in premature infants. Very-low-birth-weight infants are generally intolerant of enteral feeding and require PN during the first 24 hours after birth. Signs of starvation may be seen in underfed premature infants in as few as 1 to 2 days. Although older children and adults generally do not require PN unless periods of starvation extend beyond 7 to 10 days, infants require PN if periods of starvation extend beyond 4 to 5 days.

Very-low-birth-weight infants are born with limited nutritional reserves, lose protein in desquamated epidermal cells and urine, and quickly use their somatic protein reserves for energy when given inadequate nutrition. Providing early nutrition within 12 hours after birth is essential for the transition from fetal to extrauterine life to prevent growth failure and neurodevelopment delays. Therefore, prompt initiation of PN within a few hours after birth is essential. Further, because very-low-birth-weight infants have shown decreased plasma amino acid levels after birth, protein intake at approximately 3.8 g/kg per day improves nitrogen retention and stimulates weight gain.[47,48]

### PN Components and Requirements

Specific components of PN solution are similar to those used in adults.Specific requirements for children do exist, however. Pediatric parenteral crystalline amino acid formulas provide essential and nonessential amino acids specifically balanced to meet the needs of developing children. Neonatal-specific amino acid formulas are formulated to reproduce the plasma amino acid profile of breastfed infants closely. These formulas have led to greater weight gain and improved nitrogen balance in infants compared with standard amino acid formulas.[49] Taurine supplementation for premature infants is essential to promote bile acid conjugation and to improve bile flow[50] and has been shown to decrease the degree of PN-associated cholestasis.[20] Hydrous dextrose acts as a protein-sparing substrate by preventing breakdown of somatic protein stores via suppression of gluconeogenesis.[51] In infants, PN should be initiated at a dextrose infusion rate of 4 to 8 mg/kg per minute to maintain adequate serum glucose concentrations and advanced at a daily rate of 2 mg/kg per minute until the nutritional goal is achieved. The maximum dextrose infusion rate should not exceed 10 to 14 mg/kg per minute.[52,53] Lipid emulsions in infants and children are initiated at a dose of 1 g/kg per day and advanced by 1 g/kg per day to a maximum of 3 g/kg per day. Lipid emulsion is better cleared[54,55] and lipid use is improved[56] when lipid is infused continuously over 24 hours rather than intermittently or for part of the day. Pediatric parenteral multivitamins and trace elements have been specifically designed to meet requirements unique to a child's age. Pediatric parenteral multivitamins provide low vitamin A and high water-soluble vitamins to premature infants, although higher vitamin A intake may be essential in low-birth-weight infants who are at increased risk for lung disease.[57] Depletion of water-soluble vitamins occurs rapidly under stressful conditions. Standard pediatric trace mineral formulas contain zinc, copper, manganese, and chromium and some formulas have added selenium. Trace element formulas are designed to meet the recommendations of the American Gastroenterological Association–American Medical Association and the Society of Clinical Nutrition for daily intravenous supplements of trace minerals in the absence of deficiencies.[58] The safe practice guidelines by the American Society for Parenteral and Enteral Nutrition recently issued different guidelines with lower daily parenteral trace element requirements and supplementation.[59]

### Fluids and Electrolytes

PN solution should be not be used to manage acute fluid and electrolyte losses. Instead, patients should receive a separate intravenous solution for fluid and electrolyte supplementation (**Table 10**). Electrolyte adjustments in PN are based on serum electrolyte concentrations. Adjustments should account for all electrolyte sources and losses, acid base status, clinical conditions, and medications that affect electrolyte balance.

### Sodium

Neonates and especially premature infants develop natriuresis during the first 1 to 2 weeks after birth as a result of their immature kidney function. Because adequate sodium intake is essential for protein synthesis and tissue development, adequate sodium supplementation is necessary and is guided by serum and urine sodium levels.[60] Premature infants may require as much as 8 mEq/kg per day of sodium, and this requirement decreases with age such that in older children needs range from 1 to 2 mEq/kg per day. Maximum sodium concentration in PN solutions should not exceed normal saline solution equivalent (154 mEq of sodium/L).

### Potassium

Potassium requirements are higher during anabolism[61] and when correcting for any gastrointestinal or renal potassium losses. Potassium concentrations in the PN solution should not exceed 120 mEq/L, and potassium infusion rates in infants and children should not exceed 0.5 mEq/kg per hour[62]; in adolescents, dosing should be at 0.7 mEq/kg per hour.

### Chloride and acetate

The chloride-to-acetate ratio in the PN solution can be adjusted based on a patient's acid-base status. A high acetate–to–low chloride ratio is indicated to help correct

**Table 10**
**Daily electrolyte and mineral requirements for pediatric patients[a]**

| Electrolyte | Preterm Neonates | Infants/Children | Adolescents and Children >50 kg |
|---|---|---|---|
| Sodium | 2–5 mEq/kg | 2–5 mEq/kg | 1–2 mEq/kg |
| Potassium | 2–4 mEq/kg | 2–4 mEq/kg | 1–2 mEq/kg |
| Calcium | 2–4 mEq/kg | 0.5–4 mEq/kg | 10–20 mEq |
| Phosphorus | 1–2 mmol/kg | 0.5–2 mmol/kg | 10–40 mmol |
| Magnesium | 0.3–0.5 mEq/kg | 0.3–0.5 mEq/kg | 10–30 mEq |
| Acetate | As needed to maintain acid-base balance | | |
| Chloride | As needed to maintain acid-base balance | | |

[a] Assumes normal age-related organ function and normal losses.
*Data from* Mirtallo J, Canada T, Johnson D. Task force for the revision of safe practices for parenteral nutrition. Safe practices for parenteral nutrition. JPEN J Parenter Enteral Nutr 2004;28:S39–70.

a metabolic acidosis, such as that resulting from lower intestinal bicarbonate losses, or to help a child compensate for a respiratory acidosis. Premature infants are especially at risk for acid-base changes because of their inadequate responses, due to inefficient hydrogen ion excretion and bicarbonate reabsorption by the kidneys.[60,63] A low acetate–to–high chloride ratio minimizes the bicarbonate load in patients with metabolic alkalosis, such as that resulting from excessive gastric fluid and electrolyte losses. Great caution should be used when adjusting the chloride-to-acetate ratio, because dramatic acid-base changes may rapidly occur.

### Calcium and phosphate

Calcium and phosphate requirements in infants and children are greater than requirements in adults due to increased demands for growth. Corticosteroids and loop diuretics, which are commonly used in neonatal and pediatric intensive care patients, can further increase calcium requirements by increasing calcium losses. After birth, hypophosphatemia is commonly observed in premature infants due to high urinary phosphate excretion.[64] Calcium and phosphate should be provided in an adequate ratio and with amounts to optimize bone mineralization and prevent metabolic bone disease.[65] Bone mineralization is optimized at an intake ratio of 2.6 mEq of calcium:1 mmol of phosphorus (1.7 mg calcium:1 mg phosphorus).[66] Inadequate calcium and phosphorus supplementation is problematic due to solubility limitations. As a result, enteral calcium and phosphorus supplementation may be required. Also, cysteine hydrochloride, an acidic compound that can be added to the PN solution, can be used to lower the solution pH and allow higher calcium and phosphate amounts in PN. An acidic medium favors the formation of monovalent phosphates instead of the divalent phosphates that otherwise would bind to calcium. Cysteine hydrochloride is added to the neonatal PN solution at a dose of 40 mg/g of amino acids.[67] Calcium and phosphorus can safely be added to PN when the concentrations provided satisfy the following equation:

$$\text{Calcium (mEq)} + \text{phosphorus (mmol)} \leq 30 \text{ (per 1000 mL of PN)}$$

Because of these solubility issues, the full needs for optimal tissue and bone growth may not be met unless calcium and phosphorus are also provided enterally.

### Iron dextran

Iron deficiency anemia may occur in PN-dependent children, particularly because iron is not added to PN solutions. Although not recommend by manufacturers, it has been used safely during the first 4 months of life by many qualified groups. Daily iron dextran doses up to 1 mg/kg have been added to neonatal PN to prevent iron deficiency anemia. An iron replacement calculation can be found in **Box 1**. Additive iron has been used predominantly in renal failure patients but also seems effective in children.[68]

### Carnitine

Carnitine is required for transport of long-chain fatty acids into the mitochondria where they undergo oxidation.[69] Premature infants are at risk for carnitine deficiency because of their limited carnitine reserves and reduced ability for carnitine synthesis.[70] Supplementation of L-carnitine can improve fatty oxidation.[71] Premature infants who develop unexplained hypertriglyceridemia during lipid infusion may benefit from L-carnitine supplementation at a dose of approximately 10 mg/kg per day.[72] In neonates, L-carnitine given at 20 mg/kg per day for 8 weeks resulted in higher-than-normal plasma total carnitine concentrations. Parenteral L-carnitine doses of

---

**Box 1**
**Intravenous iron replacement therapy: calculation for total iron replacement dose**

mL of iron dextran = $0.0476 \times$ weight (kg) $\times$ ($Hb_n - Hb_o$) + 1 mL per 5 kg of body weight (up to a maximum of 14 mL),

where *1 mL of iron dextran* = 50 mg of elemental iron; $Hb_n$ = desired hemoglobin (g/dL)—the desired hemoglobin is 12 if patient weighs <15 kg or 14.8 if patient weighs >15 kg; and $Hb_o$ = measured hemoglobin (g/dL).

Maximal daily iron replacement dose:

Infants weighing <5 kg: 25 mg

Children weighing 5–10 kg: 50 mg

Children >10 kg: 100 mg

---

48 mg/kg per day in low-birth-weight infants increased protein oxidation, decreased nitrogen balance, and increased the time to regain birth weight.[73]

### Complications of Parenteral Nutrition

Despite more than 40 years of experience with PN, complications continue to be a major obstacle in the care of pediatric patients. Complications of PN can be classified as metabolic, respiratory, hepatobiliary, and infectious.

#### Metabolic complications

Metabolic complications are not unique to pediatric patients and thus are discussed on a limited basis in this article. The most prevalent complications include hyperglycemia. Although uncontrolled hyperglycemia is unacceptable, there is disparity in practice of glycemic control in pediatric ICUs, and the long-term outcomes and optimal blood glucose targets in these children remain unknown.[74] The first attempt in managing hyperglycemia is to decrease the dextrose load or reduce the infusion rate. If reducing dextrose does not improve hyperglycemia, insulin therapy is then indicated. Because infants have a variable response to insulin therapy,[75] adding insulin to the PN solution should be avoided. Instead, a regular insulin drip should be initiated and titrated based on serial glucose measurements. Hypoglycemia with PN is usually the result of a sudden reduction of the PN infusion rate. Premature infants are at increased risk for hypoglycemia due to their underdeveloped metabolic response[76]; cycling of PN in this group of patients is typically not performed safely. Hypertriglyceridemia is not uncommon, may be due to excessive carbohydrate intake, and may occur commonly in prematurity,[77] lipid overfeeding,[78,79] critical illness, and sepsis.[80] Although the tendency might be to reduce lipid infusion, a reduction in dextrose would be far more effective. Dextrose infusion rate should not be decreased, however, below 4 mg/kg per minute in infants, the minimum rate required for protein sparing. If hypertriglyceridemia persists despite reducing glucose intake, the lipid emulsion dose and rate should be decreased to keep triglyceride levels below 275 mg/dL. A lipid dose of 0.5 to 1 g/kg per day in children should prevent essential fatty acid deficiency.

Metabolic acidosis may result from excessive chloride (hyperchloremic acidosis may occur with serum chloride levels >130 mEq/L) or high amino acid load in PN. The addition of cysteine hydrochloride to the PN solution to improve calcium and phosphate solubility may also cause acidemia.[81] Premature infants and patients with liver or renal disease are at increased risk for metabolic acidosis and should be closely monitored for acid-base changes.

Metabolic bone disease, including osteopenia, osteomalacia, and rickets, is a complication in PN-dependent patients. Diagnosis is often difficult and may not be evident until a pathologic fracture is observed. Biochemical markers may reveal elevated serum alkaline phosphatase concentrations, hypercalciuria, low to normal plasma parathyroid hormone, and low 1,25 dihydroxyvitamin D.[82,83] Several factors predispose to PN-associated metabolic bone disease, including calcium and phosphorus deficiency, excessive losses of calcium due to diuretics, excessive vitamin D intake,[84] and aluminum toxicity.[85] Maximizing calcium and phosphorus intake is most important to improve bone mineralization.

### Hepatobiliary complications

Hepatobiliary complications include cholestasis, steatosis, and cholelithiasis. Because this is one of the most devastating complications of neonatal PN, a separate article is dedicated to this subject so for a discussion of hepatobiliary complications please see the article by Puder elsewhere in this issue.

### Infectious

Catheter-related infections remain the main cause of sepsis in patients receiving PN. Factors that correlate with catheter-related infections include prolonged catheterization, use of the catheter for multiple purposes, manipulation of the catheter hub, and chronic PN therapy. Most series report an incidence of 0.5 to 2.0 infections per 1000 catheter-days for nonimmunosuppressed patients with a central venous catheter.[86,87] A considerably higher rate of infection is found in children with short bowel syndrome; this rate ranges from 7 to 9 infections per 1000 catheter-days.[88-91] Use of chlorhexidine-impregnated dressings has been shown to reduce pediatric catheter infections.[92] Guidelines for the prevention and management of catheter-related infections are published elsewhere.[93,94] In general, nonpermanent polyvinyl chloride lines should be removed for treatment of catheter sepsis; however, more than 80% of patients with a silastic catheter (eg, Broviac or Hickman) are able to have the infection cleared with intravenous antibiotics. Another technique to treat such infections is the antibiotic lock technique. More recently, the use of ethanol lock therapy, which can reduce infections by almost 10-fold, is being used. Ethanol can cause a precipitation with heparin or citrate, requiring that these two agents not be used during this treatment.[95] Also, ethanol may weaken plastics in the catheter and should not be used if the infusion device is made of polyurethane.[95,96] Due to the high failure rate of antibiotics, most patients with a tract infection should have the line removed. Attempting to maintain a catheter with a *Candida* infection is associated with a mortality of up to 25% and a low chance of clearing the infection with the line in place (13%).[97] Only a short course of antifungal agents needs to be given after the catheter is removed (7 to 14 days); however, the results of blood cultures must be negative.[98] For rare cases in which venous access has been nearly exhausted, a trial of antifungal agents and ethanol lock while retaining the line may be attempted.

### Complications from overfeeding

Overfeeding can lead to several adverse consequences and for a discussion of overfeeding see the article by Palesty elsewhere in this issue. Recent data in children, however, show similar trends of benefit in prevention of hyperglycemia in ICUs (see hyperglycemia).[99]

### Administration of PN

PN is generally begun in neonates within the first 12 hours after birth, and many centers now stock a premade D10% solution, often with crystalline amino acids, for such use in their units. Neonates tend to be somewhat intolerant of large amounts of dextrose or amino acids for the first 2 to 3 days of life. Dextrose solution concentrations are generally initiated at 10% to 12.5%, and the concentration is slowly increased on a daily basis to between 20% and 25%. Monitoring a patient's blood glucose levels and electrolyte balance and checking for glucosuria confirm whether a child can tolerate this level of dextrose administration. The maximum dextrose concentration in peripherally infused solutions in infants and children is 12.5%. Because lipid emulsions are isotonic solutions, co-infusion of lipids with peripheral PN protects the veins and prolongs the viability of peripheral intravenous catheters.[100] PN should be initiated as a continuous infusion over 24 hours. For patients receiving long-term PN, delivery may be given over a shortened period of time (eg, 16 hours). Importantly, to avoid hypoglycemia or hyperglycemia, the rate of infusion should be reduced by half for 1 to 2 hours before terminating or starting up infusion each day. A suggested guideline for ordering neonatal PN is given in **Fig. 1**.

## SPECIAL PROBLEMS IN THE NUTRITIONAL SUPPORT OF THE PEDIATRIC SURGICAL PATIENT

### Nutrition in the Pediatric Surgical Patient

Pediatric surgical patients respond to surgical stress differently from older children or adults.[101] The metabolism of children is markedly affected by operative stress. The time period of increased energy expenditure, however, is much shorter than it is in adults.[102] Induction of anesthesia has profound effects on body metabolism, with agents, such as fentanyl, having a beneficial effect in reducing the catabolic effect.[103] Moreover, protein turnover and catabolism seem not to be affected by major operative procedures in neonates. PN, however, in surgical neonates is associated with increased production of oxygen-free radicals, and this may contribute to a suppression of the immune status. Thus, use must be tempered by potential benefit. The use of nutritional support both preoperatively and postoperatively is discussed.

### Indications for Preoperative Nutrition

In malnourished adults, provision of enteral feedings preoperatively for 2 to 3 weeks may reduce postoperative wound infections, anastomotic leakage, hepatic and renal failure, and length of hospital stay.[104,105] Data for PN support are less clear. A meta-analysis demonstrated little benefit and possibly an increase in complications in mildly or moderately malnourished patients.[106] The most significant benefit has been documented in severely malnourished patients who have developed fewer noninfectious complications if receiving perioperative PN (PN presurgery for 7 to 15 days and postsurgery for 3 days).[107] PN patients were noted, however, to have increased infection rates, which could not totally be explained by the use of central venous catheters. This suggests that the use of PN may predispose patients to increased infectious complications. Thus, unless there are clear indications of severe malnutrition, a delay in operative management to provide preoperative PN is not indicated.[3] An extrapolation of these findings to neonatal patients is difficult because of their limited nutritional stores.

### Indications for Postoperative Nutrition

Use of aggressive postoperative nutritional support is even more controversial. In critically ill adult patients, early EN within 24 to 48 hours of admission to an ICU has been

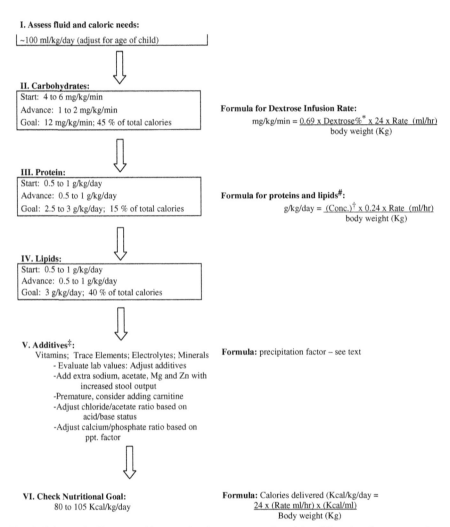

**I. Assess fluid and caloric needs:**

~100 ml/kg/day (adjust for age of child)

**II. Carbohydrates:**
Start: 4 to 6 mg/kg/min
Advance: 1 to 2 mg/kg/min
Goal: 12 mg/kg/min; 45 % of total calories

**Formula for Dextrose Infusion Rate:**

$$mg/kg/min = \frac{0.69 \times Dextrose\%^* \times 24 \times Rate \; (ml/hr)}{body \; weight \; (Kg)}$$

**III. Protein:**
Start: 0.5 to 1 g/kg/day
Advance: 0.5 to 1 g/kg/day
Goal: 2.5 to 3 g/kg/day; 15 % of total calories

**Formula for proteins and lipids#:**

$$g/kg/day = \frac{(Conc.)^\dagger \times 0.24 \times Rate \; (ml/hr)}{body \; weight \; (Kg)}$$

**IV. Lipids:**
Start: 0.5 to 1 g/kg/day
Advance: 0.5 to 1 g/kg/day
Goal: 3 g/kg/day; 40 % of total calories

**V. Additives‡:**
Vitamins; Trace Elements; Electrolytes; Minerals
- Evaluate lab values: Adjust additives
-Add extra sodium, acetate, Mg and Zn with
    increased stool output
-Premature, consider adding carnitine
-Adjust chloride/acetate ratio based on
    acid/base status
-Adjust calcium/phosphate ratio based on
    ppt. factor

**Formula: precipitation factor – see text**

**VI. Check Nutritional Goal:**
80 to 105 Kcal/kg/day

**Formula:** Calories delivered (Kcal/kg/day =
$$\frac{24 \times (Rate \; ml/hr) \times (Kcal/ml)}{Body \; weight \; (Kg)}$$

**Fig. 1.** Schematic diagram of how to begin to approach writing PN orders for a neonate or young infant. Fluids should be adjusted based on the infant's gestation age and body weight. *Dextrose concentration should be used as the percent number (ie, 20 for 20%). †The concentration in this formula should be written as the percent number (ie, 4.25 for 4.25%). ‡See relevant tables for each of these additives. #If the amino acid concentration is greater than 1.5%, the precipitation factor should be less than 3. If the final amino acid concentration is greater than 1% and less than 1.5%, a precipitation factor should be less than 2, and for an amino acid concentration less than 1%, calcium and phosphate should not be added. Adjustments to this formulation need to be done if additives (eg, cysteine) are placed in the parenteral nutrition.

shown to reduce infectious complications.[108,109] Gastrointestinal complications and feeding intolerance, however, can be a considerable limitation to the adequate delivery of enteral nutrition.[110] These data suggest that, when used, postoperative nutrition should be started early using a combination of PN and EN until the gastrointestinal tract fully recovers. A controlled study examining the effect of postoperative PN in children demonstrated a positive effect on nitrogen balance and levels of insulinlike growth factor 1; however, no clinical benefit was noted.[111] The effect of PN on postoperative healing has been negligible. In the postoperative period, there are higher infection rates in patients on PN. Meta-analysis studies show that there is an adverse effect to postoperative PN.[106] Although prolonged starvation postoperatively places patients at adverse risk,[112] postoperative PN should be restricted to infants who do not tolerate even a short period of starvation or older children who probably cannot tolerate EN for at least 5 to 7 days. In well-nourished adolescents, this period of time can be increased to 7 to 10 days.[3]

### Nutritional Support in Critically Ill Surgical Patients

Nutritional care of critically ill or septic postoperative patients represents a much greater challenge than the general pediatric surgical patient. Clinically, critically ill children manifest poor enteral feeding, anorexia, and often a paralytic ileus. Insulin resistance results in hyperglycemia and hypertriglyceridemia. Estimates of energy needs during this time are important. Energy needs of postoperative or septic critically ill infants have not uncommonly been overestimated. Almost one-third of an infant's energy needs is provided to support growth (30 to 35 kcal/kg/d). Because a cessation of growth occurs during periods of sepsis and critical illness, a marked decrease in energy needs may ensue. In a study of critically ill postoperative infants, the mean measured basal energy expenditure was only 43 kcal/kg per day.[17] Results are extraordinarily variable, however, further emphasizing the utility of performing indirect calorimetry. Although data from meta-analyses in adult patients suggest that PN has little proved benefit for most critically ill surgical patients, and thus supplementation should be used sparingly,[113] potentially a more aggressive approach may benefit neonates and children. Energy and nutrient deficiencies occur rapidly in a pediatric ICU, and this highlights the need for aggressive nutritional support.[114] High lipid infusion may also have benefit in neonates and results in achieving significantly higher energy delivery, and a reduction in need for insulin therapy; other potential benefits include a reduced rate of retinopathy of prematurity and NEC.[115] A 3-fold reduction in NEC can also be seen in neonates receiving human milk.[116] This somewhat aggressive nutritional support must be balanced with recent data that suggest physicians overestimate energy needs in critically ill children and support more accurate measurements of these needs, including the use of indirect calorimetry.[117] Recent data have supported the use of tight glucose control in an ICU setting, which has been shown to improve short-term outcomes.[99] Such support must be performed carefully, because up to 25% of children developed hypoglycemia. Recent guidelines should be used when caring for this complex group of children.[118]

### Biliary Atresia

Infants with biliary atresia, even after a clinically successful hepatic portoenterostomy, typically have lower than normal amounts of bile flow into the intestine. This subsequently leads to an inadequate absorption of fat-soluble vitamins.[119] As a consequence; this leads to a lack of bone mineralization as well as failure to thrive (FTT). The essential goals for such infants are to provide adequate calories using a formula that maximizes fat intake. Commonly used formulas have increased MCTs and include Pregestimil (Mead Johnson) or Enfaport (Mead Johnson) (see **Table 7**). Use of these formulas has been shown to increase growth in such patients.[120] Breastfeeding, although generally ideal in infancy, should be used cautiously in patients with biliary atresia secondary to the increased fat content. Vitamin supplementation is critical in patients with biliary atresia (**Table 11**). Frequent monitoring of vitamin levels is essential to ensure sufficient supplementation is achieved. Many formulas use a combination

**Table 11**
**Vitamin therapy in cholestasis**

| Name | Dose | Supplied As |
|------|------|-------------|
| Vitamin A (Aquasol A, Centeon) | 10,000–15,000 IU/d (50,000 IU = 15 mg) | 3-mg tablets 3-mg, 7.5-mg, or 15-mg capsules 50,000-IU/mL drops |
| Vitamin D (25OH) (Calderal, Organon Teknika) | 2–4 µg/kg/d | 20-µg and 50-µg capsules |
| Vitamin D [1,25 (OH)] (Rocaltral, Roche) | 0.01–0.05 µg/kg/d | 0.25-µg and 0.5-µg capsules 0.1-µg/mL/liquid |
| Vitamin E (TPGS) (Liqui-E, Twinlab) | 25 IU/kg/d | 26.7-IU/mL liquid |
| Vitamin K | 2.5–5 mg/d | 5-mg tablets |

*Abbreviation:* TPGS, d-alpha tocopheryl polyethylene glycol 1000 succinate.

form of fat-soluble vitamins (A, D, E and K 0.5 mL/kg); however, vitamin K may be inadequate in this formulation, and additional supplementation (2.5 mg/d) should be given. Protein metabolism is impaired in children with biliary atresia, increasing from 4% to 9% of energy expenditure in healthy infants to 17% in patients with biliary atresia.[121] REE was approximately 29% higher than expected in biliary atresia infants, and only 35% of the metabolizable energy intake was retained for growth.[122] Optimal growth and nutrition in infants with biliary atresia has recently been associated with improved outcomes and should be a major goal for pediatric surgeons.[123]

### Short Bowel Syndrome

Readers are referred to see article by Thompson elsewhere in this issue on short bowel syndrome; however, pertinent aspects to neonates are discussed. Neonates, particularly those with ostomies, may have high stool output, which is associated with excessive losses of zinc, magnesium, sodium, bicarbonate, and potassium.[124] These losses must be monitored. Total body sodium depletion has been shown to be associated with FTT, despite the administration of adequate amounts of calories.[125] A simple way to detect such a deficit is to measure a spot urine sodium. A urine sodium of less than 10 mEq/L may indicate total body sodium depletion and supplementation (sodium chloride or sodium bicarbonate, as indicated) should be given on a daily basis.[126] Stool or ostomy volume should be 45 mL/kg per day, and a major obstacle to advancing feeds may be high stool output. The cause of this high output may include infections, malabsorption, or rapid transit as well as bile acid irritation of the colonic epithelium.[127] Measurement of stool pH, reducing substances, and qualitative fecal fats should be obtained and may pinpoint the etiology of high stool output. Stool pH less than or equal to 5.5 and an elevated reducing substance level (>0.5%) indicates carbohydrate malabsorption. Formulas with sucrose as the carbohydrate do not yield a positive reducing substance test despite carbohydrate malabsorption. Elevation in fecal fats suggests fat malabsorption, which may require modification of a child's enteral diet (ie, increase the percentage of MCTs). An increase in stool α1-antitrypsin indicates a protein malabsorption, although this is less commonly encountered. Use of a resin binder (eg, cholestyramine) markedly reduces bile acid irritation and has proved effective in many infants who have their small bowel in continuity with a portion of the colon. Excessive use of bile acid binders, however, such as cholestyramine, may result in depletion of the circulating bile acid pool, and thereby further limit fatty acid absorption. Because many infants with short bowel syndrome have dysmotility, it is only after all other causes have been eliminated (ie, infectious, bacterial overgrowth, bile acid irritation, and potentially correctable malabsorption) that an agent to reduce motility (eg, Imodium) should be considered.

### Obesity

Pediatric obesity has become a worldwide issue,[128,129] and more than 50% of children who are diagnosed with obesity carry this excess weight into adulthood. Several secondary complications are manifested in these children, including the prediabetic condition of syndrome X, type 2 diabetes mellitus, coronary artery disease, and obstructive sleep apnea.[130,131] Additional problems include bone and joint disease and cholelithiasis. Although a National Institutes of Health consensus has established a BMI of greater than 40 as morbid obesity,[132] BMIs change dramatically during adolescence and do not follow a linear curve. A more consistent diagnosis is based on number of SDs from the mean using Centers for Disease Control and Prevention standardized growth curves.[133] In this regard, at risk for overweight is defined as being at the 84th percentile, and overweight is defined as greater than or equal to 94th percentile.[128] Factors influencing development of obesity are environmental as well as genetic.[134] Should surgical intervention be used in children, it is important for families to understand the life-long implications of this decision, as well as the willingness to participate in follow-up for the rest of their lives. Vitamin and nutrient deficiencies, especially protein, vitamin $B_{12}$, folate, iron, calcium, vitamin D, and thiamine are common in such patients and require monitoring every 6 months.[135]

### Failure to Thrive

Malnutrition in childhood is associated with poor growth and development. The diagnosis of FTT is based on a weight greater than 2 SDs below the mean weight percentile ($z$ score of 2.0), resulting in a child falling on the 2.3rd percentile.[136] FTT is symmetric, in which height, length, and development of other body organs (eg, head circumference) fall to less than the 5th percentile, or asymmetric, in which the weight is less than the 5th percentile but length and head circumference are within normal limits. In general, patients with symmetric FTT have more profound malnutrition and suffer from greater neurologic underdevelopment than those with asymmetric FTT; the latter patients have normal cognitive development.[137,138] The approach to feeding patients with FTT should include a multidisciplinary assessment of medical, social, and psychological factors. Nutritional support for an infant should begin at approximately 50 kcal/kg per day and be increased by 20 to 25 kcal/kg per day as long as gastrointestinal tolerance to the feeding is adequate. Stool weight should be less than 150 g per day in young infants. Feedings may increase to 150 to 240 kcal/kg per day to achieve adequate catch-up growth,[139] but overshooting is not uncommon, and such high-energy delivery states demands close clinical observation. Levels of potassium, magnesium, and phosphate must be closely monitored because they may drop rapidly after the initiation of feedings in profoundly malnourished children. One simple method to calculate caloric needs is that for each gram of weight gain desired per day, 5 additional calories should be provided.

### Children with Special Care Needs

Between 10% and 20% of children in the United States have special health care needs because of chronic illness and developmental disorders.[140] For several of these disorders, pediatric surgeons take an active part in the nutritional care. Some

**Table 12**
**Guidelines for estimating caloric requirements based on height in children with developmental disabilities**

| Condition | Caloric Recommendation |
|---|---|
| Ambulatory, ages 5 to 12 years | 13.9 kcal/cm height |
| Nonambulatory, ages 5 to 12 years | 11.1 kcal/cm height |
| Cerebral palsy with severely restricted activity | 10 kcal/cm height |
| Cerebral palsy with mild to moderate activity | 15 kcal/cm height |
| Athetoid cerebral palsy, adolescence | Up to 6000 kcal/d |
| Down syndrome, boys, ages 1 to 14 years | 16.1 kcal/cm height |
| Down syndrome, girls, ages 1 to 14 years | 14.3 kcal/cm height |
| Myelomeningocele | Approximately 50% of recommended daily allowance for age after infancy May need as little as 7 kcal/cm height to maintain normal weight |
| Prader-Willi syndrome | 10–11 kcal/cm height (maintenance) 9 kcal/cm height (to promote weight loss) |

*From* Nelson JK, Jenson M, Gastineau C, et al. Mayo clinic diet manual: a handbook of nutrition practice. 7th edition. St Louis (MO): Mosby–Year Book; 1994; with permission.

of the disorders include severe neurologic impairment, developmental delay, cerebral palsy, and some genetic syndromes. Pediatric surgeons are often responsible for providing nutritional access in some of these patients as well as for maintaining nutritional care before and after surgery. Estimates of energy needs (**Table 12**) are challenging. Children with spastic-type (hypertonia) cerebral palsy may have lower energy needs than normal; adolescents require approximately 1200 to 1300 kcal per day, or even less with lower activity.[141,142] Children with athetosis may require a higher-than-normal calorie intake—sometimes more than twice the recommended daily allowance. Children with myelomeningocele are far less active than their peers; for that reason, their energy needs are approximately only 50% to 60% that of normal children (see **Table 12**). Close follow-up is critical to maintain a child on target for growth objectives.

## ACKNOWLEDGMENTS

The authors thank Megan Perkowski, RD, for her contributions and editing of **Tables 7** and **8**.

## REFERENCES

1. Marian M. Pediatric nutrition support. Nutr Clin Pract 1993;8:199–209.
2. Rose J, Gibbons K, Carlson SE, et al. Nutrient needs of the preterm infant. Nutr Clin Pract 1993;8:226–32.
3. August D, Teitelbaum D. Guidelines for the use of parenteral and enteral nutrition in adult and pediatric patients. JPEN J Parenter Enteral Nutr 2002;26:1SA–137SA.
4. Cooper A, Jakobowski D, Spiker J, et al. Nutrition assessment: an integral part of the preoperative pediatric surgical evaluation. J Pediatr Surg 1982;16:554.
5. Hendricks K, Duggan C, Gallagher I. Malnutrition in hospitalized pediatric patients: current prevalence. Arch Pediatr Adolesc Med 1995;149:1118–20.

6. Guigoz Y, Vellas B, Garry P. Mini nutritional assessment: a practical assessment tool for grading the nutritional state of elderly patients. Facts Res Gerontol 1994; 4:15–59.

7. Sermet-Gaudelus I, Poisson-Salomon A, Colomb V. Simple pediatric nutritional risk score to identify children at risk of malnutrition. Am J Clin Nutr 2000;72: 64–70.

8. Van Riper C, Wallace L. Position of the American Dietetic Association: providing nutrition services for people with developmental disabilities and special health care needs; American Dietetic Association. J Am Diet Assoc 2010;110: 296–307.

9. Zlotkin SH, Bryan MH, Anderson GH. Intravenous nitrogen and energy intakes required to duplicate in utero nitrogen accretion in prematurely born human infants. J Pediatr 1981;99:115–20.

10. Dreizen S, Spirakis CN, Stone RE. A comparison of skeletal growth in maturation in under nourished and well nourished girls before and after menarche. J Pediatr 1967;70:256.

11. Otten JJ, Hellwig JP, Meyers LD, editors. Dietary Reference Intakes: The Essential Guide to Nutrient Requirements. Washington, DC: The National Academies Press; 2006.

12. Baker J, Detsky A, Wesson D. Nutritional assessment: a comparison of clinical judgement and objective measurements. N Engl J Med 1982;306:969–72.

13. Kaplan AS, Zemel BS, Neiswender KM, et al. Resting energy expenditure in clinical pediatrics: measured versus prediction equations. J Pediatr 1995;127:200–5.

14. Mendeloff E, Wesley J, Deckert R. Comparison of measured resting energy expenditure (REE) versus estimated energy expenditure (EEE) in infants. JPEN J Parenter Enteral Nutr 1986;10(Suppl):65.

15. Mitchell IM, Davies PSW, Day JME, et al. Energy expenditure in children with congenital heart disease, before and after cardiac surgery. J Thorac Cardiovasc Surg 1994;107:374–80.

16. Chwals WJ, Lally KP, Woolley MM. Indirect calorimetry in mechanically ventilated infants and children: measurement accuracy with absence of audible airleak. Crit Care Med 1992;20:768–70.

17. White MS, Shepherd RW, McEniery JA. Energy expenditure measurements in ventilated critically ill children: within- and between-day variability. JPEN J Parenter Enteral Nutr 1999;23:300–4.

18. Letton RW, Chwals WJ, Jamie A, et al. Early postoperative alterations in infant energy use increase the risk of overfeeding. J Pediatr Surg 1995;30:988–93.

19. Btaiche I, Khalidi N, Kovacevich D. The parenteral and enteral nutrition manual. 9th edition. Ann Arbor (MI): University of Michigan; 2010. The University of Michigan Hospitals and Health Centers. Ann Arbor.

20. Spencer A, Yu S, Tracy T, et al. Effect of taurine on cholestasis in neonates on parenteral nutrition. JPEN J Parenter Enteral Nutr 2005;29(5):337–43.

21. Sangild P, Petersen Y, Schmidt M, et al. Preterm birth affects the intestinal response to parenteral and enteral nutrition in newborn pigs. J Nutr 2002;132: 3786–94.

22. Denne S, Poindexter B. Evidence supporting early nutritional support with parenteral amino acid infusion. Semin Perinatol 2007;31(2):56–60.

23. Ziegler EE. Protein in premature feeding. Nutrition 1994;10:69–71.

24. Zelikovic I, Chesney RW, Friedman AL, et al. Taurine depletion in very low birth weight infants receiving total parenteral nutrition: role of renal immaturity. J Pediatr 1990;116:301–6.

25. Friedman Z, Danon A, Stahlman MT, et al. Rapid onset of essential fatty acid deficiency in the newborn. Pediatrics 1976;58:640–9.
26. Leung FY. Nutrient needs and feeding of premature infants. nutrition committee, canadian paediatric society. Trace elements in parenteral micronutrition [see comments]. CMAJ 1995;152:1765–85.
27. Feuerstein G, Hallenbeck JM. Leukotrienes in health and disease. FASEB J 1987;1:186–92.
28. Kelly D. Guidelines and available products for parenteral vitamins and trace elements. JPEN J Parenter Enteral Nutr 2002;26:S34–6.
29. Mertz W. The essential trace elements. Science 1981;18:1332–8.
30. Tasman-Jones C, Kay RG, Lee SP. Zinc and copper deficiency, with particular reference to parenteral nutrition. Surg Annu 1978;10:23–52.
31. Karpel JT, Peden VH. Copper deficiency in long-term parenteral nutrition. J Pediatr 1972;80:32–4.
32. Spiegel J, Willenbucher R. Rapid development of severe copper deficiency in a patient with Crohn's disease receiving parenteral nutrition. JPEN J Parenter Enteral Nutr 1999;23:169–72.
33. Hankins DA, Riella MC, Scribner BH, et al. Whole blood trace element concentrations during total parenteral nutrition. Surgery 1976;79:674–7.
34. Beasley SW, Catto-Smith AG, Davidson PM. How to avoid complications during percutaneous endoscopic gastrostomy. J Pediatr Surg 1995;30:671–3.
35. Braunschweig CL, Wesley JR, Clark SF, et al. Rationale and guidelines for parenteral and enteral transition feeding of the 3- to 30-kg child. J Am Diet Assoc 1988;88:479–82.
36. Silvestre MAA, Morbach CA, Brans YW, et al. A prospective randomized trial comparing continuous versus intermittent feeding methods in very low birth weight neonates. J Pediatr 1996;128:748–52.
37. Akintorin SM, Kamat M, Pildes RS, et al. A prospective randomized trial of feeding methods in very low birth weight infants. Pediatrics 1997;100:e4.
38. Schanler RJ, Shulman RJ, Lau C, et al. Feeding strategies for premature infants: randomized trial of gastrointestinal priming and tube-feeding method. Pediatrics 1999;103:434–9.
39. Kleinman RE, editor. American Academy of Pediatrics CoN Pediatric nutrition handbook. 4th edition. Elk Grove Village (IL): AAP; 1998.
40. Pittard WBI. Breast milk immunology: a frontier in infant nutrition. Am J Dis Child 1987;133:83–7.
41. Taylor R, Preedy V, Baker A, et al. Nutritional support in critically ill children. Clin Nutr 2003;22:365–9.
42. Rogers E, Gilbertson H, Heine R, et al. Barriers to adequate nutrition in critically ill children. Nutrition 2003;19:865–8.
43. Montecalvo M, Steger K, Farber H, et al. Nutritional outcome and pneumonia in critical care patients randomized to gastric versus jejunal tube feedings. Crit Care Med 1992;20:1377–87.
44. Meert KL, Daphtary KM, Metheny NA. Gastric vs small-bowel feeding in critically ill children receiving mechanical ventilation: a randomized controlled trial. Chest 2004;126:872–8.
45. Strong R, Condon S, Soling M, et al. Equal aspiration rates from postpylorus and intragastric-placed small bore nasoenteric feeding tubes: a randomized prospective study. JPEN J Parenter Enteral Nutr 1992;16:59–63.
46. Bankhead R, Boullata J, Brantley S, et al. Enteral nutrition practice recommendations. JPEN J Parenter Enteral Nutr 2009;33:122–67.

47. Stephens B, Walden R, Gargus R. First-week protein and energy intakes are associated with 18-month developmental outcomes in extremely low birth weight infants. Pediatrics 2009;123:1337–43.

48. Premji S, Fenton T, Sauve R. Higher versus lower protein intake in formula-fed low birth weight infants. Cochrane Database Syst Rev 2006;1:CD003959.

49. Beck R. Use of a pediatric parenteral amino acid mixture in a population of extremely low birth weight neonates: frequency and spectrum of direct bilirubinemia. Am J Perinatol 1990;7:84–6.

50. Okamoto E, Rassin DK, Zucker CL, et al. Role of taurine in feeding the low-birth-weight infant. J Pediatr 1984;104:936–40.

51. Shaw JH, Holdaway CM. Protein-sparing effect of substrate infusion in surgical patients is governed by the clinical state, and not by the individual substrate infused. JPEN J Parenter Enteral Nutr 1988;12:433–40.

52. Farrag HM, Nawrath LM, Healey JE, et al. Persistent glucose production and greater peripheral sensitivity to insulin in the neonate vs the adult. Am J Physiol 1997;272:E86–93.

53. Stonestreet BS, Rubin L, Pollak A, et al. Renal functions of low birth infants with hyperglycemia and glucosuria produced by glucose infusions. Pediatrics 1980; 66:561–7.

54. Brans YW, Andrew DS, Carrillo DW, et al. Tolerance of fat emulsions in very-low-birth-weight neonates. Am J Dis Child 1988;142:145–52.

55. Kao LC, Cheng MH, Warburton D. Triglycerides, free fatty acids, free fatty acids/albumin molar ratio, and cholesterol levels in serum of neonates receiving long-term lipid infusions: controlled trial of continuous vs intermittent regimens. J Pediatr 1984;104:429–35.

56. Ghisolfi J, Garcia J, Thouvenot JP, et al. Plasma phospholipid fatty acids and urinary excretion of prostaglandins $PGE_1$ and $PGE_2$ in infants during total parenteral nutrition, with continuous or sequential administration of fat emulsion. JPEN J Parenter Enteral Nutr 1986;10:631–4.

57. Kennedy KA, Stoll BJ, Ehrenkranz RA, et al. Vitamin A to prevent bronchopulmonary dysplasia in very-low-birth-weight infants: has the dose been too low? Early Hum Dev 1997;49:19–31.

58. American Medical Association. NAG Department of food and nutrition: multivitamin preparations for parenteral use. A statement by the nutrition advisory group. JPEN J Parenter Enteral Nutr 1979;3:258.

59. Mirtallo J, Canada T, Johnson D. Task force for the revision of safe practices for parenteral nutrition. Safe practices for parenteral nutrition. JPEN J Parenter Enteral Nutr 2004;28:S39–70.

60. Chevalier RL. Developmental renal physiology of the low birth weight pre-term newborn. J Urol 1996;156:714–9.

61. Brooks MJ, Melnik G. The refeeding syndrome: an approach to understanding its complications and preventing its occurrence. Pharmacotherapy 1995;15:713–26.

62. Taketomo CK, Hodding JH, Kraus DM. Pediatric dosage handbook. In: Pediatric dosage handbook: including neonatal dosing. 8th edition. Hudson (OH): Lexi-Comp; 2001. p. 816–8.

63. Kalhoff H, Wiese B, Kunz C, et al. Increased renal net acid excretion in prematures below 1,600 g body weight compared with prematures and small-for-date newborns above 2,100 g on alimentation with commercial preterm formula. Biol Neonate 1994;66:10–5.

64. Karlen J, Aperia A, Zetterstorm R. Renal excretion of calcium and phosphate in preterm and term infants. J Pediatr 1985;106:814–9.

65. Prestridge LL, Schanler RJ, Shulman R, et al. Effect of parenteral calcium and phosphorus on mineral retention and bone mineral content in very low birth weight infants. J Pediatr 1993;122:761–8.
66. Pelegano JF, Rowe JC, Carey DE, et al. Effect of calcium/phosphorus ratio on mineral retention in parenterally fed premature infants. J Pediatr Gastroenterol Nutr 1991;12:351–5.
67. Fitzgerald KA, MacKay MW. Calcium and phosphate solubility in neonatal parenteral nutrient solutions containing TrophAmine. Am J Hosp Pharm 1986; 43:88–93.
68. Nissenson A, KLindsay R, Swan S, et al. Sodium ferric gluconate complex in sucrose is safe and effective in hemodialysis patients: North American clinical trial. Am J Kidney Dis 1999;35:360–1.
69. Boehm KA, Helms RA, Christensen ML, et al. Carnitine: a review for the pharmacy clinician. Hosp Pharm 1993;28:843–50.
70. Schmidt-Sommerfeld E, Penn D. Carnitine and parenteral nutrition of the neonate. Biol Neonate 1990;58:81–8.
71. Bonner CM, DeBrie KL, Hug G, et al. Effects of parenteral L-carnitine supplementation on fat metabolism and nutrition in premature infants. J Pediatr 1995;126:287–92.
72. Tibboel D, Delemarre FMC, Przyrembel H, et al. Carnitine deficiency in surgical neonates receiving total parenteral nutrition. J Pediatr Surg 1990;25:418–21.
73. Crill C, Helms R. The use of carnitine in pediatric nutrition. Nutr Clin Pract 2007; 22:204–13.
74. van den Heuvel I, Vlasselaers D. Clinical benefits of tight glycaemic control: focus on the paediatric patient. Best Pract Res Clin Anaesthesiol 2009;23:441–8.
75. Pollack A, Cowett RM, Schwartz R, et al. Glucose disposal in low-birth-weight infants during steady-state hyperglycemia: effects of exogenous insulin administration. Pediatrics 1978;61(4):546–9.
76. Cornblath M, Hawdon JM, Williams AF, et al. Controversies regarding the definition of neonatal hypoglycemia: suggested operational thresholds. Pediatrics 2000;105:1141–5.
77. Shennan AT, Bryan MH, Angel A. The effect of gestational age on Intralipid tolerance in newborn infants. J Pediatr 1977;91:134–7.
78. Andrew F, Chan G, Schiff D. Lipid metabolism in the neonate. I. The effects of Intralipid infusion on plasma triglyceride and free fatty acid concentrations in the neonate. J Pediatr 1976;88:273–8.
79. Andrew F, Chan G, Schiff D. Lipid metabolism in the neonate. II. The effects of Intralipid on bilirubin binding in vitro and in vivo. J Pediatr 1976;88: 279–84.
80. Park W, Paust H, Schroder H. Lipid infusion in premature infants suffering from sepsis. JPEN J Parenter Enteral Nutr 1984;8:290–2.
81. Heird WC, Gomez MR. Parenteral nutrition in low-birth-weight infants. Annu Rev Nutr 1996;16:471–99.
82. Shike M, Shils ME, Heller A, et al. Bone disease in prolonged parenteral nutrition: osteopenia without mineralization defect. Am J Clin Nutr 1986;44:89–98.
83. de Vernejoul MC, Messing B, Modrowski D, et al. Multifactorial low remodeling bone disease during cyclic total parenteral nutrition. J Clin Endocrinol Metab 1985;60:109.
84. Shike M, Sturtridge WC, Tam CS, et al. A possible role of vitamin D in the genesis of parenteral nutrition-induced metabolic bone disease. Ann Intern Med 1981;95:560–8.

85. Ott SM, Maloney NA, Klein GL, et al. Aluminum is associated with low bone formation in patients receiving chronic parenteral nutrition. Ann Intern Med 1983;98:910–4.

86. King DR, Komer M, Hoffman J, et al. Broviac catheter sepsis: the natural history of an iatrogenic infection. J Pediatr Surg 1985;20:728–33.

87. Wurzel CL, Halom K, Feldman JG, et al. Infection rates of Broviac-Hickman catheters and implantable venous devices. Am J Dis Child 1988;142:536–40.

88. Caniano D, Starr J, Ginn-Pease M. Extensive short-bowel syndrome in neonates: outcome in the 1980s. Surgery 1989;105:119–24.

89. Kurkchubasche AG, Smith SD, Rowe MI. Catheter sepsis in short-bowel syndrome. Arch Surg 1992;127:21–5.

90. Moukarzel AA, Haddad I, Ament ME, et al. 230 Patient years of experience with home long-term parenteral nutrition in childhood: natural history and life of central venous catheters [review] [32 refs]. J Pediatr Surg 1994;29:1323–7.

91. Piedra P, Dryja D, LaScolea L Jr. Incidence of catheter-associated gram-negative bacteremia in children with short bowel syndrome. J Clin Microbiol 1989;6: 1317–9.

92. Levy I, Katz J, Solter E, et al. Chlorhexidine-impregnated dressing for prevention of colonization of central venous catheters in infants and children: a randomized controlled study. Pediatr Infect Dis J 2005;24:676–9.

93. O'Grady NP, Alexander M, Dellinger EP, et al. Guidelines for the prevention of intravascular catheter-related infections. Centers for disease control and prevention. MMWR Morb Mortal Wkly Rep 2002;51:1–29.

94. Mermel L. Prevention of intravascular catheter-related infections. Ann Intern Med 2000;132:391–402.

95. Cober M, Kovacevich D, Teitelbaum DH. Ethanol-lock therapy for the prevention of central venous access device infections in pediatric intestinal failure patients. JPEN J Parenter Enteral Nutr 2011;35(1):67–73.

96. Crnich C, Halfmann J, Crone W, et al. The effects of prolonged ethanol exposure on the mechanical properties of polyurethane and silicone catheters used for intravascular access. Infect Control Hosp Epidemiol 2005;26:708–14.

97. Eppes SC, Troutman JL, Gutman LT. Outcome of treatment of candidemia in children whose central catheters were removed or retained. Pediatr Infect Dis J 1989;8:99–104.

98. Donowitz LG, Hendley JO. Short-course amphotericin B therapy for candidemia in pediatric patients. Pediatrics 1995;95:888–91.

99. Vlasselaers D, Milants I, Desmet L, et al. Intensive insulin therapy for patients in paediatric intensive care: a prospective, randomised controlled study. Lancet 2009;373:547–56.

100. Matsusue S, Nishimura S, Koizumi S, et al. Preventive effect of simultaneously infused lipid emulsion against thrombophlebitis during postoperative peripheral parenteral nutrition. Surg Today 1995;25:667–71.

101. Pierro A. Metabolism and nutritional support in the surgical neonate. J Pediatr Surg 2002;37:811–22.

102. Jones MO, Pierro A, Hammond P, et al. Glucose utilization in the surgical newborn infant receiving total parenteral nutrition. J Pediatr Surg 1993;28:1121–5.

103. Anand K, Sippell M, Aynsley-Green A. Randomised trial of fentanyl anaesthesia in preterm babies undergoing surgery: effects on the stress response. Lancet 1987;1:243–8.

104. Campos ACL, Meguid MM. A critical appraisal of the usefulness of perioperative nutritional support. Am J Clin Nutr 1992;55:117–30.

105. Detsky JM, Baker JP, O'Rourke K, et al. Perioperative parenteral nutrition: a meta-analysis. Ann Intern Med 1987;107:195–203.

106. Klein S, Kinney J, Jeejeebhoy K, et al. Nutrition support in clinical practice: review of published data and recommendations for future research directions. JPEN J Parenter Enteral Nutr 1997;21:133–56.

107. Buzby GP, Williford WO, Peterson OL, et al. A randomized clinical trial of total parenteral nutrition in malnourished surgical patients: the rationale and impact of previous clinical trials and pilot study on protocol design. Am J Clin Nutr 1988;47:357–65.

108. Marik P, Zaloga G. Early enteral nutrition in acutely ill patients: a systematic review. Crit Care Med 2001;29:2264–70.

109. Lewis S, Egger M, Sylvester P, et al. Early enteral feeding versus "nil by mouth" after gastrointestinal surgery: systematic review and meta-analysis of controlled trials. BMJ 2001;323:773–6.

110. Btaiche I, Chan L, Pleva M, et al. Critical illness, gastrointestinal complications, and medication therapy during enteral feeding in critically ill adult patients. Nutr Clin Pract 2010;25:32–49.

111. Marvin V, Rebollo M, Castillo-Duran C, et al. Controlled study of early postoperative parenteral nutrition in children. J Pediatr Surg 1999;34:1330–5.

112. Sandstrom R, Drott C, Hyltander A, et al. The effect of postoperative intravenous feeding (TPN) on outcome following major surgery evaluated in a randomized study. Ann Surg 1993;217:185–95.

113. Heyland DK, MacDonald S, Keefe L, et al. Total parenteral nutrition in the critically ill patient: a meta-analysis. JAMA 1998;280:2013–9.

114. Hulst JM, van Goudoever JB, Zimmermann LJ, et al. The effect of cumulative energy and protein deficiency on anthropometric parameters in a pediatric ICU population. Clin Nutr 2004;23:1381–9.

115. Drenckpohl D, McConnell C, Gaffney S, et al. Randomized trial of very low birth weight infants receiving higher rates of infusion of intravenous fat emulsions during the first week of life. Pediatrics 2008;122:743–51.

116. Sisk PM, Lovelady CA, Dillard RG, et al. Early human milk feeding is associated with a lower risk of necrotizing enterocolitis in very low birth weight infants. J Perinatol 2007;27:428–33.

117. Mehta NM, Bechard LJ, Dolan M, et al. Energy imbalance and the risk of overfeeding in critically ill children. Pediatr Crit Care Med 2010. [Epub ahead of print].

118. Mehta NM, Compher CASPEN. Clinical Guidelines: nutrition support of the critically ill child. JPEN J Parenter Enteral Nutr 2009;33:260–76.

119. Kaufman S, Murray N, Wood R. Nutritional support for the infant with extrahepatic biliary atresia. J Pediatr 1987;110:679–85.

120. Cohen M, Gartner L. The use of medium chain triglycerides in the management of biliary atresia. J Pediatr 1971;79:379–81.

121. Pierro A, Koletzko B, Carnielli V. Resting energy expenditure is increased in infants and children with extrahepatic biliary atresia. J Pediatr Surg 1989;24:534–9.

122. Pierro A, Jones MO, Hammond P, et al. A new equation to predict the resting energy expenditure of surgical infants. J Pediatr Surg 1994;29:1103–8.

123. DeRusso P, Ye W, Shepherd R, et al. Growth failure and outcomes in infants with biliary atresia: a report from the biliary atresia research consortium. Hepatology 2007;46:1632–8.

124. Sundaram A, Koutkia P, Apovian C. Nutritional management of short bowel syndrome in adults. J Clin Gastroenterol 2002;34:207–20.

125. Schwarz K, Ternberg J, Bell M, et al. Sodium needs of infants and children with ileostomy. J Pediatr 1983;102:509–13.
126. Sacher P, Hirsig J, Gresser J, et al. The importance of oral sodium replacement in ileostomy patients. Prog Pediatr Surg 1989;24:226–31.
127. Potter G. Bile acid diarrhea. Dig Dis 1998;16:118–24.
128. Ball G, Willows N. Definitions of pediatric obesity. CMAJ 2005;172:309–10.
129. Cole T, Bellizzi M, Flegal K, et al. Establishing a standard definition for child overweight and obesity worldwide: international survey. BMJ 2000;320:1240–3.
130. Pinhas-Hamiel O, Dolan LM, Daniels SR, et al. Increased incidence of non-insulin-dependent diabetes mellitus among adolescents [see comments]. J Pediatr 1996;128:608–15.
131. Must A, Jacques P, Dallal G, et al. Long-term morbidity and mortality of overweight adolescents. A follow-up of the Harvard Growth Study of 1922 to 1935. N Engl J Med 1992;327:1350–5.
132. Howard L, editor. North American home parenteral and enteral nutrition patient registry Annual Reports 1985 to 1992. Albany (NY): Oley Foundation; 1987–1994.
133. Barden EM, Zemel BS, Kawchak DA, et al. Total and resting energy expenditure in children with sickle cell disease. J Pediatr 2000;136:73–9.
134. Maffeis C. Childhood obesity: the genetic-environmental interface [review] [116 refs]. Baillieres Best Pract Res Clin Endocrinol Metab 1999;13:31–46.
135. Kushner R. Managing the obese patient after bariatric surgery: a case report of severe malnutrition and review of the literature. JPEN J Parenter Enteral Nutr 2000;24:126–32.
136. Anonymous Report of the Dietary Guidelines. Advisory Committee for the 2000 Dietary Guidelines for Americans. 2000.
137. Levitsky DA, Strupp BJ. Malnutrition and the brain: changing concepts, changing concerns. J Nutr 1995;125:2212S–20S.
138. Strupp BJ, Levitsky DA. Enduring cognitive effects of early malnutrition: a theoretical reappraisal. J Nutr 1995;125:2221S–32S.
139. Peterson KE, Washington J, Rathbun JM. Team management of failure to thrive. J Am Diet Assoc 1984;84:810–5.
140. Roche A. Growth and assessment of handicapped children. Diet Curr 1970;6:25.
141. Krick J, Murphy P, Markham J, et al. A proposed formula for calculating energy needs of children with cerebral palsy. Dev Med Child Neurol 1992;34:481–7.
142. Eddy T, Nicholson A, Wheeler E. Energy expenditures and dietary intakes in cerebral palsy. Dev Med Child Neurol 1965;7:377–80.

# The Prevention and Treatment of Intestinal Failure-associated Liver Disease in Neonates and Children

Deepika Nehra, MD[a], Erica M. Fallon, MD[a], Mark Puder, MD, PhD[b],*

**KEYWORDS**

- Parenteral nutrition • Intestinal failure • Short bowel syndrome
- Liver disease • Cholestasis • Neonate • Children

Short bowel syndrome (SBS) is a malabsorptive state that occurs as a result of surgical resection or congenital disease involving a significant portion of the small intestine. These patients suffer from a variety of conditions, all of which result in either insufficient intestinal length or function, with the most common being necrotizing enterocolitis, midgut volvulus, intestinal atresia, gastroschisis, and extensive aganglionosis.[1] The length and function of the remaining small bowel determine the degree of enteral absorption possible and thus dictate the need for supplemental enteral nutrition (EN) and parenteral nutrition (PN). Intestinal failure (IF) occurs with severe SBS and, in children, is defined as the critical reduction of functional gut mass to less than the amount necessary to obtain the minimal energy and fluid requirements necessary to sustain growth. Children with IF are often dependent on PN to meet their nutritional needs.[1,2] Successful bowel adaptation in these patients refers to the ability to sustain growth while only receiving EN. This adaptation is

Disclosure: a license agreement for the use of Omegaven has been signed by Children's Hospital Boston and Fresenius Kabi and a patent has been submitted by Children's Hospital Boston on behalf of Mark Puder.
[a] The Vascular Biology Program, Department of Surgery, Children's Hospital Boston, 1 Blackfan Circle, Boston, MA 02215, USA
[b] The Vascular Biology Program, Department of Surgery, Children's Hospital Boston, Harvard Medical School, Fegan 3, 300 Longwood Avenue, Boston, MA 02115, USA
* Corresponding author.
*E-mail address:* mark.puder@childrens.harvard.edu

Surg Clin N Am 91 (2011) 543–563
doi:10.1016/j.suc.2011.02.003
0039-6109/11/$ – see front matter © 2011 Elsevier Inc. All rights reserved.

both a structural and physiologic process that is often long term, and some children never attain successful bowel adaptation.

The management of children with SBS was revolutionized by the clinical introduction of PN by Wilmore and Dudrick[3] in 1968, when they published a case report of an infant whose growth and development was maintained with PN alone. Over the past 40 years, PN has become a life-saving therapy for children unable to absorb adequate enteral nutrients. Before the advent of PN, these patients frequently died of severe dehydration and malnutrition, a phenomenon that has been virtually eliminated with the use of PN. Today, PN has become an integral component of the care of these patients, and more than 30,000 patients in the United States are now permanently dependent on PN for survival. However, long-term PN has its own complications including blood stream infections, metabolic abnormalities, and organ dysfunction. One of the most prevalent and severe complications of PN is hepatobiliary dysfunction, commonly referred to as PN-associated liver disease (PNALD) or intestinal failure–associated liver disease (IFALD). This article refers to this entity as IFALD.

## PREVALENCE AND PROGNOSIS

The reported prevalence of IFALD varies widely, but is estimated to be 40% to 60% in children and as high as 85% in neonates receiving PN for prolonged periods of time.[4–7] IFALD can be a lethal complication of SBS and PN-dependence. The clinical spectrum of IFALD includes hepatic steatosis, cholestasis, fibrosis, and, ultimately, progression to hepatic cirrhosis with portal hypertension and end-stage liver disease.[7] Recent studies have shown that liver disease in patients on long-term PN is strongly correlated with survival; in a cohort of 78 children with SBS, the survival rate among those with cholestasis (conjugated bilirubin >2 mg/dL), was close to 20% compared with 80% in those without cholestasis.[8] In addition, the degree of liver dysfunction has also been correlated with outcome. A recent study evaluating a cohort of 66 patients with IFALD reported that, although 38% of infants with a maximum conjugated bilirubin greater than or equal to 10 mg/dL died or were referred for intestinal transplantation, only 7% of infants with a maximum conjugated bilirubin less than 10 mg/dL died during the first year of life.[9] Other studies report that the mortality of patients with end-stage liver disease while on PN approaches 100%, as does the mortality of neonates with IFALD within a year of diagnosis if they are unable to be weaned off PN or fail to receive a liver/small bowel transplant.[10] Overall, approximately 15% of patients with IFALD progress to end-stage liver disease requiring either isolated or combined liver–small bowel transplantation, a treatment that is associated with a high morbidity and mortality.[8,10–12]

## CAUSE

The cause of IFALD is complex, multifactorial, and poorly understood. There is some evidence that certain components of PN may be harmful, but bacterial endotoxins and the lack of enteral feeding are also believed to play significant roles.[13] Severe and progressive liver disease is more common in infants and neonates than in adults, which suggests that the liver disease seen in infants and neonates may have a pathophysiology different from that seen in adults, or that the neonatal liver may be more susceptible to injury.

## RISK FACTORS

There are a myriad of established risk factors associated with IFALD. They include premature birth, low birth weight, prolonged duration of PN, intestinal stasis with subsequent bacterial overgrowth, early and/or recurrent catheter-related sepsis, and a diagnosis of gastroschisis or jejunal atresia.[14,15] Previous studies have shown that, in the neonatal age group, the most important factor in the development of PN-related cholestasis is prematurity, which may be largely attributable to the physiologic immaturity of the hepatobiliary system.[14,16,17] These children often require PN for survival, and thus the impact of other factors on the development of IFALD must be carefully considered. The avoidance of catheter-related sepsis has been shown to be the second most important factor in the prevention of IFALD, because successive episodes of sepsis have been shown to result in a 30% increase in the serum bilirubin level.[14]

## DIAGNOSIS
### Clinical Features

All children in whom the diagnosis of IFALD is considered should be carefully examined for signs of liver disease. Clinical features of liver disease include jaundice, hepatomegaly, splenomegaly, ascites, edema, spider nevi, palmar erythema, and dilated veins in the anterior abdominal wall (caput medusae).

### Laboratory Studies

The diagnosis of IFALD has historically been established by routine biochemical tests of hepatic function. These tests include conjugated/direct bilirubin (cholestasis), albumin and international normalized ratio (INR; hepatic synthetic function), γ-glutamyl transferase (GGT; cholestasis), alanine aminotransferase (ALT; hepatic injury), platelet count, and absolute neutrophil count (ANC; portal hypertension). These laboratory values are pivotal in the diagnosis of IFALD, commonly defined as a direct bilirubin of greater than or equal to 2.0 mg/dL. An increase in the conjugated bilirubin is often the earliest sign of IFALD and is a surrogate for cholestasis as well as a relative indicator of liver excretory function. The plasma albumin is a relative biochemical indicator of liver synthetic function and is also a marker of overall nutritional status and anabolic/catabolic balance. However, given that the plasma albumin is also an acute phase reactant, it can sometimes be unreliable or misleading. In the appropriate clinical setting, the conjugated bilirubin and albumin levels can be used to estimate the degree of liver function and nutritional status.

Regularly scheduled laboratory studies are routinely obtained on PN-dependent patients because it is important to monitor them for electrolyte disturbances, signs of dehydration, evidence of sepsis, and liver function over time. These laboratory values can be predictive of the progression of liver disease and, subsequently, the overall condition of the patient. A recent study by Kaufman and colleagues[18] found that progressively worsening hyperbilirubinemia, thrombocytopenia, and hypoalbuminemia were all independent predictors of liver failure; for every 1 mg/dL increase in the serum bilirubin, the odds of developing liver failure increased by 20%; for every 1000/μL decrease in platelet count, the odds of developing liver failure increased by 1%; and for every 1.0 g/dL decrease in albumin, the odds of liver failure increased by 75%. Sepsis can have a confounding effect on these laboratory values, specifically causing increases in serum bilirubin, INR, and aminotransferase concentrations while lowering the platelet count. Thus, the presence of an infection at the time of laboratory studies should be taken into consideration.[19]

### Liver Biopsy

The gold standard for diagnosis of IFALD is definitive histopathology from a liver biopsy specimen, but the invasive nature of this test, in combination with the young age, small size, and often critical condition of many of the children with suspected IFALD, makes routine and serial liver biopsies impractical and often unsafe.

Pathologic review of liver specimens shows a clear progression of disease starting with periportal inflammation and cholestasis, progressing to bile duct proliferation, fibrosis, and cirrhosis.[20] However, it seems that the correlation between the biochemical reversal of PN-associated cholestasis and liver histology is not clear, and that some patients may experience normalization of the conjugated bilirubin despite persistent liver fibrosis.[21–23] Although alternative methods of assessing liver fibrosis in patients with normalized indirect measures of hepatic function are not currently available, hopefully future advances in medical techniques will allow clinicians to assess the degree of liver fibrosis accurately in a noninvasive fashion.

### Differential Diagnosis

Cholestasis should be attributed to PN only after other major causes have been excluded. A common cause of neonatal transient conjugated hyperbilirubinemia is sepsis, or infection, which can lead to shock liver, and for this reason the possibility of infection should always be considered in any patient receiving PN who develops hyperbilirubinemia. All infants with sustained conjugated hyperbilirubinemia should be evaluated for biliary obstruction (ie, biliary atresia, choledochal cyst, neonatal sclerosing cholangitis) in addition to metabolic and genetic liver disease (ie, Alagille syndrome, nonsyndromic paucity of the interlobular bile ducts, progressive familial intrahepatic cholestasis, Caroli disease, $\alpha$-1 antitrypsin deficiency, neonatal hemochromatosis, cystic fibrosis, mitochondrial disorders, disorders of carbohydrate, lipid, or amino acid metabolism), infection (ie, human immunodeficiency virus, cytomegalovirus, herpes, rubella, parvovirus B19, sepsis, syphilis, Toxoplasma), and toxicity secondary to pharmacologic agents. Several of these disorders require urgent intervention, and the management of these conditions overall is different from the management of IFALD, making it essential to differentiate these entities from IFALD.

## PREVENTION/TREATMENT
### PN

PN is typically administered in conjunction with an intravenous lipid emulsion, to provide a calorically dense source of nonprotein calories, and to prevent essential fatty acid deficiency (EFAD).[24–26] Lipid emulsions provide what have traditionally been known as the 2 essential fatty acids, linoleic acid (LA) and $\alpha$-linolenic acid (ALA). These fatty acids are important precursors of eicosanoids and prostaglandins,[27] and are imperative essentials in many biochemical pathways. Components of both the PN solution and lipid emulsion have been associated with the development of IFALD.

### Lipid type

Lipid emulsions derived from soybean oils are the standard of care in the United States and have been shown to cause liver injury both in vitro and in vivo in rodent models.[28–30] In general, lipid emulsions differ primarily in the composition of the long-chain polyunsaturated fatty acids (PUFAs). The only lipid emulsion approved for use in the United States is soybean oil-based (Intralipid, Baxter Health care/ Fresenius Kabi, Deerfield, IL, USA). This lipid emulsion contains a high concentration of $\omega$-6 fatty acids and phytosterols, which are associated with impaired biliary secretion and are hypothesized to contribute to liver injury.[31]

Outside the United States, several alternatives to the conventional soybean oil–based lipid emulsion are available, including Lipofundin (50% soybean oil, 50% coconut oil; B Braun Melsungen AG, Melsungen, Germany) and ClinOleic (20%

soybean oil, 80% oleic oil; Baxter/Clintec Parenteral SA, Cedex, France). Although not approved by the Food and Drug Administration in the United States, ClinOleic has been shown to be a safe alternative to soybean oil–based lipid emulsions.[32,33] Other emulsions approved for use in Europe include SMOFlipid and Omegaven (Fresenius Kabi Deutschland GmbH, Bad Homburg, Germany). SMOFlipid is composed of 30% soybean oil and 15% fish oil, with the remaining oils provided as olive oil and medium-chain triglycerides, whereas Omegaven is composed of 100% fish oil. Fish oil contains docosahexaenoic acid (DHA) and eicosapentaenoic acid (EPA), and has anti-inflammatory properties believed to be secondary to the inhibition of the arachidonic acid (AA) pathway and the production of certain 5-series leukotrienes (leukotriene B5, C5, D5), 3-series prostaglandins (prostaglandin E3, prostacyclin I3), and thromboxane A3.[34–39]

In part, the development of IFALD seems to be associated with the composition of the soybean oil–based lipid emulsion administered with PN, likely a result of the proinflammatory metabolites of $\omega$-6 fatty acids[40,41] and hepatotoxic phytosterols.[42,43] We reported a fish oil–based lipid emulsion (Omegaven) to be effective in preventing IFALD and reversing cholestasis caused by IFALD.[44–47] Fish oil has been introduced as a supplement to the soybean oil–based lipid emulsion, as an ingredient in a combination emulsion, and as monotherapy.[48] As monotherapy, fish oil–based lipid emulsions have been used in patients with IFALD, with promising results.[44–56] Gura and colleagues[44] described the first case in which Omegaven was used as the sole intravenous lipid source in a patient who was allergic to soy and who was previously unable to tolerate any parenteral fat emulsion. Subsequently, Gura and colleagues[45] also reported the reversal of PN-cholestasis and normalization of serum bilirubin levels within 60 days of institution of a fish oil–based lipid emulsion substituted for a soy oil–based lipid emulsion in 2 pediatric patients.[47] Since these case reports, Omegaven monotherapy has been used at our institution in a compassionate use protocol, with 163 PN-dependent patients treated to date.[46,48] A recent review of 42 patients enrolled within the open-label trial of Omegaven showed that patients who received the fish oil–based lipid emulsion experienced reversal of cholestasis approximately 6 times faster (95% confidence interval, 2.0–37.3) than those receiving a soybean oil–based lipid emulsion.[47] The reversal of cholestasis allowed for eventual discontinuation of PN and subsequent development of enteral tolerance. The provision of the fish oil–based lipid emulsion was not associated with hypertriglyceridemia, EFAD, coagulopathy, growth impairment, or an increased number of central venous catheter infections.[50] Recent evidence has shown that the frequency of hypertriglyceridemic events was more common among patients who did not receive the fish oil–based emulsions.[47,52] Similar results have been reported by other centers,[53,56] and are consistent with the results from multiple animal experiments.[57–59] Fish oil monotherapy has additionally been shown to result in significant improvement in all major serum lipid panels.[60]

However, the use of fish oil–based lipid emulsions as the sole source of fat energy is not recommended by its manufacturer because there remains some skepticism regarding its ability to prevent EFAD and maintain adequate growth, and concern that it may contribute to an increased risk of coagulopathy and infection. Although some data suggest that dietary $\omega$-3 fatty acids provoke a hypocoagulant effect in adults,[61] clinical pediatric experience to date does not show similar findings with the use of intravenous fish oil emulsions in children. Thus far, there has been no reported increased incidence of coagulopathy and/or EFAD even in patients completely dependent on PN with a fish oil–based lipid emulsion.[44,46–49] At the authors' institution, children who received the fish oil–based emulsion had lower mean INR and overall rate of bloodstream infections than those who received the soybean oil–based emulsion.[47] Nonetheless, an ongoing randomized, controlled, double-blind clinical trial comparing Intralipid (soybean oil–based lipid emulsion) with Omegaven (fish oil–based lipid emulsion) is imperative, and likely to be definitive, in resolving the current debate regarding the efficacy and safety of parenteral fish oil–based intravenous lipid emulsions in the prevention of IFALD.

### Lipid dosing
Standard guidelines recommend administering lipid emulsions at a dose of less than 2.5 g/kg/d. However, a dose greater than 1 g/kg/d has been associated with the development of IFALD,[62–64] whereas a dose less than or equal to 1 g/kg/d has been shown to be effective in preventing IFALD.[62,63,65] In neonates, the enzymatic pathways are not adequately developed and cannot efficiently convert ALA and LA to their active moieties, DHA and AA, thus making supplementation of downstream fatty acids extremely important.[66,67] Premature infants require at least 3% of total calories from essential fatty acids.[68] Because biochemical changes associated with EFAD can occur within days in neonates, decreasing or withholding lipids for extended periods can be detrimental, especially the potential for growth retardation and/or inadequate brain development. Lipid emulsions, dosed appropriately, are therefore an essential nutritional component for PN-dependent neonates.

### PN cycling
Cycling of PN involves the provision of total daily PN volume in less than 24 hours. Cycling PN is recommended for patients who are expected to be nourished with prolonged courses of PN (ie, >30 days) and whose cardiac, renal, and endocrine function can tolerate shifts in fluid and dextrose infusion rates.[69] Advantages include intermittent disconnection from an intravenous line, improvement in visceral protein stores, reduction of the incidence of hyperinsulinemia, and promotion of the cyclic release of gastrointestinal hormones.[4,70,71] Cycling should be adjusted as enteral intake increases and should be tailored to patient age, because neonates often have diminished glycemic reserve.[72,73] In a recent retrospective study by Jensen and colleagues,[74] infants with gastroschisis who received cycled PN were approximately one-third less likely to develop IFALD compared with infants who received continuous PN.

### PN-associated toxins
Elements involved in PN administration and compounding, specifically di(2-ethylhexyl) phthalate (DEHP) and aluminum, have been linked to IFALD. DEHP is an industrial additive plasticizer present in polyvinylchloride (PVC)[75] and infusion systems,[76] which has been consistently detected in human plasma, urine, amniotic fluid, and breast milk,[77] and has been shown to increase oxidative stress and toxicity in preterm neonates and infants.[24] Von Rettberg and colleagues[76] found that changing to PVC-free infusion systems decreased the incidence of cholestasis from 50% to 13%, and that the use of PVC infusion sets strongly correlated with the development of cholestasis. Aluminum is another element found in raw materials and incorporated into parenteral products during the manufacturing process.[78] Aluminum toxicity can occur in PN-dependent neonates and infants as a result of immature kidneys and bones.[79] The US Food and Drug Administration has stated that the amount of aluminum provided by PN should be less than 5 μg/kg/d.[80] However, low-aluminum PN component alternatives, such as organic phosphate salts, are not currently available in the United States.

### PN supplementation

Antioxidant therapy has been suggested as a therapeutic option for the prevention of IFALD, because oxidative stress has been proposed as the second hit leading to the steatohepatitis-associated cell injury and death pathway of hepatocytes.[81] Although animal models have shown that vitamin E is hepatoprotective,[82] a comparable benefit has not been shown in humans. Nonetheless, the high concentration of vitamin E in Omegaven is believed to be a contributing factor to its success in the prevention and reversal of IFALD.[83,84]

Taurine supplementation may be beneficial in preventing IFALD, because deficiency of this sulfonic amino acid can cause liver dysfunction. Taurine can increase taurocon-jugated bile acids,[85,86] enhance bile flow,[87] and is involved in overall osmoregulation, membrane stability, and antioxidation within the liver. Deficiency of taurine has been reported in infants and children with severe IFALD.[88–90] Spencer and colleagues[91] recently found that taurine supplementation lowered direct bilirubin levels in premature infants and those with necrotizing enterocolitis. However, an earlier study by Cooke and colleagues[92] did not find any differences in IFALD development associated with taurine supplementation. From these results, it is evident that further studies are needed to elucidate whether taurine supplementation is beneficial in the PN-dependent neonatal population before recommendations can be made regarding implementation of taurine supplementation in clinical practice.

Supplementation of zinc, especially in infants and children with enterostomies, fistulas, and/or drains, is especially important to compensate for losses and prevent associated complications of deficiency, including retarded growth and impaired wound healing.[93–96]

### EN

Despite the benefits of PN, achievement of full enteral tolerance is the underlying goal in the nutritional management of children with IFALD. Enteral feeding stimulates physiologic processes, exposes the gastrointestinal tract to nutrient and hormonal stimuli that promote intestinal adaptation, and can protect against stress-induced gastropathy and gastrointestinal hemorrhage.[69,97,98]

### Early institution of enteral feeds

Even minimal EN, often referred to as trophic feeding or gut-priming, promotes human intestinal epithelial cell growth and brush border enzyme activity and motility.[99] Enteral feeding, when administered continuously, can promote saturation of the intestinal transporters, thereby maximizing gut absorption[100] while gradually increasing enteral tolerance and advancement of feeds. Studies have shown that EN, when tolerated, may help to protect against the development of IFALD.[101,102]

Because intraluminal nutrients and luminal substrates are essential for optimal intestinal adaptation,[97] the initiation of enteral feeding is strongly recommended early in the postoperative period. Typically, feedings are begun at a low rate and gradually advanced as tolerated until goal volumes are achieved, and held back if stool output exceeds 30 to 40 $cm^3$/kg/d.[69] Dilute elemental tube feeding (eg, 0.5kcal/$cm^3$) is generally implemented to decrease intraluminal residual, facilitate absorption, and reduce the risk of gastrointestinal allergy. Retrospective reviews have shown that the percentage of calories fed within 6 weeks after surgery and 3-months adjusted age in neonates following intestinal resection correlate with decreased PN duration, risk of bacteremia, and liver dysfunction.[12,103] Withdrawal of PN with implementation of full EN, has been shown to result in normalization of hyperbilirubinemia and improvement in liver function in approximately a 4-month period in PN-dependent infants with

SBS.[104] These findings support an aggressive wean of PN to EN, although feedings can only be advanced as clinical status and alimentary tract capability permit.

In some cases, patients can develop significant oral aversion from ongoing illness, noxious oral stimuli (eg, ventilation, nasogastric tubes), and prolonged periods of nonoral nutrition. Non-nutritive sucking can facilitate the development of sucking behavior, lessen aversion, and may improve tolerance of enteral feedings.[105]

### Enteral type and route

The type and route of EN can influence duration and success of weaning PN. For example, the use of breast milk (BM) has been shown to correlate with shorter PN courses and to promote intestinal adaptation.[12,106] Beneficial components of BM include high levels of nucleotides, amino acids, and immunologic and growth factors.[107–110] BM also has anti-infectious properties, and glycoproteins in BM deliver iron to the intestinal epithelium, stimulate proliferation and differentiation of crypt cells, influence brush border enzyme activity, and function as scavengers to prevent free radical–mediated tissue damage.

Aside from BM, amino acid–based formulas, such as Elecare (Ross, Columbus, OH, USA) and Neocate (SHS, Gaithersburg, MD, USA) have similarly been associated with a shorter duration of PN-dependence.[12,111] Proposed explanations for improved outcomes with these formulas include a reduced incidence of food allergy and a high percentage of long-chain triglycerides (LCT), which have been shown to stimulate mucosal adaptation better than medium-chain triglycerides (MCT).[112–114] In patients with a colon in continuity, it has been shown that a mixture of MCT and LCT may improve energy and fat absorption. Although Neocate has only about 5% MCT as a fat source, Elecare has 33% MCT, thus favoring Elecare as the amino acid–based formula of choice for a child with intestinal/colonic continuity.[4]

Elemental diets containing amino acids may enhance nutrient absorption; however, they may not be as effective as hydrolyzed or whole-protein formulas in maximizing adaptation.[115] Semielemental formulas include Alimentum (Ross, Columbus, OH, USA), and Pregestimil and Nutramigen (Mead Johnson, Evansville, IN, USA). These hypoallergenic formulas contain hydrolyzed casein as the protein source as opposed to mixtures of individual amino acids.

In pediatric patients requiring enteral access, surgically, endoscopically, or radiologically placed percutaneous feeding tubes are commonly used. Whenever possible, nutrition should be provided orally, as this may help to stimulate epidermal growth factor, in addition to other factors important for intestinal growth and adaptation. Tube feeding should be considered when there is an inability to consume calculated energy needs by mouth, inadequate growth, or prolonged feeding time.[116] Feeding delivery regimens widely vary according to the nutritional needs of the infant, type of enteral access, and degree of intestinal adaptation. EN can be provided in continuous gastric feedings to saturate carrier proteins maximally and to use intestinal function optimally.[117] Tube and oral feedings can be administered simultaneously as long as spontaneous oral intake is insufficient, and parenteral administration can be adjusted accordingly to maintain nutritional needs, control fluid losses, and promote intestinal adaptation.

### Pharmacologic Strategies

#### Ursodeoxycholic acid

Ursodeoxycholic acid (Ursodiol), a dihydroxy bile acid and choleretic agent developed according to the structure of bile in Chinese black bears, functions to improve bile flow and reduce the formation of biliary sludge, and has been widely used in various chronic cholestatic conditions. This drug may be helpful in correcting the liver biochemical abnormalities seen with prolonged PN use in humans; however, the data available to date on the efficacy of this drug for neonates and children with IFALD remain inconclusive.

An initial pilot study conducted by Spagnuolo and colleagues[118] was encouraging; they found the disappearance of signs of cholestatic liver disease and normalization of biochemical markers of cholestasis within 4 to 8 weeks in 7 children receiving long-term PN treated with Ursodiol. Two subsequent retrospective reports supported this conclusion and found that treatment with Ursodiol led to an early sustained decrease in serum bilirubin levels after 2 weeks of therapy in premature infants,[119] reduced the duration of cholestasis, and decreased the peak conjugated bilirubin in very low birth weight infants with IFALD.[120] Other alternative choleretic agents (ie, cholecystekinin-octapeptide and tauroursodeoxycholic acid) have also been tested, but have shown no significant benefit in the prevention of IFALD.[121–123] A systematic review confirmed that the administration of Ursodiol generally led to short-term improvement in biochemical indices, but it highlighted the serious limitations of the currently available studies, including small sample sizes, absence of randomization and controls, short duration, and lack of control for confounding variables.[124] Large, prospective, randomized, placebo-controlled, clinical trials evaluating the efficacy, optimal dosing, and duration of Ursodiol therapy for IFALD are necessary.

Based on the limited evidence available, our institution currently administers urso-deoxycholic acid (10 mg/kg/dose twice or 3 times daily) in infants with IFALD who are able to tolerate some enteral intake. If the conjugated bilirubin improves, but the serum aminotransferase activity remains increased, the ursodeoxycholic acid is continued.

### Drug-induced liver disease

Liver injury can occur with many drugs through a variety of mechanisms. When considering the diagnosis of IFALD, it is prudent to review the child's medication list for potentially hepatotoxic drugs. There is a spectrum of liver disease that can be caused by drugs, with acute presentations ranging from asymptomatic mild biochemical abnormalities to acute illnesses with jaundice and acute fulminant liver failure.[125,126] Examples of drugs known to cause liver injury, although not inclusive, that are frequently used in the pediatric population, include certain antibiotics (eg, ampicillin, amoxicillin-clavulanate, nafcillin, dicloxacillin, trimethoprim-sulfamethoxazole, rifampin, erythromycin, tetracycline), acetaminophen, phenytoin, ranitidine, and halo-peridol.[127–130] Withdrawal of these drugs typically leads to reversal of the liver injury; however, some types of toxicity can be associated with a progressive course and may result in fibrosis or cirrhosis despite discontinuation of the offending agent.

### Management of Sepsis

Recurrent episodes of sepsis are an important risk factor for IFALD, and sepsis is one of the leading causes of death in patients with IFALD.[131] As such, one of the most important preventative strategies for children at risk for IFALD is the prevention of sepsis. The risk of sepsis is largely attributed to the risk of catheter-related blood stream infection (CRBSI) and bacterial translocation as a result of enteral bacterial overgrowth.[132] The effects of sepsis on the liver may be exacerbated by the exaggerated inflammatory response in patients with SBS. For these reasons, the prevention and prompt management of sepsis are of pivotal importance in both PN-dependent children who are at risk for developing IFALD and in those who have already developed IFALD. Important clinical features to recognize as potential indicators of sepsis in the neonate or child include fever or low/unstable temperature, feeding difficulty, emesis, irritability, lethargy, tachypnea, apneic episodes, decreased urination, and changes in skin color (jaundice, pallor).

### Catheter-related bloodstream infection

Maintaining the integrity of the central venous catheter (CVC) is of pivotal importance for the PN-dependent child. Not only is catheter-related sepsis associated with significant morbidity and mortality, but these septic episodes are also known to have a significant negative impact on the liver. Despite this, the incidence of CRBSI in children remains high, approaching 60% for the life-span of a CVC.[133] Vigilant daily catheter care is important, and newer strategies such as antibiotic-coated catheters as well as antibiotic and ethanol locks may also help to decrease the incidence of catheter-associated sepsis.

### CVC insertion

The Centers for Disease Control and Prevention (CDC) have published guidelines with recommendations for the prevention of a central venous CRBSI.[134] To reduce the rates of central venous CRBSI, maximal sterile barrier precautions must be observed during line placement. These precautions consist of strict compliance with sterile hand washing and the use of a surgical gown, mask, cap, gloves, and a large sterile drape in combination with aseptic CVC insertion technique. Strict adherence to maximal sterile barrier precautions is an independent factor associated with a reduced risk of acquiring a central venous CRBSI.[135] In addition, the CDC recommends the use of a 2% chlorhexidine preparation rather than both 10% povidone-iodine and 70% alcohol for skin antisepsis because of the reduced incidence of infection associated with the use of this preparation.[134]

### Antibiotic-coated catheter

Antibiotic-coated catheters have been studied in the prevention of CRBSI primarily in the adult population. However, minocycline-rifampin–coated CVCs have been shown to delay the onset of catheter-related infection in pediatric patients without increasing the incidence of thrombosis or resistance,[136] and have also been shown to decrease the incidence of both femoral and subclavian catheter-related infections in adults.[137] These impregnated catheters are not widely used because of the associated increased cost and because of the CDC recommendation that these catheters should only be implemented for short-term use, particularly when there remains a need to enhance prevention of CRBSI after standard evidence-based strategies have been executed. In addition, antibiotic-impregnated catheters are not currently available for the use in neonates weighing less than 3 kg.[134] Further studies are necessary to define the role of these catheters in pediatric patients, particularly those who require long-term central venous access.

### Antibiotic and ethanol locks

Antibiotic locks including vancomycin, ciprofloxacin, gentamicin, and amphotericin B have been studied, with the reported efficacy in the prevention of adult CRBSI ranging from 30% to 100%.[138] Data in the pediatric age group are limited, but one randomized controlled study evaluating the use of an antibiotic lock containing vancomycin and heparin showed no significant decrease in the incidence of CRBSI compared with a standard heparin lock.[139] The CDC does not recommend the use of antibiotic locks because of the potential risk of promoting resistant organisms.[134]

Recently, there has also been a growing interest in ethanol locks. The primary advantage of an ethanol lock compared with an antibiotic lock is the putative elimination of the potential for the development of resistant organisms. Ethanol, because of its ability to rapidly degrade proteins, is both bactericidal and fungicidal.[140] A pilot study in adults documented the safety and potential efficacy of ethanol locks in treating CVC-associated infections,[141] and a subsequent small study in children with SBS found that the use of daily ethanol locks for the prevention of CRBSI was both safe and effective.[142] Although a subsequent randomized controlled trial in adult hematology patients showed a nonsignificant 41% reduction of CRBSI in patients with ethanol locks,[143] further studies are necessary, particularly in the pediatric age group to determine the overall efficacy and safety of ethanol lock therapy for CRBSI prevention and treatment.

### Bacterial overgrowth

Rotating, short courses of antibiotics have been suggested to reduce enteral bacterial overgrowth and subsequently reduce the risk of sepsis in patients with SBS. However, the data on the effectiveness of this treatment are limited and, despite reports of a reduction in the rate of IFALD with this intervention, it is often difficult to separate the effects of this intervention from other measures simultaneously taken to manage IFALD.[102,144,145] When short courses of antibiotics are given, metronidazole is most commonly used because of its broad anaerobic coverage and inherent anti-inflammatory properties.[146] Some institutions prefer to alternate metronidazole with enteral gentamicin or kanamycin, with or without 1 or more intervening weeks without antibiotics.[102,144]

## Operative Intervention

### Timing of operative intervention

Patients with intestinal failure who undergo frequent operative procedures have been shown to have a greater likelihood to develop IFALD, suggesting that the inflammatory cytokine state caused by a major surgical procedure may be hepatotoxic for the PN-dependent patient.[147,148] Recent work by our group has shown that patients with IFALD receiving an intravenous fish oil–based lipid emulsion, who undergo major abdominal operations before the resolution of cholestasis, are more likely to experience an acute increase in serum bilirubin after surgery compared with patients who undergo similar operative procedures following the resolution of cholestasis. These findings suggest that abdominal operations are a risk factor not only for the development of IFALD, as previously described, but also for the exacerbation of established cholestasis in PN-dependent patients.[149]

Progression to full enteral feeds remains the primary goal for all patients with IFALD. Thus, it may be in the patient's best interest to perform certain operative procedures likely to result in a substantial increase in enteral absorptive capacity regardless of whether cholestasis is present at the time of surgical intervention. This decision must be made on an individual patient basis. Based on the available data, it may be prudent to delay any nonurgent abdominal operation, not believed to significantly increase enteral absorptive capacity, until the degree of cholestasis or liver injury has improved.

### Options for operative intervention

Several surgical procedures may be considered useful in a patient with SBS or associated IFALD. These children may require placement of a feeding tube (ie, gastrostomy or jejunostomy tube) to allow for enteral feeds if the child's enteral intake is limited by an ineffective swallowing mechanism and/or gastric/duodenal dysmotility. Such feeding tubes allow for the continuous administration of EN, which may be better tolerated than bolus feeding in children with SBS.[150] Children with significantly dilated segments of intestine and resultant complications secondary to bacterial overgrowth may benefit from a procedure to reduce the caliber of the intestine, such as a tapering enteroplasty. In addition, intestinal lengthening procedures have been described to increase the length of the intestine in patients with SBS with the goal of improving enteral tolerance. The longitudinal intestinal lengthening procedure, which involves the division of symmetrically dilated segments of small bowel in half longitudinally, was first described in 1980 by Bianchi.[151] Although initial results with this procedure were considered favorable,[152] it has proved to be a challenging operation associated with a risk of vascular compromise and resultant further bowel loss in addition to significant overall morbidity and mortality.[153] The serial transverse enteroplasty procedure (STEP) was subsequently described and involves the application of a stapler at right angles to the bowel, successively alternating sides to create a zigzag longer and narrower channel.[154] Although a recently created STEP registry reported improved enteral tolerance in patients with SBS following a STEP procedure, this study is limited by its small sample size and retrospective nature, which results in the lack of an appropriate control group or a SBS cohort not treated with the STEP procedure. A prospective, randomized, controlled trial would be necessary to show the true benefit or potential detriment of the STEP procedure for patients with IFALD.

### Transplantation

Liver and intestinal transplantation are considerations in PN-dependent children who develop impending or overt liver failure. However, the importance of taking all steps possible to prevent the development of overt liver failure cannot be overestimated, because outcomes following transplantation remain dismal. The University of Pittsburgh, a large transplant center, has recently reported its 5-year patient survival (for isolated intestinal transplants and combined liver/small intestinal transplants) at 77% with a corresponding graft survival rate of only 58%.[155]

Patients with liver and intestinal failure who are not predicted to achieve intestinal rehabilitation and for whom death is otherwise unavoidable may be offered a combined liver and intestinal transplant despite the formidable immediate and long-term risks. Recent studies report that isolated liver transplant may be a successful strategy for select infants with SBS and IFALD in whom the residual bowel has the potential for intestinal adaptation. In these situations, it is believed that significant liver disease may hamper intestinal adaptation, and, thus, an isolated liver transplant may allow for more complete intestinal adaptation.[156] Accurately identifying children who have the potential for bowel adaptation remains difficult, and although there is no set of definitive criteria, important considerations include bowel length and maximal enteral tolerance.[157] Although an isolated liver transplant may be an option for some children, the outcome of an isolated liver transplant in a child with IFALD is dismal, having a 3-year survival of only 64%.[158] In addition, there is no protective effect of a mature donor liver on the recurrence of IFALD. The increased risk of sepsis resulting from immunosuppressive medications in combination with poor enteral feeding tolerance and the ischemia/reperfusion injury associated with organ transplantation may render the transplant liver as vulnerable to IFALD as an original neonatal liver.[159] Some studies report that IFALD recurs in all transplanted livers in children transplanted for IFALD. Although the liver disease did stabilize and regress in children successfully weaned from PN, it progressed to end-stage liver disease in all children with poor enteral tolerance and all of these children subsequently died of multisystem organ failure.[158]

These data clearly highlight the absolute importance of the early institution of aggressive prevention and treatment strategies for IFALD in neonates and children to minimize liver injury during bowel adaptation and thus prevent the development of overt liver failure. Once overt liver failure develops, both isolated liver and combined liver/intestinal transplantation may be considered, but the outcomes associated with both procedures remain dismal in the pediatric population.

## SUMMARY

IFALD is a common and potentially life-threatening problem for pediatric patients receiving long-term PN. With a solid understanding of IFALD, the associated risk factors, and the available therapies for the prevention and treatment of the condition, there exists the potential for decreasing its incidence and thus improving the outcome of children with SBS on prolonged PN. Risk factors for IFALD that should be recognized include premature birth, low birth weight, prolonged duration of PN, intestinal stasis, and early and/or recurrent catheter-related sepsis. Preventative strategies are the cornerstone of improving outcomes in IFALD and include institution of enteral feedings, early weaning and cycling of PN, and reduction in the dose of lipid emulsions administered with PN. Recent work also shows the efficacy of fish oil–based lipid emulsions in both the prevention and treatment of IFALD and should also be strongly considered in children with IFALD. The importance of early recognition, aggressive treatment, and prevention of sepsis cannot be overstated. Although there may be a role for surgical intervention, the risks and benefits involving the exact timing and nature of the surgical procedure must be carefully considered. While transplantation remains an option for children with end-stage liver disease, it is still associated with significant morbidity and mortality.

## REFERENCES

1. Goulet O, Ruemmele F. Causes and management of intestinal failure in children. Gastroenterology 2006;130(2 Suppl 1):S16–28.
2. Duro D, Kamin D, Duggan C. Overview of pediatric short bowel syndrome. J Pediatr Gastroenterol Nutr 2008;47(Suppl 1):S33–6.
3. Wilmore DW, Dudrick SJ. Growth and development of an infant receiving all nutrients exclusively by vein. JAMA 1968;203(10):860–4.
4. Ching YA, Gura K, Modi B, et al. Pediatric intestinal failure: nutrition, pharmacologic, and surgical approaches. Nutr Clin Pract 2007;22(6):653–63.
5. Btaiche IF, Khalidi N. Parenteral nutrition-associated liver complications in children. Pharmacotherapy 2002;22(2):188–211.
6. Buchman A. Total parenteral nutrition-associated liver disease. JPEN J Parenter Enteral Nutr 2002;26(Suppl 5):S43–8.
7. Kelly DA. Liver complications of pediatric parenteral nutrition–epidemiology. Nutrition 1998;14(1):153–7.
8. Quiros-Tejeira RE, Ament ME, Reyen L, et al. Long-term parenteral nutritional support and intestinal adaptation in children with short bowel syndrome: a 25-year experience. J Pediatr 2004;145(2):157–63.
9. Willis TC, Carter BA, Rogers SP, et al. High rates of mortality and morbidity occur in infants with parenteral nutrition-associated cholestasis. JPEN J Parenter Enteral Nutr 2010;34(1):32–7.
10. Chan S, McCowen KC, Bistrian BR, et al. Incidence, prognosis, and etiology of end-stage liver disease in patients receiving home total parenteral nutrition. Surgery 1999;126(1):28–34.
11. Diamanti A, Basso MS, Castro M, et al. Prevalence of life-threatening complications in pediatric patients affected by intestinal failure. Transplant Proc 2007; 39(5):1632–3.

12. Andorsky DJ, Lund DP, Lillehei CW, et al. Nutritional and other postoperative management of neonates with short bowel syndrome correlates with clinical outcomes. J Pediatr 2001;139(1):27–33.

13. Moss RL, Amii LA. New approaches to understanding the etiology and treatment of total parenteral nutrition-associated cholestasis. Semin Pediatr Surg 1999;8(3):140–7.

14. Beath SV, Davies P, Papadopoulou A, et al. Parenteral nutrition-related cholestasis in postsurgical neonates: multivariate analysis of risk factors. J Pediatr Surg 1996;31(4):604–6.

15. Christensen RD, Henry E, Wiedmeier SE, et al. Identifying patients, on the first day of life, at high-risk of developing parenteral nutrition-associated liver disease. J Perinatol 2007;27(5):284–90.

16. Beale EF, Nelson RM, Bucciarelli RL, et al. Intrahepatic cholestasis associated with parenteral nutrition in premature infants. Pediatrics 1979;64(3):342–7.

17. Kubota A, Okada A, Nezu R, et al. Hyperbilirubinemia in neonates associated with total parenteral nutrition. JPEN J Parenter Enteral Nutr 1988; 12(6):602–6.

18. Kaufman SS, Pehlivanova M, Fennelly EM, et al. Predicting liver failure in parenteral nutrition-dependent short bowel syndrome of infancy. J Pediatr 2010; 156(4):580.e1–585.e1.

19. Wu PA, Kerner JA, Berquist WE. Parenteral nutrition-associated cholestasis related to parental care. Nutr Clin Pract 2006;21(3):291–5.

20. Zambrano E, El-Hennawy M, Ehrenkranz RA, et al. Total parenteral nutrition induced liver pathology: an autopsy series of 24 newborn cases. Pediatr Dev Pathol 2004;7(5):425–32.

21. Dahms BB, Halpin TC Jr. Serial liver biopsies in parenteral nutrition-associated cholestasis of early infancy. Gastroenterology 1981;81(1):136–44.

22. Fitzgibbons SC, Jones BA, Hull MA, et al. Relationship between biopsy-proven parenteral nutrition-associated liver fibrosis and biochemical cholestasis in children with short bowel syndrome. J Pediatr Surg 2010;45(1):95–9 [discussion: 99].

23. Moss RL, Das JB, Raffensperger JG. Total parenteral nutrition-associated cholestasis: clinical and histopathologic correlation. J Pediatr Surg 1993;28(10):1270–4 [discussion: 1274–5].

24. Wretlind A. Development of fat emulsions. JPEN J Parenter Enteral Nutr 1981; 5(3):230–5.

25. Edgren B, Wretlind A. The theoretical background of the intravenous nutrition with fat emulsions. Nutr Dieta Eur Rev Nutr Diet 1963;13:364–86.

26. Schuberth OWA. Intravenous infusion of fat emulsions, phosphatides and emulsifying agents. Acta Chir Scand 1961;13(Suppl):S278–84.

27. Das UN. Essential fatty acids: biochemistry, physiology and pathology. Biotechnol J 2006;1(4):420–39.

28. Chen WJ, Yeh SL, Huang PC. Effects of fat emulsions with different fatty acid composition on plasma and hepatic lipids in rats receiving total parenteral nutrition. Clin Nutr 1996;15(1):24–8.

29. Aksnes J, Eide TJ, Nordstrand K. Lipid entrapment and cellular changes in the rat myocard, lung and liver after long-term parenteral nutrition with lipid emulsion. A light microscopic and ultrastructural study. APMIS 1996;104(7–8):515–22.

30. Zaman N, Tam YK, Jewell LD, et al. Effects of intravenous lipid as a source of energy in parenteral nutrition associated hepatic dysfunction and lidocaine

elimination: a study using isolated rat liver perfusion. Biopharm Drug Dispos 1997;18(9):803–19.

31. Clayton PT, Whitfield P, Iyer K. The role of phytosterols in the pathogenesis of liver complications of pediatric parenteral nutrition. Nutrition 1998;14(1):158–64.

32. Thomas-Gibson S, Jawhari A, Atlan P, et al. Safe and efficacious prolonged use of an olive oil-based lipid emulsion (ClinOleic) in chronic intestinal failure. Clin Nutr 2004;23(4):697–703.

33. Palova S, Charvat J, Kvapil M. Comparison of soybean oil- and olive oil-based lipid emulsions on hepatobiliary function and serum triacylglycerols level during realimentation. J Int Med Res 2008;36(3):587–93.

34. Fallon EM, Le HD, Puder M. Prevention of parenteral nutrition-associated liver disease: role of omega-3 fish oil. Curr Opin Organ Transplant 2010;15(3):334–40.

35. Lee S, Gura KM, Puder M. Omega-3 fatty acids and liver disease. Hepatology 2007;45(4):841–5.

36. Prescott SM. The effect of eicosapentaenoic acid on leukotriene B production by human neutrophils. J Biol Chem 1984;259(12):7615–21.

37. Camandola S, Leonarduzzi G, Musso T, et al. Nuclear factor kB is activated by arachidonic acid but not by eicosapentaenoic acid. Biochem Biophys Res Commun 1996;229(2):643–7.

38. Chen MF, Lee YT, Hsu HC, et al. Effects of dietary supplementation with fish oil on prostanoid metabolism during acute coronary occlusion with or without reperfusion in diet-induced hypercholesterolemic rabbits. Int J Cardiol 1992; 36(3):297–304.

39. Lee S, Gura KM, Kim S, et al. Current clinical applications of omega-6 and omega-3 fatty acids. Nutr Clin Pract 2006;21(4):323–41.

40. Alwayn IP, Gura K, Nose V, et al. Omega-3 fatty acid supplementation prevents hepatic steatosis in a murine model of nonalcoholic fatty liver disease. Pediatr Res 2005;57(3):445–52.

41. Grimminger F, Wahn H, Mayer K, et al. Impact of arachidonic versus eicosapen-taenoic acid on exotonin-induced lung vascular leakage: relation to 4-series versus 5-series leukotriene generation. Am J Respir Crit Care Med 1997; 155(2):513–9.

42. Carter BA, Shulman RJ. Mechanisms of disease: update on the molecular etiology and fundamentals of parenteral nutrition associated cholestasis. Nat Clin Pract Gastroenterol Hepatol 2007;4(5):277–87.

43. Carter BA, Taylor OA, Prendergast DR, et al. Stigmasterol, a soy lipid-derived phytosterol, is an antagonist of the bile acid nuclear receptor FXR. Pediatr Res 2007;62(3):301–6.

44. Gura KM, Parsons SK, Bechard LJ, et al. Use of a fish oil-based lipid emulsion to treat essential fatty acid deficiency in a soy allergic patient receiving parenteral nutrition. Clin Nutr 2005;24(5):839–47.

45. Gura KM, Duggan CP, Collier SB, et al. Reversal of parenteral nutrition-associated liver disease in two infants with short bowel syndrome using paren-teral fish oil: implications for future management. Pediatrics 2006;118(1): e197–201.

46. Gura KM, Lee S, Valim C, et al. Safety and efficacy of a fish-oil-based fat emul-sion in the treatment of parenteral nutrition-associated liver disease. Pediatrics 2008;121(3):e678–86.

47. Puder M, Valim C, Meisel JA, et al. Parenteral fish oil improves outcomes in patients with parenteral nutrition-associated liver injury. Ann Surg 2009;250(3): 395–402.

48. de Meijer VE, Gura KM, Le HD, et al. Fish oil-based lipid emulsions prevent and reverse parenteral nutrition-associated liver disease: the Boston experience. JPEN J Parenter Enteral Nutr 2009;33(5):541–7.

49. de Meijer VE, Le HD, Meisel JA, et al. Parenteral fish oil as monotherapy prevents essential fatty acid deficiency in parenteral nutrition-dependent patients. J Pediatr Gastroenterol Nutr 2010;50(2):212–8.

50. de Meijer VE, Gura KM, Meisel JA, et al. Parenteral fish oil as monotherapy for patients with parenteral nutrition-associated liver disease. Pediatr Surg Int 2009; 25(1):123–4.

51. Diamond IR, Sterescu A, Pencharz PB, et al. Changing the paradigm: omegaven for the treatment of liver failure in pediatric short bowel syndrome. J Pediatr Gastroenterol Nutr 2009;48(2):209–15.

52. Lee SI, Valim C, Johnston P, et al. The impact of fish oil-based lipid emulsion on serum triglyceride, bilirubin, and albumin levels in children with parenteral nutrition-associated liver disease. Pediatr Res 2009;66(6):698–703.

53. Calhoun AW, Sullivan JE. Omegaven for the treatment of parenteral nutrition associated liver disease: a case study. J Ky Med Assoc 2009;107(2):55–7.

54. de Meijer VE, Gura KM, Meisel JA, et al. Parenteral fish oil monotherapy in the management of patients with parenteral nutrition-associated liver disease. Arch Surg 2010;145(6):547–51.

55. Ekema G, Falchetti D, Boroni G, et al. Reversal of severe parenteral nutrition-associated liver disease in an infant with short bowel syndrome using parenteral fish oil (Omega-3 fatty acids). J Pediatr Surg 2008;43(6):1191–5.

56. Cheung HM, Lam HS, Tam YH, et al. Rescue treatment of infants with intestinal failure and parenteral nutrition-associated cholestasis (PNAC) using a parenteral fish-oil-based lipid. Clin Nutr 2009;28(2):209–12.

57. Carlson SE, Cooke RJ, Werkman SH, et al. First year growth of preterm infants fed standard compared to marine oil n-3 supplemented formula. Lipids 1992; 27(11):901–7.

58. Carlson SE, Werkman SH, Peeples JM, et al. Arachidonic acid status correlates with first year growth in preterm infants. Proc Natl Acad Sci U S A 1993;90(3): 1073–7.

59. Carlson SE, Werkman SH, Tolley EA. Effect of long-chain n-3 fatty acid supplementation on visual acuity and growth of preterm infants with and without bronchopulmonary dysplasia. Am J Clin Nutr 1996;63(5):687–97.

60. Le HD, de Meijer VE, Zurakowski D, et al. Parenteral fish oil as monotherapy improves lipid profiles in children with parenteral nutrition-associated liver disease. JPEN J Parenter Enteral Nutr 2010;34(5):477–84.

61. Vanschoonbeek K, Feijge MA, Paquay M, et al. Variable hypocoagulant effect of fish oil intake in humans: modulation of fibrinogen level and thrombin generation. Arterioscler Thromb Vasc Biol 2004;24(9):1734–40.

62. Mirtallo J, Canada T, Johnson D, et al. Safe practices for parenteral nutrition. JPEN J Parenter Enteral Nutr 2004;28(6):S39–70.

63. Cavicchi M, Beau P, Crenn P, et al. Prevalence of liver disease and contributing factors in patients receiving home parenteral nutrition for permanent intestinal failure. Ann Intern Med 2000;132(7):525–32.

64. Wessel JJ, Kocoshis SA. Nutritional management of infants with short bowel syndrome. Semin Perinatol 2007;31(2):104–11.

65. Colomb V, Jobert-Giraud A, Lacaille F, et al. Role of lipid emulsions in cholestasis associated with long-term parenteral nutrition in children. JPEN J Parenter Enteral Nutr 2000;24(6):345–50.

66. Crawford MA, Costeloe K, Ghebremeskel K, et al. The inadequacy of the essential fatty acid content of present preterm feeds. Eur J Pediatr 1998;157(Suppl 1):S23–7.
67. Innis SM. Omega-3 Fatty acids and neural development to 2 years of age: do we know enough for dietary recommendations? J Pediatr Gastroenterol Nutr 2009; 48(Suppl 1):S16–24.
68. Kleinman RE, editor. Pediatric nutrition handbook. 6th edition. Elk Grove Village (IL): American Academy of Pediatrics; 2009.
69. Le HD, Fallon EM, de Meijer VE, et al. Innovative parenteral and enteral nutrition therapy for intestinal failure. Semin Pediatr Surg 2010;19(1):27–34.
70. Chwals WJ. The metabolic response to surgery in neonates. Curr Opin Pediatr 1994;6:330–40.
71. Schiller WR. Burn management in children. Pediatr Ann 1996;25:434–8.
72. Collier S, Crouch J, Hendricks K, et al. Use of cyclic parenteral nutrition in infants less than 6 months of age. Nutr Clin Pract 1994;9(2):65–8.
73. Takehara H, Hino M, Kameoka K, et al. A new method of total parenteral nutrition for surgical neonates: it is possible that cyclic TPN prevents intrahepatic chole-stasis. Tokushima J Exp Med 1990;37(3–4):97–102.
74. Jensen AR, Goldin AB, Koopmeiners JS, et al. The association of cyclic nutrition and decreased incidence of cholestatic liver disease in patients with gastroschi-sis. J Pediatr Surg 2009;44:183–9.
75. Sjoberg P, Bondesson U, Sedin G, et al. Dispositions of di- and mono-(2-ethyl-hexyl) phthalate in newborn infants subjected to exchange transfusions. Eur J Clin Invest 1985;15(6):430–6.
76. Von Rettberg H, Hannman T, Subotic U, et al. Use of di(2-ethylhexyl)phthalate containing infusion systems increases the risk for cholestasis. Pediatrics 2009; 124:710–6.
77. Silva MJ, Barr DB, Reidy JA, et al. Urinary levels of seven phthalate metabolites in the U.S. population from the National Health and Nutrition Examination Survey (NHANES) 1999–2000. Environ Health Perspect 2004;112:331–3.
78. Bohrer D, Cicero do Nascimento P, Binotto R, et al. Contribution of the raw mate-rial to the aluminum contamination in parenterals. JPEN J Parenter Enteral Nutr 2002;26:382–8.
79. Poole RL, Hintz SR, Mackenzie NI, et al. Aluminum exposure from pediatric parenteral nutrition: meeting the new FDA regulation. JPEN J Parenter Enteral Nutr 2008;32:242.
80. Aluminum in large and small volume parenterals used in total parenteral nutri-tion–FDA. Proposed rule. Fed Regist 1998;63(2):176–85.
81. Day CP, James OF. Steatohepatitis: a tale of two "hits"? Gastroenterology 1998; 114(4):842–5.
82. Becvarova I, Saker KE, Swecker WS Jr, et al. Peroxidative protection of paren-teral admixture by D-alpha-tocopherol. Vet Ther 2005;6(4):280–90.
83. Soden JS, Devereaux MW, Haas JE, et al. Subcutaneous vitamin E ameliorates liver injury in an in vivo model of steatocholestasis. Hepatology 2007;46(2):485–95.
84. Goulet O, Joly F, Corriol O, et al. Some new insights in intestinal failure-associated liver disease. Curr Opin Organ Transplant 2009;14(3):256–61.
85. Sweeny DJ, Barnes S, Diasio RB. Bile acid conjugation pattern in the isolated perfused rat liver during infusion of an amino acid formulation. JPEN J Parenter Enteral Nutr 1991;15(3):303–6.
86. Yousef IM, Tuchweber B, Vonk RJ, et al. Lithocholate cholestasis-sulfated glyco-lithocholate-induced intrahepatic cholestasis in rats. Gastroenterology 1981;80: 233–41.

87. Guertin F, Roy CC, Lepage G, et al. Effect of taurine on total parenteral nutrition-associated cholestasis. JPEN J Parenter Enteral Nutr 1991;15(3):247–51.

88. Cooper A, Betts JM, Pereira GR, et al. Taurine deficiency in the severe hepatic dysfunction complicating total parenteral nutrition. J Pediatr Surg 1984;19(4): 462–6.

89. Vinton NE, Laidlaw SA, Ament ME, et al. Taurine concentrations in plasma, blood cells, and urine of children under-going long-term parenteral nutrition. Pediatrics 1987;21:399–403.

90. Dahlstrom KA, Ament ME, Laidlaw SA, et al. Plasma amino acid concentrations in children receiving long-term parenteral nutrition. J Pediatr Gastroenterol Nutr 1988;7:748–54.

91. Spencer AU, Yu S, Tracy TF, et al. Parenteral nutrition-associated cholestasis in neonates: multivariate analysis of the potential protective effect of taurine. JPEN J Parenter Enteral Nutr 2005;29(5):337–43 [discussion: 343–4].

92. Cooke RJ, Whitington PF, Kelts D. Effect of taurine supplementation on hepatic function during short-term parenteral nutrition in the premature infant. J Pediatr Gastroenterol Nutr 1984;3(2):234–8.

93. Friel JK, Gibson RS, Peliowski A, et al. Serum zinc, copper, and selenium concentrations in preterm infants receiving enteral nutrition or parental nutrition supplemented with zinc and copper. J Pediatr 1984;104(5):763–8.

94. Zlotkin SH, Buchanan BE. Meeting zinc and copper intake requirements in the parenterally fed preterm and full-term infant. J Pediatr 1983;103(3):441–6.

95. Latimer JS, McClain CJ, Sharp HL. Clinical zinc deficiency during zinc-supplemented parenteral nutrition. J Pediatr 1980;97(3):434–7.

96. Weber TR, Sears N, Davies B, et al. Clinical spectrum of zinc deficiency in pediatric patients receiving total parenteral nutrition (TPN). J Pediatr Surg 1981;16(3):236–40.

97. Goulet O. Short bowel syndrome in pediatric patients. Nutrition 1998;14(10): 784–7.

98. Jeejeebhoy KN. Management of short bowel syndrome: avoidance of total parenteral nutrition. Gastroenterology 2006;130(2 Suppl 1):S60–6.

99. Perdikis DA, Basson MD. Basal nutrition promotes human intestinal epithelial (Caco-2) proliferation, brush border enzyme activity, and motility. Crit Care Med 1997;25(1):159–65.

100. Parker P, Stroop S, Greene H. A controlled comparison of continuous versus intermittent feeding in the treatment of infants with intestinal disease. J Pediatr 1981;99(3):360–4.

101. Zamir O, Nussbaum MS, Bhadra S, et al. Effect of enteral feeding on hepatic steatosis induced by total parenteral nutrition. JPEN J Parenter Enteral Nutr 1994;18(1):20–5.

102. Meehan JJ, Georgeson KE. Prevention of liver failure in parenteral nutrition-dependent children with short bowel syndrome. J Pediatr Surg 1997;32(3): 473–5.

103. Sondheimer JM, Cadnapaphornchai M, Sontag M, et al. Predicting the duration of dependence on parenteral nutrition after neonatal intestinal resection. J Pediatr 1998;132(1):80–4.

104. Javid PJ, Collier S, Richardson D, et al. The role of enteral nutrition in the reversal of parenteral nutrition-associated liver dysfunction in infants. J Pediatr Surg 2005;40(6):1015–8.

105. Pimenta HP, Moreira ME, Rocha AD, et al. Effects of non-nutritive sucking and oral stimulation on breastfeeding rates for preterm, low birth weight infants:

a randomized clinical trial. J Pediatr (Rio J) 2008;84(5):423–7 [in English, Portuguese].

106. Playford RJ, Macdonald CE, Johnson WS. Colostrum and milk-derived peptide growth factors for the treatment of gastrointestinal disorders. Am J Clin Nutr 2000;72(1):5–14.

107. Xanthou M, Bines J, Walker WA. Human milk and intestinal host defense in newborns: an update. Adv Pediatr 1995;42:171–208.

108. Byrne TA, Morrissey TB, Nattakom TV, et al. Growth hormone, glutamine, and a modified diet enhance nutrient absorption in patients with severe short bowel syndrome. JPEN J Parenter Enteral Nutr 1995;19(4):296–302.

109. Stern LE, Falcone RA Jr, Huang F, et al. Epidermal growth factor alters the bax:bcl-w ratio following massive small bowel resection. J Surg Res 2000; 91(1):38–42.

110. Cummins AG, Thompson FM. Effect of breast milk and weaning on epithelial growth of the small intestine in humans. Gut 2002;51(5):748–54.

111. Bines J, Francis D, Hill D. Reducing parenteral requirement in children with short bowel syndrome: impact of an amino acid-based complete infant formula. J Pediatr Gastroenterol Nutr 1998;26(2):123–8.

112. Vanderhoof JA. New and emerging therapies for short bowel syndrome in children. J Pediatr Gastroenterol Nutr 2004;39(Suppl 3):S769–71.

113. Vanderhoof JA, Grandjean CJ, Kaufman SS, et al. Effect of high percentage medium-chain triglyceride diet on mucosal adaptation following massive bowel resection in rats. JPEN J Parenter Enteral Nutr 1984;8(6):685–9.

114. Kollman KA, Lien EL, Vanderhoof JA. Dietary lipids influence intestinal adaptation after massive bowel resection. J Pediatr Gastroenterol Nutr 1999;28(1): 41–5.

115. Lai HS, Chen WJ, Chen KM, et al. Effects of monomeric and polymeric diets on small intestine following massive resection. Taiwan Yi Xue Hui Za Zhi 1989; 88(10):982–8.

116. Axelrod D, Kazmerski K, Iyer K. Pediatric enteral nutrition. JPEN J Parenter Enteral Nutr 2006;30(Suppl 1):S21–6.

117. Serrano MS, Schmidt-Sommerfeld E. Nutrition support of infants with short bowel syndrome. Nutrition 2002;18(11–12):966–70.

118. Spagnuolo MI, Iorio R, Vegnente A, et al. Ursodeoxycholic acid for treatment of cholestasis in children on long-term total parenteral nutrition: a pilot study. Gastroenterology 1996;111(3):716–9.

119. Levine A, Maayan A, Shamir R, et al. Parenteral nutrition-associated cholestasis in preterm neonates: evaluation of ursodeoxycholic acid treatment. J Pediatr Endocrinol Metab 1999;12(4):549–53.

120. Chen CY, Tsao PN, Chen HL, et al. Ursodeoxycholic acid (UDCA) therapy in very-low-birth-weight infants with parenteral nutrition-associated cholestasis. J Pediatr 2004;145(3):317–21.

121. Heubi JE, Wiechmann DA, Creutzinger V, et al. Tauroursodeoxycholic acid (TUDCA) in the prevention of total parenteral nutrition-associated liver disease. J Pediatr 2002;141(2):237–42.

122. Teitelbaum DH, Tracy TF Jr, Aouthmany MM, et al. Use of cholecystokinin-octapeptide for the prevention of parenteral nutrition-associated cholestasis. Pediatrics 2005;115(5):1332–40.

123. Tsai S, Strouse PJ, Drongowski RA, et al. Failure of cholecystokinin-octapeptide to prevent TPN-associated gallstone disease. J Pediatr Surg 2005;40(1):263–7.

124. San Luis VA, Btaiche IF. Ursodiol in patients with parenteral nutrition-associated cholestasis. Ann Pharmacother 2007;41(11):1867–72.
125. Chang CY, Schiano TD. Review article: drug hepatotoxicity. Aliment Pharmacol Ther 2007;25(10):1135–51.
126. de Abajo FJ, Montero D, Madurga M, et al. Acute and clinically relevant drug-induced liver injury: a population based case-control study. Br J Clin Pharmacol 2004;58(1):71–80.
127. Chang CC, Petrelli M, Tomashefski JF Jr, et al. Severe intrahepatic cholestasis caused by amiodarone toxicity after withdrawal of the drug: a case report and review of the literature. Arch Pathol Lab Med 1999;123(3):251–6.
128. Stieger B, Fattinger K, Madon J, et al. Drug- and estrogen-induced cholestasis through inhibition of the hepatocellular bile salt export pump (Bsep) of rat liver. Gastroenterology 2000;118(2):422–30.
129. Larrey D, Erlinger S. Drug-induced cholestasis. Baillieres Clin Gastroenterol 1988;2(2):423–52.
130. Zimmerman HJ, Lewis JH. Drug-induced cholestasis. Med Toxicol 1987;2(2):112–60.
131. Sondheimer JM, Asturias E, Cadnapaphornchai M. Infection and cholestasis in neonates with intestinal resection and long-term parenteral nutrition. J Pediatr Gastroenterol Nutr 1998;27(2):131–7.
132. O'Brien DP, Nelson LA, Kemp CJ, et al. Intestinal permeability and bacterial translocation are uncoupled after small bowel resection. J Pediatr Surg 2002; 37(3):390–4.
133. Fratino G, Molinari AC, Mazzola C, et al. Prospective study of indwelling central venous catheter-related complications in children with broviac or clampless valved catheters. J Pediatr Hematol Oncol 2002;24(8):657–61.
134. O'Grady NP, Alexander M, Dellinger EP, et al. Guidelines for the prevention of intravascular catheter-related infections. Centers for Disease Control and Prevention. MMWR Recomm Rep 2002;51(RR-10):1–29.
135. Lee DH, Jung KY, Choi YH. Use of maximal sterile barrier precautions and/or antimicrobial-coated catheters to reduce the risk of central venous catheter-related bloodstream infection. Infect Control Hosp Epidemiol 2008;29(10):947–50.
136. Chelliah A, Heydon KH, Zaoutis TE, et al. Observational trial of antibiotic-coated central venous catheters in critically ill pediatric patients. Pediatr Infect Dis J 2007;26(9):816–20.
137. Lorente L, Lecuona M, Ramos MJ, et al. The use of rifampicin-miconazole-impregnated catheters reduces the incidence of femoral and jugular catheter-related bacteremia. Clin Infect Dis 2008;47(9):1171–5.
138. Segarra-Newnham M, Martin-Cooper EM. Antibiotic lock technique: a review of the literature. Ann Pharmacother 2005;39(2):311–8.
139. Rackoff WR, Weiman M, Jakobowski D, et al. A randomized, controlled trial of the efficacy of a heparin and vancomycin solution in preventing central venous catheter infections in children. J Pediatr 1995;127(1):147–51.
140. Metcalf SC, Chambers ST, Pithie AD. Use of ethanol locks to prevent recurrent central line sepsis. J Infect 2004;49(1):20–2.
141. Broom J, Woods M, Allworth A, et al. Ethanol lock therapy to treat tunnelled central venous catheter-associated blood stream infections: results from a prospective trial. Scand J Infect Dis 2008;40(5):399–406.
142. Mouw E, Chessman K, Lesher A, et al. Use of an ethanol lock to prevent catheter-related infections in children with short bowel syndrome. J Pediatr Surg 2008;43(6):1025–9.

143. Slobbe L, Doorduijn JK, Lugtenburg PJ, et al. Prevention of catheter-related bacteremia with a daily ethanol lock in patients with tunnelled catheters: a randomized, placebo-controlled trial. PLoS One 2010;5(5):e10840.

144. Sigalet D, Boctor D, Robertson M, et al. Improved outcomes in paediatric intestinal failure with aggressive prevention of liver disease. Eur J Pediatr Surg 2009; 19(6):348–53.

145. Vanderhoof JA, Langnas AN. Short-bowel syndrome in children and adults. Gastroenterology 1997;113(5):1767–78.

146. Freund HR, Muggia-Sullam M, LaFrance R, et al. A possible beneficial effect of metronidazole in reducing TPN-associated liver function derangements. J Surg Res 1985;38(4):356–63.

147. Drongowski RA, Coran AG. An analysis of factors contributing to the development of total parenteral nutrition-induced cholestasis. JPEN J Parenter Enteral Nutr 1989;13(6):586–9.

148. Ginn-Pease ME, Pantalos D, King DR. TPN-associated hyperbilirubinemia: a common problem in newborn surgical patients. J Pediatr Surg 1985;20(4):436–9.

149. Arsenault DA, Potemkin AK, Robinson EM, et al. Surgical intervention in the setting of parenteral nutrition associated cholestasis may exacerbate liver injury. J Pediatr Surg 2011;46(1):122–7.

150. Weizman Z, Schmueli A, Deckelbaum RJ. Continuous nasogastric drip elemental feeding. Alternative for prolonged parenteral nutrition in severe prolonged diarrhea. Am J Dis Child 1983;137(3):253–5.

151. Bianchi A. Intestinal loop lengthening–a technique for increasing small intestinal length. J Pediatr Surg 1980;15(2):145–51.

152. Bianchi A. Longitudinal intestinal lengthening and tailoring: results in 20 children. J R Soc Med 1997;90(8):429–32.

153. Modi BP, Javid PJ, Jaksic T, et al. First report of the international serial transverse enteroplasty data registry: indications, efficacy, and complications. J Am Coll Surg 2007;204(3):365–71.

154. Kim HB, Fauza D, Garza J, et al. Serial transverse enteroplasty (STEP): a novel bowel lengthening procedure. J Pediatr Surg 2003;38(3):425–9.

155. Mazariegos GV, Squires RH, Sindhi RK. Current perspectives on pediatric intestinal transplantation. Curr Gastroenterol Rep 2009;11(3):226–33.

156. Goulet O, Kamin D. Intestinal failure, short bowel syndrome, and intestinal transplantation. In: Duggan C, Watkins JB, Walker WA, editors. Nutrition in pediatrics. 4th edition. Hamilton (ON): BC Decker; 2007. p. 641–62.

157. Horslen SP, Sudan DL, Iyer KR, et al. Isolated liver transplantation in infants with end-stage liver disease associated with short bowel syndrome. Ann Surg 2002; 235(3):435–9.

158. Dell-Olio D, Beath SV, de Ville de Goyet J, et al. Isolated liver transplant in infants with short bowel syndrome: insights into outcomes and prognostic factors. J Pediatr Gastroenterol Nutr 2009;48(3):334–40.

159. Santra S, McKiernan P, Lander A, et al. Ischemic hepatitis is a risk factor for progression of liver disease associated with parenteral nutrition in intestinal failure. J Pediatr Gastroenterol Nutr 2008;47(3):367–9.

# Adjuvant Nutrition Management of Patients with Liver Failure, Including Transplant

Andrew J. Kerwin, MD[a,b,*], Michael S. Nussbaum, MD[b,c]

**KEYWORDS**

• Liver failure • Malnutrition • Nutrition support • Liver transplant

Liver failure is a complex disorder that presents physicians with difficult challenges. This condition can be classified based on duration, extent, pathophysiology, and etiology.[1] Liver failure can also be classified as acute, chronic, or acute on chronic. Acute liver failure is characterized by acute loss of liver function with associated hepatic encephalopathy and coagulopathy, which occurs within 26 weeks of the onset of jaundice or other symptoms in a patient who previously did not manifest any symptoms of liver disease. Acute liver failure can be further classified as hyperacute (jaundice to encephalopathy in ≤7 days), acute (jaundice to encephalopathy in 8–28 days), and subacute (jaundice to encephalopathy in >28 days).[2]

The liver is a complex organ that has many functions that are vital to everyday healthy living. The major functions of the liver include energy metabolism, synthesis of blood proteins, secretion and excretion of bile, detoxification and excretion of both exogenous and endogenous substances, and reticuloendothelial system clearance of old or damaged blood cells, fibrin degradation products, infectious agents, and endotoxin. Thus, liver dysfunction results in multisystem effects having the potential for a multitude of complications.[3] Nutritional support is of paramount importance in an effort to alleviate some of these complications and to improve survival.[1,4,5]

The authors have nothing to disclose.

[a] Acute Care Surgery, Department of Surgery, University of Florida College of Medicine-Jacksonville, 655 West 8th Street, Jacksonville, FL 32209, USA

[b] Shands Jacksonville, 655 West 8th Street, Jacksonville, FL 32209, USA

[c] Department of Surgery, University of Florida College of Medicine-Jacksonville, 653 West 8th Street, Jacksonville, FL 32209, USA

* Corresponding author. Acute Care Surgery, Department of Surgery, University of Florida College of Medicine-Jacksonville, 655 West 8th Street, Jacksonville, FL 32209.

*E-mail address:* andy.kerwin@jax.ufl.edu

Surg Clin N Am 91 (2011) 565–578

doi:10.1016/j.suc.2011.02.010

surgical.theclinics.com

## ETIOLOGY OF MALNUTRITION

Protein-calorie malnutrition is a common complication in patients with liver disease. Malnutrition is seen in up to 90% of patients with cirrhosis.[6,7] The cause of malnutrition in liver disease is multifactorial (**Fig. 1**). Patients with liver disease have decreased caloric intake. This decreased caloric intake may be related to specialized diets (low salt and low protein) that are unpalatable as well as to the altered gustatory sensation that develops in cirrhosis.[8] This problem can be exacerbated when patients with liver

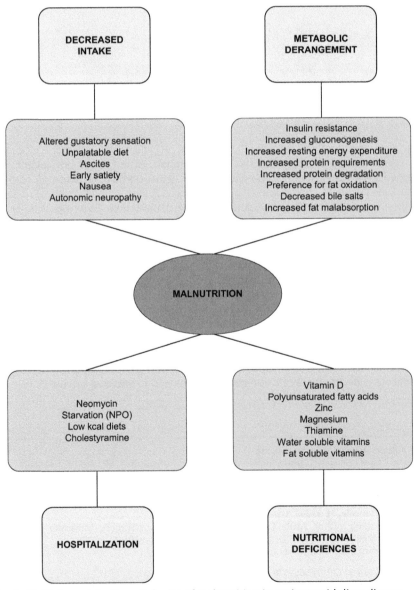

**Fig. 1.** Multiple contributing etiologies of malnutrition in patients with liver disease.

disease are admitted to the hospital for diagnostic or therapeutic procedures and have their intake withheld or limited in preparation for, during, and after the procedures. Autonomic dysfunction in liver disease is common[9–11] and leads to gastroparesis,[12] a delay in small bowel motility,[13] and ultimately a delay in orocecal transit,[14] which subsequently causes decreased nutrient intake as well.[15–17] This autonomic dysfunction along with tense ascites and bacterial overgrowth[17] leads to nausea and early satiety, which further contribute to decreased oral intake.[18,19] Ascites is also responsible for increased protein loss as well as early satiety because of increased intra-abdominal pressure and delayed gastric emptying.[12,13,18,20,21]

The derangements in the physiology of metabolism that occur in patients with liver failure are complex and further add to malnutrition. Studies have shown that many patients with liver disease are hypermetabolic, with an increase in their resting energy expenditure (REE). The incidence of hypermetabolism is estimated to occur in 18% to 34% of patients with liver failure,[22] and the cause of this condition is unclear but may be related to increased sympathetic nervous system activity. In liver disease, there is a decrease in glycogen stores, with a resultant increase in gluconeogenesis. This increase in gluconeogenesis leads to a shift from carbohydrate metabolism to a preference for fat metabolism. The key abnormality is glucose intolerance. Patients with liver disease are resistant to insulin, even though an elevation of circulating insulin occurs in these patients. The cause of this insulin resistance and hyperinsulinemia is not well understood, but it seems to be multifactorial.[23] Moreover, frank diabetes mellitus is seen in as many as 38% of patients with liver disease.

Protein metabolism is also altered in liver disease. Patients with liver disease have increased protein requirements as evidenced by the increased amount of protein intake needed to maintain a positive nitrogen balance compared with normal healthy people.[24] One hypothesis to explain the increased protein requirement is that patients with liver disease have increased protein synthesis and increased protein breakdown along with low glycogen stores that lead to gluconeogenesis from amino acids and resultant amino acid loss.[25] Branched-chain amino acids (BCAA: leucine, isoleucine, and valine) do not require the liver for metabolism and are thus preferentially used by the liver in liver failure, whereas aromatic amino acids (AAA: phenylalanine, tryptophan, and tyrosine) are not metabolized effectively in liver failure and accumulate excessively in the body fluids. This altered protein metabolism leads to a reduction in the BCAAs and an increase in the circulating levels of the AAA. This imbalance between the AAA and the BCAA may play a role in the hepatic encephalopathy that accompanies severe liver disease by creating weak false neurotransmitters.[26] Both the BCAAs and AAAs share a common pathway across the blood-brain barrier, and with elevated levels of AAAs, preferential transport of the AAAs occur across the blood-brain barrier. Once AAAs cross the blood-brain barrier, the metabolism of phenylalanine and tyrosine produces octopamine. Octopamine inhibits excitatory stimulation of the brain by acting as a weak false neurotransmitter that competes with the other neurotransmitters normally occurring in the brain. In addition, the tryptophan that is present is metabolized to 5-hydroxytryptophan (serotonin), which can produce further lethargy.

There are multiple vitamin and micronutrient deficiencies that accompany liver disease. Deficiencies in both the water-soluble and fat-soluble vitamins have been described. Both magnesium and zinc deficiencies have been described as well. Zinc deficiency has been shown to contribute to glucose intolerance[27] and also at times to precipitate hepatic encephalopathy.[28] However, it remains controversial as to whether or not zinc supplementation is beneficial to clinical management or outcome in patients with liver failure.

## NUTRITIONAL ASSESSMENT

Despite malnutrition being nearly ubiquitous in liver disease, determining an accurate assessment of a patient's nutritional status is difficult. Traditional assessment tools are not accurate in patients with liver disease, and no gold standard for assessment exists at this time. Given the association between malnutrition, complications, and mortality,[6,29,30] it is important to obtain an accurate and reliable assessment. The initial assessment should begin with a careful history taking to elucidate relevant signs and symptoms and pertinent information, such as nausea, vomiting, diarrhea, early satiety, changes in taste, weight loss, specialized diets and supplements, and recent dietary intake. A complete physical examination should elicit and document signs of peripheral edema, ascites, palmar erythema, spider angiomas, loss of subcutaneous fat, and muscle wasting.

Protein malnutrition is the predominant feature of advanced liver disease. Biochemical tests of nutritional status include serum levels of prealbumin, transferrin, and retinol binding protein, plus urine nitrogen excretion and creatinine height index. Given the catabolic nature of liver disease and the associated protein turnover, however, these measurements have not been shown to be accurate or dependable indices of nutrition status. In fact, one study demonstrated that levels of serum visceral proteins did not correlate with malnutrition but rather correlated with severity of liver damage.[31] The most important measure of nutritional status in this patient population is the serum albumin level.

Objective measurements have been suggested as a more reliable and accurate way to assess nutritional status. Body mass index (BMI) is one such measure, although the accuracy of this measure has been questioned especially in the presence of peripheral edema or ascites. However, a recent study validated that BMI was reliable when evaluating the nutritional status of patients with liver disease with ascites or peripheral edema.[6] This study defined optimal cutoff values for BMI in patients with no ascites, mild ascites, and tense ascites that had good correlation with other anthropometric measures of nutritional status. The optimal BMI values were 22 $kg/m^2$ in patients with no ascites, 23 $kg/m^2$ in those with mild ascites, and 25 $kg/m^2$ in those with tense ascites.

Anthropometric measurements, such as midarm muscle circumference and triceps skin fold thickness, have also been used as part of a nutritional assessment. When compared with a clinical assessment based on history taking and physical examination, the clinical assessment from the anthropometric measurements differed in 23% of patients.[7] The clinical assessment underestimated the nutritional abnormalities. Based on this finding, the investigators suggested that anthropometric measurements be incorporated into the nutritional assessment of patients with liver disease. However, these measures have been called into question over concerns of interrater reliability and their reliability in patients with ascites.

Subjective global assessment (SGA) is a clinical tool first described more than 2 decades ago and has been used to assess nutritional status in patients with liver disease as well as other disease states.[32] It combines a thorough history taking and physical examination to evaluate and quantify evidence of muscle wasting and loss of subcutaneous fat to classify patients as well nourished, moderately malnourished, or severely malnourished. Although this tool seems simple, it has been criticized because of concerns over its accuracy. However, Duerksen[33] has shown that SGA can be taught to medical students and that these students were able to classify patients reliably as either moderately or severely malnourished using this assessment methodology.

## NUTRITIONAL THERAPY

Because it seems that malnutrition is nearly universal in patients with liver disease, nutritional support is essential in its management. This observation is especially true, given the association between protein-calorie malnutrition and mortality.[6,29,30] Despite this association, consensus has not been achieved to date regarding the amount of nutritional support, use of supplements, and method of delivery of nutrition support. This lack of consensus was demonstrated in a European survey of 33 hepatology units evaluating the practice of nutritional support of patients with acute liver failure in 11 different European countries.[34] Even though some centers had extensive experience with acute liver failure, little consensus was reached with regard to use of enteral versus parental nutrition, amount of glucose and fat infusions in patients receiving parental nutrition, the amount of protein that should be supplied, and the type and amount of amino acid supplementation.

Some of these factors have been addressed in the recently published guidelines from the Society of Critical Care Medicine (SCCM), the American Society for Parenteral and Enteral Nutrition[35] (ASPEN), and the European Society for Clinical Nutrition and Metabolism[36] (ESPEN). The recommendations from the ESPEN have been included in **Tables 1–3**. Enteral nutrition is the preferable route of delivery of nutrition for all patients who are not able to maintain adequate oral intake. It is well accepted that the use of enteral nutrition is less costly and associated with fewer complications and decreased hospital length of stay compared with parenteral nutrition. The goals for caloric intake and protein intake should be 35 to 40 kcal/kg body weight per day and 1.2 to 1.5 g/kg body weight per day, respectively.[36] Protein intake should not be limited as previously thought because it has been shown that doing so increases mortality.

The dogma that protein should be restricted in the diets of patients with liver disease comes from early studies dating back to the 1890s showing that protein-rich blood diverted away from the liver produced neurologic changes that are now recognized

**Table 1**
**Recommendations for enteral nutrition support in patients with alcoholic hepatitis**

| Subject | Recommendation |
|---|---|
| General | Use simple bedside methods such as the SGA or anthropometry to identify patients at risk of undernutrition<br>Recommended energy intake: 35–40 kcal/kg body weight/d<br>Recommended protein intake: 1.2–1.5 g/kg body weight/d |
| Application | Use supplementary enteral nutrition when patients cannot meet their caloric requirements through normal food<br>In general, oral nutritional supplements are recommended |
| Route | Use tube feeding if patients are not able to maintain adequate oral intake (even when esophageal varices are present)<br>Percutaneous endoscopic gastrostomy placement is associated with a higher risk of complications and is not recommended |
| Type of formula | Whole protein formulas are generally recommended<br>Consider using more concentrated high-energy formulas in patients with ascites<br>Use BCAA-enriched formulas in patients with hepatic encephalopathy arising during enteral nutrition |

*Adapted from* Plauth M, Cabre E, Riggio O, et al. ESPEN guidelines on enteral nutrition: liver disease. Clin Nutr 2006;25:286; with permission from Elsevier.

**Table 2**
**Recommendations for enteral nutrition support in patients with liver cirrhosis**

| Subject | Recommendation |
|---------|----------------|
| General | Use simple bedside methods such as the SGA or anthropometry to identify patients at risk of undernutrition |
|         | Use phase angle– or body cell mass–measured bioelectric impedance analysis to quantitate undernutrition despite some limitations in patients with ascites |
|         | Recommended energy intake: 35–40 kcal/kg body weight/d |
|         | Recommended protein intake: 1.2–1.5 g/kg body weight/d |
| Application | Use supplementary enteral nutrition when patients cannot meet their caloric requirements through normal food despite adequate nutritional advice |
|             | In general, oral nutritional supplements are recommended |
| Route | If patients are not able to maintain adequate oral intake from normal food, use oral nutritional supplements or tube feeding (even when esophageal varices are present) |
|       | Percutaneous endoscopic gastrostomy placement is associated with a higher risk of complications and is not recommended |
| Type of formula | Whole protein formulas are generally recommended |
|                 | Consider using more concentrated high-energy formulas in patients with ascites |
|                 | Use BCAA-enriched formulas in patients with hepatic encephalopathy arising during enteral nutrition |
|                 | The use of oral BCAA supplementation can improve clinical outcome in advanced cirrhosis |
| Outcome | Enteral nutrition improves nutritional status and liver function, reduces complications, and improves survival in patients with cirrhosis and is, therefore, recommended |

*Adapted from* Plauth M, Cabre E, Riggio O, et al. ESPEN guidelines on enteral nutrition: liver disease. Clin Nutr 2006;25:286, 287; with permission from Elsevier.

as hepatic encephalopathy.[37–39] It was later determined that ammonia was the causative factor for these neurologic changes.[40] Hyperammonemia results from the production of ammonia in the gut and kidney as well as the decreased breakdown by skeletal muscle[41] caused by loss of skeletal muscle mass in malnourished patients with liver disease. It is well known that ammonia has a direct toxic effect on the brain, specifically the astrocytes. This effect definitely contributes to the neurologic changes seen when patients develop hepatic encephalopathy. In addition, recent research has shown that inflammation, infection, and oxidative stress also play a role in exacerbating the effects of ammonia.[42] Future studies to define the role of antiinflammatory and antioxidative strategies are needed to identify treatment options for hepatic encephalopathy, but protein restriction should not be part of the armamentarium.

The great debate has centered on the use of BCAA-enriched formulations based on the hypothesis that the imbalance between BCAA and AAA contributes to hepatic encephalopathy. This topic has generated a great deal of research and many reviews[43] over the past 30 years since it was initially brought to light by Fischer and Baldessarini.[44] The results of the studies comparing formulas enriched with BCAA versus standard amino acid formulas have been variable. These studies have examined the effect of BCAA on mortality and hepatic encephalopathy. A recent Cochrane review[45] addressed the utility of BCAA as a nutritional adjunct for patients with liver disease. Eleven randomized trials consisting of a total of 556 patients were reviewed.

| Table 3 |
|---|
| **Recommendations for enteral nutrition support in patients undergoing transplant and surgery** |

| Subject | Recommendation |
|---|---|
| General | Use simple bedside methods such as the SGA or anthropometry to identify patients at risk of undernutrition |
| | Use phase angle– or body cell mass–measured bioelectric impedance analysis to quantitate undernutrition despite some limitations in patients with ascites |
| | Recommended energy intake: 35–40 kcal/kg body weight/d |
| | Recommended protein intake: 1.2–1.5 g/kg body weight/d |
| Indication | Preoperative |
| |   Follow recommendations for cirrhosis |
| | Postoperative |
| |   Initiate normal food/enteral nutrition within 12–24 h postoperatively |
| |   Initiate early normal food or enteral nutrition after other surgical procedures |
| Application | Preoperative |
| |   Follow recommendations for cirrhosis |
| |   For children awaiting transplantation, consider BCAA administration |
| | Postoperative |
| |   Recommended energy intake: 35–40 kcal/ kg body weight/d |
| |   Recommended protein intake: 1.2–1.5 g/ kg body weight/d |
| Route | Preoperative |
| |   Follow recommendations for cirrhosis |
| | Postoperative |
| |   Use nasogastric tubes or catheter jejunostomy for early enteral nutrition |
| Type of formula | Preoperative |
| |   Follow recommendations for cirrhosis |
| | Postoperative |
| |   Whole protein formulas are generally recommended |
| |   In patients with ascites, prefer concentrated high-energy formulas for reasons of fluid balance |
| |   Use BCAA-enriched formulas in patients with hepatic encephalopathy arising during enteral nutrition |
| Outcome | Preoperative |
| |   An improvement of perioperative mortality or complication rate by preoperative tube feeding or oral nutritional supplements has not yet been shown |
| |   However, a clear recommendation for nutritional therapy in undernourished patients with liver cirrhosis is supported |
| | Postoperative |
| |   Early normal food or enteral nutrition is recommended for patients with liver cirrhosis undergoing transplant and surgery to minimize perioperative complications (especially infectious complications) |

*Adapted from* Plauth M, Cabre E, Riggio O, et al. ESPEN guidelines on enteral nutrition: liver disease. Clin Nutr 2006;25:287, 288; with permission from Elsevier.

When all of these studies were reviewed, it seemed that there was modest improvement in hepatic encephalopathy but no improvement in mortality or adverse events in the BCAA-supplemented group. However, most studies were of low quality, and when the low-quality studies were not considered in the analysis, there was no significant effect of BCAA on patients with hepatic encephalopathy. In addition, the guidelines from the SCCM and the ASPEN[35] did not recommend using specialized formulas with BCAA in critically ill patients with liver disease. On the other hand, there is some evidence that long-term supplementation with oral BCAA supplements in patients with advanced cirrhosis may be useful in slowing progression of hepatic failure and in improving event-free survival.[46–49] The problem with the use of oral BCAA supplements is long-term compliance, given their poor palatability.[47] Incorporation of the BCAA supplement into granules and capsules may improve palatability,[48] which in turn could lead to greater compliance and better results.

Even though enteral nutrition is the preferred route of nutritional supplementation in patients with liver disease who are not able to maintain adequate oral intake, there are still situations in which parenteral nutrition must be used as an alternative route. The indications for the use of parental nutrition in liver disease have recently been reviewed and published by the ESPEN.[50] These recommendations are shown in **Tables 4–6**. For patients who are moderately or severely malnourished and cannot achieve adequate caloric intake either orally or through enteral feedings, parenteral nutrition should be started immediately. In patients who require fasting for more than 72 hours, it is appropriate to start parenteral nutrition also. Given the low glycogen stores in patients with liver disease, it is important to provide a glucose infusion in these patients if they are not able to take oral nutrients or enteral nutrition for more than 12 hours. The glucose infusion should be used to supply 2 to 3 g/kg body weight per day of glucose.

If parenteral nutrition is required, then the energy goal should be $1.3 \times REE$. Carbohydrates should comprise 50% to 60% of the total nonprotein energy requirements, whereas lipids should make up the other 40% to 50%. Just as when using enteral nutrition, parenteral nutrition should provide 1.2 to 1.5 g amino acids per kilogram body weight per day. For patients with compensated cirrhosis, 1.2 g amino acids

| Table 4 | |
|---|---|
| **Recommendations for parenteral nutrition support in patients with alcoholic hepatitis** | |
| **Subject** | **Recommendation** |
| General | Use simple bedside methods such as the SGA or anthropometry to identify patients at risk of undernutrition |
| | Start parenteral nutrition immediately in moderately or severely malnourished patients who cannot be fed sufficiently either orally or enterally |
| | Give intravenous glucose (2–3 g/kg body weight/d) when patients have to abstain from food for more than 12 h |
| | Give parenteral nutrition when the fasting period lasts longer than 72 h |
| Energy | Provide energy to cover $1.3 \times REE$ |
| | Give glucose to cover 50%–60% of nonprotein energy requirements |
| | Use lipid emulsions with a content of n-6 unsaturated fatty acids lower than in traditional pure soybean oil emulsions |
| Amino acids | Provide amino acids at 1.2–1.5 g/kg body weight/d |
| Micronutrients | Give water-soluble vitamins and trace elements daily from first day of parenteral nutrition |
| | Administer vitamin B1 before starting glucose infusion to reduce the risk of Wernicke encephalopathy |
| Monitoring | Employ repeat blood sugar determinations to detect hypoglycemia and to avoid parenteral nutrition–related hyperglycemia |
| | Monitor phosphate, potassium, and magnesium levels when refeeding malnourished patients |

*Adapted from* Plauth M, Cabre E, Riggio O, et al. ESPEN guidelines on enteral nutrition: liver disease. Clin Nutr 2006;25:436; with permission from Elsevier.

**Table 5**
**Recommendations for parenteral nutrition support in patients with liver cirrhosis**

| Subject | Recommendation |
|---------|----------------|
| General | Use simple bedside methods such as the SGA or anthropometry to identify patients at risk of undernutrition |
| | Start parenteral nutrition immediately in moderately or severely malnourished patients who cannot be fed sufficiently either orally or enterally |
| | Give intravenous glucose (2–3 g/kg body weight/d) when patients have to abstain from food for more than 12 h |
| | Give parenteral nutrition when the fasting period lasts longer than 72 h |
| | Consider parenteral nutrition in patients with unprotected airways and encephalopathy when cough and swallow reflexes are compromised |
| | Use early postoperative parenteral nutrition if patients cannot be nourished sufficiently by either oral or enteral route |
| | After liver transplantation, use early postoperative nutrition; parenteral nutrition is second choice to enteral nutrition |
| Energy | Provide energy to cover 1.3 × REE |
| | Give glucose to cover 50%–60% of nonprotein energy requirements |
| | Use lipid emulsions with a content of n-6 unsaturated fatty acids lower than in traditional pure soybean oil emulsions |
| Amino acids | Provide amino acids at 1.2–1.5 g/kg body weight/d |
| | In patients with grade III or IV encephalopathy consider the use of solutions rich in BCAA and low in AAA, methionine and tryptophan |
| Micronutrients | Give water-soluble vitamins and trace elements daily from first day of parenteral nutrition |
| | In alcoholic liver disease, administer vitamin B1 before starting glucose infusion to reduce the risk of Wernicke encephalopathy |
| Monitoring | Use repeat blood sugar determinations to detect hypoglycemia and to avoid parenteral nutrition–related hyperglycemia |
| | Monitor phosphate, potassium, and magnesium levels when refeeding malnourished patients |

*Adapted from* Plauth M, Cabre E, Riggio O, et al. ESPEN guidelines on enteral nutrition: liver disease. Clin Nutr 2006;25:437; with permission from Elsevier.

per kilogram body weight per day is sufficient, but for those with decompensated cirrhosis, the protein infusion should be increased to 1.5 g/kg body weight per day.

There are some additional considerations for patients who present with acute liver failure, although the data in this area are limited. If these patients are not likely to resume normal oral intake within 5 to 7 days, they should be started on parental nutrition. Amino acids should be administered in acute or subacute liver failure but are not mandatory in hyperacute liver failure. The goal for these patients is 0.8 to 1.2 g amino acid per kilogram body weight per day.

## NUTRITION IN LIVER TRANSPLANT

Protein-calorie malnutrition is present in nearly all patients with liver disease; thus, unless a patient has acute liver failure requiring immediate liver transplant, those other patients on the waiting list for a long period for a liver transplant will be faced with progressive malnutrition and the associated problems described earlier. Malnutrition may be compounded by hypermetabolism as well.[22] A plethora of studies have shown that patients with cirrhosis are at risk for a multitude of complications, decompensation of their liver disease, and increased mortality after elective and emergent surgical

**Table 6**
**Recommendations for parenteral nutrition support in patients with acute liver failure**

| Subject | Recommendation |
|---|---|
| General | Commence artificial nutrition when the patient is unlikely to resume normal oral nutrition within the next 5–7 d |
| | Use parenteral nutrition when patients cannot be fed adequately by enteral nutrition |
| Energy | Provide energy to cover 1.3 × REE |
| | Consider using indirect calorimetry to measure individual energy expenditure |
| | Give intravenous glucose (2–3 g/kg body weight/d) for prophylaxis or treatment of hypoglycemia |
| | In case of hyperglycemia, reduce glucose infusion rate to 2–3 g/kg body weight/d and consider use of intravenous insulin |
| | Consider using lipid (0.8–1.2 g/kg/d) together with glucose to cover energy needs in the presence of insulin resistance |
| Amino acids | In acute or subacute liver failure, provide amino acids at 0.8 g/kg body weight/d |
| Monitoring | Use repeat blood sugar determinations to detect hypoglycemia and to avoid parenteral nutrition–related hyperglycemia |
| | Use repeat blood ammonia determinations to adjust amino acid provision |

*Adapted from* Plauth M, Cabre E, Riggio O, et al. ESPEN guidelines on enteral nutrition: liver disease. Clin Nutr 2006;25:437; with permission from Elsevier.

procedures.[51–54] Liver transplant is certainly no exception.[55] The challenge has been in attempting to define preoperative factors that portend complications, deterioration, and mortality and in developing ways to ameliorate these factors before transplant. Because nutritional support has been shown to benefit patients undergoing liver resection for hepatocellular carcinoma,[56] it is one factor that has been examined to determine if there was a link to outcomes after liver transplant. However, the data in this regard have been sparse and widely varied. Some studies have shown that preoperative malnutrition in liver recipients leads to increases in infectious complications, hospital length of stay, intensive care unit length of stay, blood usage, hospital charges, and mortality,[55,57–59] whereas others have not been able to confirm malnutrition as an independent risk factor for some or all of these bad outcome measures.[60,61]

All patients preparing for liver transplant should have a complete nutritional assessment. Given the well-known benefits associated with adequate nutritional intake, physicians should ensure that patients waiting for a liver transplant receive adequate nutrient intake whether it is via the oral, enteral, or parenteral route. The ESPEN recently published guidelines for nutritional support of patients awaiting liver transplant.[36] As in other patients with liver disease, these patients should be receiving an energy intake of 35 to 40 kcal/kg body weight per day. Because reduced protein intake can actually worsen hepatic encephalopathy, the protein intake should be 1.2 to 1.5 g/kg body weight per day. Any vitamin or micronutrient deficiencies should be corrected as well. For patients in the posttransplant period, if they are unable to resume normal oral intake promptly, then enteral nutrition should begin as early as 12 hours posttransplant. Resuming enteral nutrition within 12 hours of transplant has been shown to reduce postoperative viral infections and to produce better nitrogen retention. Ensuring adequate nutritional intake and correction of vitamin and micronutrient deficiencies may help reduce perioperative morbidity and mortality after liver transplant. Until these questions are resolved, physicians who provide care for patients awaiting liver transplant should pay close attention to nutritional status and intervene appropriately as needed. Starvation is not a reasonable option in these seriously ill and compromised patients.

## SUMMARY

Liver disease is complex and presents difficult challenges for physicians. Malnutrition is nearly universal in patients with liver disease. The physiologic derangements of metabolism are characterized by low glycogen stores, glucose intolerance, insulin resistance, increased protein turnover, and an imbalance between BCAA and AAA that may play a role in encephalopathy. A thorough nutritional assessment is important to unmask signs of malnutrition, but there is no gold standard for making such an assessment. An SGA may be the best technique available to date. For patients who cannot achieve adequate oral intake, enteral nutrition via a nasoenteric tube is the preferred route of delivery, with goals of 35 to 40 kcal/kg body weight per day and 1.2 to 1.5 g protein/kg body weight per day. These same goals should be targeted for patients who have undergone liver transplant whether in the preoperative or postoperative period.

There has been a great deal of interest in nutritional support of patients with liver disease over the past 4 decades. However, many questions are still unanswered regarding nutritional assessment and support of these seriously ill, nutritionally and metabolically complex patients. Future research should be directed at addressing these questions.

## REFERENCES

1. Dudrick SJ, Kavic SM. Hepatobiliary nutrition: history and future. J Hepatobiliary Pancreat Surg 2002;9(4):459–68.
2. O'Grady JG, Schlam SW, Williams R. Acute liver failure: redefining the syndromes. Lancet 1993;342:273–5.
3. Bernal W, Auzinger G, Dhawan A, et al. Acute liver failure. Lancet 2010;376:190–201.
4. Cabre E, Gassull MA. Nutrition in liver disease. Curr Opin Clin Nutr Metab Care 2005;8(5):545–51.
5. O'Brien A, Williams R. Nutrition in end-stage liver disease: principles and practice. Gastroenterology 2008;134(6):1729–40.
6. Campillo B, Richardet JP, Bories PN. Validation of body mass index for the diagnosis of malnutrition in patients with liver cirrhosis. Gastroenterol Clin Biol 2006; 30:1137–43.
7. Italian Multicentre Cooperative Project on nutrition in liver cirrhosis. Nutritional status in cirrhosis. J Hepatol 1994;21:317–25.
8. Madden AM, Bradbury W, Morgam MY. Taste perception in cirrhosis: its relationship to circulating, micronutrients and food preferences. Hepatology 1997;26:40–8.
9. Thuluvath PJ, Triger DR. Autonomic neuropathy and chronic liver disease. Q J Med 1989;72(268):737–47.
10. Chaudhry V, Corse AM, O'Brian R, et al. Autonomic and peripheral (sensorimotor) neuropathy in chronic liver disease: a clinical and electrophysiologic study. Hepatology 1999;29(6):1698–703.
11. Fleckenstein JF, Frank SM, Thuluvath PJ. Presence of autonomic neuropathy is a poor prognostic indicator in patients with advanced liver disease. Hepatology 1996;23(3):471–5.
12. Schoonjans R, Van Vlem B, Vandamme W, et al. Gastric emptying of solids in cirrhotic and peritoneal dialysis patients: influence of peritoneal volume load. Eur J Gastroenterol Hepatol 2002;14(4):395–8.

13. Chesta J, Defilippi C, Defilippi C. Abnormalities in proximal small bowel motility in patients with cirrhosis. Hepatology 1993;17(5):828–32.

14. Galati JS, Holdeman KP, Bottjen PL, et al. Gastric emptying and orocecal transit in portal hypertension and end-stage chronic liver disease. Liver Transpl Surg 1997;3(1):34–8.

15. Maheshwari A, Thuluvath PJ. Autonomic neuropathy may be associated with delayed orocaecal transit time in patients with cirrhosis. Auton Neurosci 2005; 118:135–9.

16. Nagasako CK, de Oliveira Figuerido MJ, de Souza Almeida JR, et al. Investigation of autonomic function and orocecal transit time in patients with nonalcoholic cirrhosis and the potential influence of these factors on disease outcome. J Clin Gastroenterol 2009;43:884–9.

17. Quigley EM. Gastrointestinal dysfunction in liver disease and portal hypertension. Dig Dis Sci 1996;41:557–61.

18. Aqel BA, Scolapio JS, Dickson RC, et al. Contribution of ascites to impaired gastric function and nutritional intake in patients with cirrhosis and ascites. Clin Gastroenterol Hepatol 2005;3(11):1095–100.

19. Kondrup J, Muller MJ. Energy and protein requirements of patients with chronic liver disease. J Hepatol 1997;27(1):239–47.

20. Galati JS, Holdeman KP, Dalrymple GV, et al. Delayed gastric emptying of both the liquid and solid components of a meal in chronic liver disease. Am J Gastroenterol 1994;89(5):708–11.

21. Isobe H, Sakai H, Satoh M, et al. Delayed gastric emptying in patients with liver cirrhosis. Dig Dis Sci 1994;39(5):983–7.

22. Muller MJ, Lautz HU, Plogmann B, et al. Energy expenditure and substrate oxidation in patients with cirrhosis: the impact of cause, clinical staging and nutritional state. Hepatology 1992;15(5):782–94.

23. Petrides AS, DeFronzo RA. Glucose metabolism in cirrhosis: a review with some perspective for the future. Diabetes Metab Rev 1989;5(8):691–709.

24. Swart GR, van den Berg JW, van Vuure JK, et al. Minimum protein requirements in liver cirrhosis determined by nitrogen balance measurements at three levels of protein intake. Clin Nutr 1989;8(6):329–36.

25. Swart GR, Van den Berg JWO, Wattimena JL, et al. Elevated protein requirements in cirrhosis of the liver investigated by whole body protein turnover studies. Clin Sci (Lond) 1988;75(1):101–7.

26. Hiyama DT, Fischer JE. Nutritional support in hepatic failure: the current role of disease-specific therapy. In: Fischer JE, editor. Total Parenteral Nutrition. 2nd Edition. Boston/Toronto/London: Little, Brown and Company; 1991. p. 263–78.

27. Marchesini G, Bugianesi E, Ronchi M, et al. Zinc supplementation improves glucose disposal in patients with cirrhosis. Metabolism 1998;47:792–8.

28. Van der Rijt CC, Schlam SW, Schat H, et al. Overt hepatic encephalopathy precipitated by zinc deficiency. Gastroenterology 1991;100(4):1114–8.

29. Mendenhall CL, Tosch T, Weesner RE, et al. VA cooperative study on alcoholic hepatitis II: prognostic significance of protein-calorie malnutrition. Am J Clin Nutr 1986;43:213–8.

30. Mendenhall CL, Moritz TE, Roselle GA, et al. A study of oral nutritional support with oxandrolone in malnourished patients with alcoholic hepatitis: results of a Department of Veterans Affairs Cooperative Study. Hepatology 1993;17: 564–76.

31. Merli M, Romiti A, Riggio O, et al. Optimal nutritional indexes in chronic liver disease. JPEN J Parenter Enteral Nutr 1987;11(Suppl 5):130S–4S.

32. Detsky AS, McLaughlin JR, Baker JP, et al. What is subjective global assessment of nutritional status? JPEN J Parenter Enteral Nutr 1987;11(1):8–13.
33. Duerksen DR. Teaching medical students the subjective global assessment. Nutrition 2002;18(4):313–5.
34. Schutz T, Bechstein WO, Neuhaus P, et al. Clinical practice of nutrition in acute liver failure—a European survey. Clin Nutr 2004;23(5):975–82.
35. Martindale RG, McClave SA, Vanek VW, et al. Guidelines for the provision and assessment of nutrition support therapy in the adult critically ill patient: Society of Critical Care Medicine and American Society for Parenteral and Enteral Nutrition. Crit Care Med 2009;37(5):1–30.
36. Plauth M, Cabre E, Riggio O, et al. ESPEN guidelines on enteral nutrition: liver disease. Clin Nutr 2006;25:285–94.
37. Hahn M, Massen O, Nencki M, et al. Eck's fistula between the inferior vena cava and the portal vein: its consequences for the organism. Naunyn Schmiedebergs Arch Pharmacol 1893;32:161–210.
38. Nencki M, Pawlow I. On the content of ammonia in blood within organs and on formation of urea in mammals. Naunyn Schmiedebergs Arch Pharmacol 1896; 37:26–51.
39. Nencki M, Zaleski J. On the quantitation of ammonia in animal fluids and tissues. Naunyn Schmiedebergs Arch Pharmacol 1895;36:385–96.
40. Matthews SA. Ammonia, a causative factor in meat poisoning in Eck fistula dogs. Am J Physiol 1922;59:459–60.
41. Shawcross D, Jalan R. The pathophysiologic basis of hepatic encephalopathy: central role for ammonia and inflammation. Cell Mol Life Sci 2005;62(19–20): 2295–304.
42. Seyan AS, Hughes RD, Shawcross DL. Changing face of hepatic encephalopathy: role of inflammation and oxidative stress. World J Gastroenterol 2010; 16(27):3347–57.
43. Charlton M. Branched-chain amino acid enriched supplements as therapy for liver disease. J Nutr 2006;136(Suppl 1):295S–8S.
44. Fischer JE, Baldessarini RJ. False neurotransmitters and hepatic failure. Lancet 1971;2(7715):75–80.
45. Als-Nielsen B, Koretz RL, Gluud LL, et al. Branched-chain amino acids for hepatic encephalopathy. Cochrane Database Syst Rev 2003;2:CD001939.
46. Horst D, Grace ND, Conn HO, et al. Comparison of dietary protein with an oral, branched chain-enriched amino acid supplement in chronic portal-systemic encephalopathy: a randomized controlled trial. Hepatology 1984;4(2):279–87.
47. Marchesini G, Bianchi G, Merli M, et al. Nutritional supplementation with branched-chain amino acids in advanced cirrhosis: a double-blind, randomized trial. Gastroenterology 2003;124:1792–801.
48. Muto Y, Sato S, Watanabe A, et al. Effects of oral branched-chain amino acid granules on event-free survival in patients with liver cirrhosis. Clin Gastroenterol Hepatol 2005;3:705–13.
49. Sato S, Watanabe A, Muto Y, et al. Clinical comparison of branched-chain amino acid (l-leucine, l-isoleucine, l-valine) granules and oral nutrition for hepatic insufficiency with decompensated liver cirrhosis (LIV-EN Study). Hepatol Res 2005; 31(4):232–40.
50. Plauth M, Cabre E, Campillo B, et al. ESPEN guidelines on parenteral nutrition: hepatology. Clin Nutr 2009;28:436–44.
51. Ziser A, Plevak DJ. Morbidity and mortality in cirrhotic patients undergoing anesthesia and surgery. Curr Opin Anaesthesiol 2001;14(6):707–11.

52. Doberneck RC, Sterling WA Jr, Allison DC. Morbidity and mortality after operation in nonbleeding cirrhotic patients. Am J Surg 1983;146(3):306–9.

53. Rice HE, O'Keefe GE, Helton WS, et al. Morbid prognostic features in patients with chronic liver failure undergoing nonhepatic surgery. Arch Surg 1997; 132(8):880–4 [discussion: 884–5].

54. Garrison RN, Cryer HM, Howard DA, et al. Clarification of risk factors for abdominal operations in patients with hepatic cirrhosis. Ann Surg 1984;199(6):648–55.

55. Selberg O, Bottcher J, Tusch G, et al. Identification of high- and low-risk patients before liver transplantation: a prospective cohort study of nutritional and metabolic parameters. Hepatology 1997;25:652–7.

56. Fan ST, Lo CM, Lai EC, et al. Perioperative nutritional support in patients undergoing hepatectomy for hepatocellular carcinoma. N Engl J Med 1994;331(23): 1547–52.

57. Stephenson GR, Moretti EW, El-Moalem H, et al. Malnutrition in liver transplant patients: preoperative subjective global assessment is predictive of outcome after liver transplantation. Transplantation 2001;72(4):666–70.

58. Merli M, Giusto M, Gentili F, et al. Nutritional status: its influence on the outcome of patients undergoing liver transplantation. Liver Int 2010;30(2):208–14.

59. Figueiredo F, Dickson ER, Pasha T, et al. Impact of nutritional status on outcomes after liver transplantation. Transplantation 2000;70(9):1347–52.

60. de Luis DA, Izaola O, Velicia MC, et al. Impact of dietary intake and nutritional status on outcomes after liver transplantation. Rev Esp Enferm Dig 2006;98(1): 6–13.

61. Shahid M, Johnson J, Nightingale P, et al. Nutritional markers in liver allograft recipients. Transplantation 2005;79(3):359–62.

# Nutritional Therapy in Critically Ill and Injured Patients

Rifat Latifi, MD[a,b,*]

**KEYWORDS**

- Critically ill • Amino acid • Acute phase protein
- Intensive care unit • Trauma • ARDS • Sepsis
- Immunonutrition

The vocabulary and practice of nutrition support of critically ill patients have changed significantly in recent years and new nutripharmaceuticals and disease-oriented nutritional support have become integral components of patient care in the new era of comprehensive management. The question to be answered is when to feed and what to feed critically ill and injured patients. Critical illness and tissue injury initiate a complex series of rapidly responding homeostatic events in an attempt to prevent ongoing tissue damage and to activate the repair process. Classically, inflammation has been recognized as the hallmark of the homeostatic response. But more recently, attention has been focused on defining the complexities of response at the cellular, metabolic, and molecular levels. There is mounting evidence regarding the multiple specific metabolic changes in critically ill and injured patients and their need for fundamental nutrients and special substrates. As there are efforts to refine and further define nutritional support for critically ill patients, pursuing a deeper understanding of this field is imperative. Specifically, to provide timely and disease-directed and disorder-directed nutritional support, the most crucial changes in acute phase proteins, cytokines, and other biochemical indices must be elucidated. Furthermore, it has already become clear that no 1 care plan or formula fits all situations in all patients. Rather, nutritional support must be based principally on each individual patient's pathophysiology and condition.

The benefit of early institution of adequate enteral or parenteral nutrition in the overall management of critically ill patients has been well established. Early nutritional support has the potential to reduce disease severity, diminish complications, and decrease the intensive care unit (ICU) length of stay. In general, whenever possible,

Author has no conflicts of interest to declare.

[a] Trauma Division, Department of Surgery, University of Arizona, PO Box 245063, 1501 North Campbell Avenue, Tucson, AZ 85724, USA

[b] Trauma Services, Hamad General Hospital, Hamad Medical Corporation, Doha, Qatar

* Trauma Division, Department of Surgery, University of Arizona, PO Box 245063, 1501 North Campbell Avenue, Tucson, AZ 85724.

E-mail address: Latifi@surgery.arizona.edu

Surg Clin N Am 91 (2011) 579–593
doi:10.1016/j.suc.2011.02.002
0039-6109/11/$ – see front matter © 2011 Elsevier Inc. All rights reserved.

surgical.theclinics.com

the gastrointestinal (GI) tract is the optimal route of providing nutrition in critically ill patients. If, on the other hand, a patient cannot receive all the needed nutrient substrates and calories enterally, nutrition should be provided parenterally.[1] Because of the recent advances in identifying and recognizing the fundamental metabolic changes of crucial nutrient substrates in critically ill patients, nutritional formulas are being designed to compensate for these changes and support the organism during critical illness, infection, trauma, and/or severe sepsis. One example of such an approach to the nutritional support of critically ill patients is the provision of immune-enhancing formulas (IEFs), which have been shown to improve immune responses both in laboratory animals and critically ill patients. These enteral formulas contain increased amounts of peptides; arginine; glutamine; vitamins E, A, and C; nucleotides and nucleosides; branched-chain amino acids (BCAAs); and ω-3 fatty acids. It is suggested that these principal nutrients can modulate and affect a variety of inflammatory, metabolic, and immune processes if given in doses higher than those ordinarily recommended or required.

## STRESS RESPONSE

The sequence of responses to stress and injury has been described as the ebb phase, the catabolic flow phase, and the anabolic flow phase.[2–4] Each of these phases induces distinct changes that require specific interventions to eliminate or minimize the untoward consequences of illness and/or injury. The ebb phase is dominated by circulatory changes that require resuscitation (with fluid, blood, and blood products) over a period of the first 8 to 24 hours. The catabolic flow phase, dominated by high levels of catabolism, typically lasts 3 to 10 days, but may last longer. The anabolic flow phase emerges more subtly as the patient's metabolism shifts to synthetic activities and reparative processes.[4] The catabolic flow phase is driven by cytokine mediators released from lymphocytes and macrophages in the cellular immune reaction, dominated by interleukin (IL)-6.[4] The release of these mediators is proportional to the intensity of the injury, but the release of the individual cytokines is also upregulated by hormonal and humoral events.[4] The early nonspecific reaction to systemic tissue injury that is responsible for the reprioritization of protein synthesis in the liver is termed the acute phase response (APR).[5–7] Depending on the magnitude and severity of the injury, APR is characterized by an exponential increase levels of positive acute phase proteins and a decrease levels of negative acute phase proteins. The regulation of APR, a complex process, depends on many factors. Tissue injury or infection leads to a local inflammatory response, which in turn leads to the release of many cytokines at the site of inflammation; the cytokines are eventually carried to the liver, where they act on the hepatocytes. These proteins reach a maximum concentration within a few days after the onset of tissue damage and return to their normal concentrations within a week.[8] A variety of cytokines have been implicated in the production of acute phase proteins from the liver, including IL-1 and IL-6 and tumor necrosis factor-α.[8] This pattern is predictable and reproducible. First, the serum concentration decreases for most of the acute phase proteins, both for positive and negative reactants. Later, the hepatic synthesis of negative acute phase proteins decreases, and the concentration of serum albumin remains depressed for days to weeks after the injury. The albumin level usually reaches the lowest point by the fifth postinjury day.[9] Whether specifically tailored nutritional support in the immediate postinjury phase can alter or blunt the APR has not been adequately answered.[6]

C-reactive protein is the earliest acute phase reactant to respond to stress, and its serum concentration peaks at 48 hours.[8] The serum protein concentration of positive acute phase proteins after minor injuries ordinarily returns to normal within the first week after injury. Continued and prolonged production of acute phase proteins in critically ill patients may be an indicator of ongoing sepsis and tissue damage and is associated with higher mortality rates.[9] Perhaps some of the changes at this stage are responsible for what is defined as compensatory antiinflammatory response syndrome.[10]

Positive acute phase proteins seem to act as a protective response to tissue injury. These proteins have diverse functions as antioxidants, proteolytic inhibitors, and mediators of coagulation. The negative acute phase proteins include albumin, prealbumin (PA), retinol-binding protein, and transferrin. Their serum concentrations decrease immediately after the injury, in proportion to the severity of the injury. These proteins are used clinically primarily to attempt to monitor the nutritional status of acutely ill patients, with a moderate degree of success.

## PROTEIN AND NITROGEN METABOLISM IN CRITICALLY ILL PATIENTS

Severely injured and critically ill patients characteristically demonstrate significant muscle losses, negative nitrogen balance, increased requirements of up to 2 to 3 times the normal, and redistribution of amino acids from the peripheral tissues to the splanchnic organs.

Metabolic response to injury is characterized by the striking increase in protein catabolism. Skeletal muscle and nitrogen losses after injury occur as a result. The process of increased nitrogen losses is complex and correlates with the increased metabolic rate, which peaks several days after injury and gradually returns toward normal over several weeks.[2,11–14] This phenomenon occurs consistently after blunt injury, burns, sepsis, and various other major injuries[15–19] and is accompanied by mobilization and increased use of nutrient substrates such as fatty acids, amino acids, and glucose.[20] Increased muscle protein catabolism after injury has also been consistently demonstrated,[18,19] seems thus far to be irreversible, and is proportional in magnitude to that of the injury.

## AMINO ACID METABOLISM

Although plasma amino acid levels have been measured in critically ill and injured patients in an effort to identify specific changes related to the catabolic response, the results have been inconsistent.[19,21] Nonetheless, the adverse consequences for the critically ill patient are a rapid loss of muscle mass and subsequent marked debility. All amino acids in the body cell mass are required for optimal protein synthesis; however, alanine and glutamine are the major carriers of nitrogen from muscle, constituting as much as 70% of the amino acids released from skeletal muscle after injury.[22]

Alanine is a major substrate for the production of glucose by the liver. Glutamine has been identified as the primary fuel for enterocytes, and for other rapidly dividing masses of cells, where it is converted to alanine. The use of glutamine by the intestine as an oxidative fuel has a sparing effect on glucose. During sepsis, glutamine depletion is even more severe and lasts longer than the generalized protein depletion associated with the hypercatabolism after injury. Furthermore, glutamine, a nonessential amino acid, serves as an important respiratory substrate not only for the enterocytes but also for other rapidly dividing cells, including the bone marrow, endothelial cells, and proliferating cells in wounds and areas of inflammation.[23,24] After surgical interventions, glutamine consumption by the GI tract is greatly increased.[25,26]

In sepsis, the lungs and kidneys, in addition to the skeletal muscle, become organs of net glutamine release.[27,28] Furthermore, during sepsis, the liver increases glutamine uptake and becomes the primary organ for glutamine use.[28]

In the presence of endotoxemia, glutamine may be used in the liver for gluconeogenesis, ureagenesis, and synthesis of proteins, nucleotides, and glutathione.[29,30] After surgery, severe injury, or sepsis, the rapid decrease in the level of glutamine in the plasma and in the intracellular pool is greater than that of any other amino acid, and plasma glutamine concentration is inversely correlated with the severity of the underlying insult. The plasma glutamine concentration is reversed toward normal only late in the course of recovery.[30] Glutamine supplementation has been shown to exert trophic effects on intestinal mucosa. Total parenteral nutrition (TPN) solutions, enriched with glutamine, increase jejunal mucosal weight, nitrogen levels, and DNA content, and significantly decrease atrophy of the villi.[31] Furthermore, glutamine prevents deterioration of gut permeability and has been proved to be beneficial for patients with intestinal mucosal injury secondary to chemotherapy and radiation.[32–34] Hepatic steatosis, pancreatic atrophy, and bacterial translocation from the gut, which are sometimes associated with standard TPN solutions, are reduced by the use of glutamine-supplemented TPN solutions.[35–37] Glutamine also improves the nitrogen balance and reduces the skeletal muscle glutamine loss in patients after elective cholecystectomy and other major surgical procedures.[38] Administration of glutamine in TPN as dipeptide glutamine complexes has decreased the incidence of infections in bone marrow transplant patients.[39]

Arginine is considered a nonessential amino acid in the diet of healthy adults because the endogenous pathways can readily synthesize adequate amounts of this amino acid from available substrates in the metabolic pool. Arginine stimulates the release of growth hormone and prolactin, and can also induce a marked release of insulin.[40] Supplementing the diet with arginine has been shown to improve weight gain, increase nitrogen retention, and accelerate wound healing in animals and human beings.[41] The trophic effects of arginine on the immune system in human beings have also been demonstrated.[41] In both animals and human beings, plasma arginine levels decrease promptly and significantly after a burn injury.[42,43]

## IMMUNONUTRITION AND IMMUNOMODULATION

Immunonutrition or immune-enhancing diets (IEDs) continue to gain wider use in the care of critically ill and injured patients. This trend follows an increasing body of literature supporting the concept that different specific nutrient substrates enhance a depressed immune system or modulate an overreactive immune system. Although the biological properties of immune-enhancing nutritional substrates have been well studied, their role in routine clinical care remains controversial. Multiple meta-analyses have shown that IED formulations when compared with standard nutritional regimens are associated with reductions in ventilator days, infectious morbidity, and hospital length of stay. However, studies have yet to show an increased survival benefit with their use. Moreover, most of those studies assessed a combination of immune-enhancing substrates, commonly in the form of a commercially available formulation. Therefore, the evidence documenting the efficacy and effect of each of the individual components is much more difficult to identify.

## KEY NUTRIENTS
### Glutamine

As stated earlier, glutamine is an amino acid that serves as the primary fuel for small bowel enterocytes and other rapidly proliferating cells, such as cells in wounds.[24] It is classified as a nonessential amino acid because the human body can ordinarily synthesize it in sufficient quantities. However, during periods of stress, the body's accentuated requirements may exceed its capacity to synthesize adequate amounts of glutamine.[44–46] Glutamine is involved in many immune functions, including the production of heat shock proteins.[47] Studies have shown that dietary supplementation with glutamine may lead to decreases in nosocomial infections in patients with systemic inflammatory response and a decrease in pneumonia, sepsis, and bacteremia in trauma patients; other studies, however, have refuted any effect of glutamine on reducing mortality.[48–51] Parenterally administered glutamine has been associated with a decrease in gram-negative bacteremia.[52] Thus, the addition of glutamine to enteral nutrition regimens has been recommended for burn and trauma patients and other patients in the ICU in the 2009 Society of Critical Care Medicine (SCCM)/American Society for Parenteral and Enteral Nutrition (A.S.P.E.N.) nutritional guidelines.[53]

## Arginine

Similar to glutamine, arginine is considered a nonessential amino acid in healthy individuals, but its role becomes much more important in critically ill patients because requirements for arginine increase during periods of stress.[54] Arginine seems to be necessary for normal T-lymphocyte function, and levels of arginine are closely regulated by specialized immune cells known as myeloid suppressor cells.[53]

Arginine may also stimulate the release of hormones such as growth hormone, prolactin, and insulin.[55] Moreover, arginine seems to have trophic effects on the immune system in humans, in addition to increasing weight gain, increasing nitrogen retention, and improving wound healing.[56–58] A systematic review of 22 randomized clinical trials (RCTs) showed in an a priori subgroup analysis that patients fed commercial formulations with high arginine levels experienced a significant reduction in infectious complications. Furthermore, surgical patients seemed to have the greatest benefits from arginine when compared with their nonsurgical counterparts.[57]

The use of arginine supplementation, however, has been linked to a potentially increased mortality rate in hemodynamically unstable septic patients when compared with those patients who received standard enteral and parenteral nutrition.[59,60] The proposed mechanism for this adverse outcome is that arginine is a biosynthetic substrate for nitric oxide (NO) production and that increased levels of NO can then lead to increased vasodilation and further hemodynamic instability.[57,60] But other studies have disputed those findings and, instead, showed a reduced mortality rate in moderately septic patients.[61] Resolution of these differences require additional, carefully controlled and monitored clinical studies. The idea that nutritional support with formulas containing arginine increases mortality is simply not logical or plausible; most hemodynamically unstable patients do not receive large enough amounts of enteral nutrition during the acute deterioration phase to induce any significant effect on their hemodynamic status.

## Nucleotides

Nucleotides are perhaps best known for their roles in the synthesis of DNA and RNA and hence, for their roles in genetic coding. However, nucleotides also play a role in ATP metabolism as components of many coenzymes involved in carbohydrate, protein, and lipid syntheses. Nucleotides may be synthesized by some cells, but it is thought that rapidly dividing cells, such as epithelial cells and T lymphocytes, are unable to produce nucleotides, and accordingly, during periods of stress, a relative deficit of nucleotides develops.[62] Nucleotides have been implicated in the modulation of immune function, and exogenous nucleotides have been found to be required for the helper/inducer T-cell response.[63] In the clinical setting, IED-containing nucleotides have been shown to reduce infections, ventilator days, and length of hospital stay significantly for both critically ill and postsurgical patients.[64] However, those studies have not addressed the isolated effects of nucleotides as substrates, so that further studies identifying their individual specific therapeutic benefits are needed to clarify this information.[65]

### Antioxidant Vitamins and Trace Minerals

Oxidative stress has been increasingly recognized as a central component of the pathophysiology of critical illness. Nutrients with antioxidant properties include vitamins E and C (ascorbic acid); trace minerals include selenium, zinc, and copper. A meta-analysis of 11 clinical trials showed overall that use of antioxidants was associated with a significant reduction in mortality (relative risk [RR], 0.65; 95% confidence interval [CI], 0.44–0.97; $P$ = .03), but had no effect on infectious complications.[66] Among the antioxidants, selenium may be the most effective.[67,68]

A systematic analysis suggested that selenium supplementation, with or without other antioxidants, was associated with a reduction in mortality (RR, 0.59; 95% CI, 0.32–1.08; $P$ = .09).[66] The current recommendation is to provide a combination of antioxidant vitamins and trace minerals, especially a regimen including selenium, to all critically ill patients receiving specialized nutrition therapy.[53,68]

## ω-3 FATTY ACIDS

Dietary ω-3 fatty acids are rapidly incorporated into the cell membranes, influencing membrane stability, membrane fluidity, cell mobility, and cell signaling pathways. Moreover, they are able to mitigate the potency of the inflammatory response and have thus been implicated in the reduction of cardiovascular disorders. In an animal model, these fatty acids protected against bacterial translocation and gut-derived sepsis whether or not the diet was also supplemented with arginine or glutamine.[69] Their role in modulating the immune system in conditions such as acute respiratory distress syndrome (ARDS) is also well known.

## BCAAS

After injury and/or sepsis, an energy deficit that may develop in skeletal muscle is met by increased oxidation of BCAAs. Ample evidence indicates that skeletal muscle is the major site of BCAA metabolism.[70–73]

A recent study demonstrated that critically ill patients who were unable to be fed enterally, but who were given TPN fortified with BCAAs at high concentrations (at either 23% or 45%) had significantly lower morbidity and mortality when compared with patients receiving standard TPN (1.5 g/kg/d of protein).[73] The decrease in mortality correlated with higher doses of BCAAs (at 0.5 g/kg/d or higher).[73]

Furthermore, BCAA-rich parenteral nutrition formulas have been shown to correct the plasma amino acid imbalance that consistently exists in critically ill patients. Such formulas also improve plasma concentrations of PA and retinol-binding protein in septic patients. In a series of trauma patients, BCAA supplementation improved nitrogen retention, transferrin levels, and lymphocyte counts. Because the concentration of BCAAs is low in septic patients, probably as a result of heavy use of BCAAs, nutritional supplementation with BCAAs may be beneficial. BCAAs are thought to be required for lymphocytes to synthesize protein, RNA, and DNA, as well as to divide in response to stimulation.[74]

## IMMUNE-MODULATING NUTRITION IN ARDS AND SEPSIS

ARDS is a constellation of clinical, radiological, and physiologic abnormalities that is observed in a variety of medical and surgical patients. It is an entity that occurs in a subset of patients with severe acute lung injury (ALI); it may coexist with left arterial or pulmonary capillary hypertension. ARDS is defined by its acute onset, bilateral infiltrates on a chest radiogram, a pulmonary artery wedge pressure less than 18 mm Hg, and a PaO2/FiO2 ratio of less than 200.[75]

Many clinical conditions and factors, direct or indirect, are associated with the development of ARDS. The direct causes of pulmonary injury include traumatic contusions, aspiration, pneumonia, and inhalation injuries from caustic substances or chemicals. Indirect causes include sepsis, polytrauma, shock, massive blood transfusion, and pancreatitis. The common clinical entity is the underlying inflammatory response in the lung itself, regardless of whether or not the primary insult occurred in the lung.

The management of ARDS has encompassed an array of supportive measures, including, most recently, low tidal volume mechanical ventilation. Other measures include aggressive pulmonary toilet, pressure control ventilation (with or without inverse ratio ventilation), and proning (prone positioning of the patient). Failure of these measures has prompted the use of others, such as tracheal gas insufflation, inhaled NO, extracorporeal membrane oxygenation, high-frequency oscillatory ventilation, and partial liquid ventilation. Most such measures, however, are merely supportive because they do not address the main issue in ARDS, which is immunologic derangement at the molecular level.

Furthermore, evidence from pulmonary lavage indicates that a neutrophil-predominant pulmonary edema fluid is partly responsible for the development of ARDS.[75] Activation of neutrophils and proinflammatory cytokines initiates or exacerbates the inflammatory response in ARDS and ALI, increasing capillary permeability, resulting in severe acute hypoxemia due to pulmonary edema, and ultimately leading to fibrosing alveolitis or fibrotic lung injury, which causes a higher mortality rate. Dietary fish oil and borage oil have been implicated in suppression of the intrapulmonary inflammatory response by modulating the eicosanoid pathway, leading to overall decreased levels of neutrophils in bronchoalveolar lavage. Moreover, fish oil and borage oil alter the fatty acid composition of lung phospholipids by decreasing the arachidonic acid level and increasing the eicosapentaenoic acid (EPA) level.[76] When fish oil and borage oil are used in combination, the dihomo-γ-linolenic acid level increases as well. It has been suggested that the incorporation of EPA into phospholipids modulates the eicosanoid metabolism, causing it to produce the less biologically active 3-series prostaglandins and 5-series leukotrienes (LTs).[77,78] In animal models, the inhibition of LTB$_4$ has been shown to reduce vascular permeability in the lungs and to decrease the response of neutrophils to endotoxins.

Experiments have also shown that supplementation of parenteral nutrition with γ-linolenic acid (GLA) increased prostaglandin E$_1$ (PGE$_1$) and the plasma arachidonic acid ratio. In an animal model, such supplementation also reduced the ratio of thromboxane B$_2$ and 6-keto-prostaglandin F1α. Those effects were induced via the increase in levels of dihomo-γ-linolenic acid (a precursor to the antiinflammatory eicosanoids) and via the increase in levels of PGE$_1$, which modulates the arachidonic acid pathway.

## EVIDENCE-BASED NUTRITIONAL SUPPORT

A prospective, multicenter, double-blinded, randomized controlled trial involving 146 patients with ARDS first showed a benefit of the EPA + GLA + antioxidants diet on pulmonary neutrophil recruitment, gas exchange, mechanical ventilation requirements, length of ICU stay, and new organ failures. In that trial, patients in the 2 randomization arms received, for at least 4 to 7 days, either an enteral formulation with EPA + GLA or an isonitrogenous isocaloric standard diet.[79]

Subsequent studies by the same authors also showed a decrease in levels of inflammatory mediators from bronchoalveolar lavage fluids (BALFs), namely, IL-8 and LTB$_4$, as well as an associated decrease in BALF neutrophils and protein permeability, suggesting a possible mechanism of the observed benefit.[80] A subsequent single-center, prospective, randomized controlled unlabeled study expanded the criteria to include patients with ALI in addition to those with ARDS; oxygenation and lung compliance improved.[81]

Subsequently, another prospective, multicenter, double-blinded, randomized controlled trial involving 165 patients showed a significant decrease in the 28-day mortality rate (absolute mortality reduction, 19.4%, $P = .037$) in patients with sepsis or septic shock, requiring mechanical ventilation, who received the EPA + GLA + antioxidants diet, when compared with the control group. Moreover, in patients receiving that diet compared with those in the control group, the number of ventilator-free days (13.4 ± 1.2 vs 5.8 ± 1.0 days) and ICU-free days (10.8 ± 1.1 vs 4.6 ± 0.9 days) also increased, and new organ dysfunction significantly decreased.[82]

A recent meta-analysis of 24 RCTs assessed the outcome of critically ill patients randomized to an immune-modulating (IM) diet, which included supplementation with arginine, glutamine, fish oil, and combinations of these components. The IM diet, when compared with the control diet, had no effect on the mortality rate or the length of hospital stay. However, a subgroup analysis showed that patients with systemic inflammatory response syndrome (SIRS), sepsis, or ARDS who received fish oil alone had a significantly improved outcome in terms of the mortality rate, the rate of secondary infections, and the length of hospital stay.[83]

The 3 RCTs mentioned in the meta-analysis that addressed fish oil alone are summarized in **Table 1**. The SCCM/A.S.P.E.N. guidelines include a grade A recommendation, for patients with ARDS and ALI, for an enteral formula with an antiinflammatory lipid profile (EPA + GLA) and with antioxidants, given the consistent evidence provided by those 3 large RCTs.[53] Grade A designates the strongest recommendation, supported by at least 2 large RCTs with clear-cut results and a low risk of false-positive (alpha error) or false-negative (beta error) results.

## IMMUNONUTRITION IN GI TRACT SURGERY

The role and effectiveness of immunonutrition in patients undergoing upper GI tract surgery have been studied and debated extensively in the literature.[83–93] According to a meta-analysis of 11 randomized controlled clinical trials of enteral nutrition with an IEF that included 1009 patients, nutritional support supplemented with key nutrients (arginine, glutamine, BCAAs, nucleotides, and ω-3 fatty acids) significantly reduced the risk of developing infectious complications and reduced the overall hospital stay in critically ill patients and in patients with GI cancer.[94] Fukuda and colleagues[87] found that the perioperative administration of immunonutrition in patients undergoing esophagectomy reduced infectious complications and shortened the length of hospital stay ($P<.05$) when compared with the control group. Similarly, Braga and colleagues,[85] in a prospective randomized study of patients with malignancy of the upper GI tract demonstrated that immunonutrition improved their outcomes. However, other investigators of the GI tract found no major differences, although major study design issues have been pointed out.[89–91]

A study of patients undergoing mastectomy found that preoperative oral IEFs supplemented with arginine and ω-3 fatty acids enhanced the patients' immune status, reduced the length of SIRS, and reduced the rate of perioperative infections.[92] Still another study of patients with cancer found that enteral nutrition enriched with

**Table 1**
Antiinflammatory IM enteral nutrition (Oxepa[a]) versus standard enteral nutrition (Stand EN) in patients with ARDS, ALI, and sepsis

| Study | Population | Study Groups | Mortality | LOS Days, Mean ± SD | Vent Days, Mean ± SD | New Organ Dysfunction |
|---|---|---|---|---|---|---|
| Gadek et al,[79] 1999 | ARDS ICU (n = 146) | Oxepa | 11/70 (16%) ICU | 11.0 ± 0.9 ICU[b] | 9.6 ± 0.9[b] | 7/70 (10%)[b] |
| | | Stand EN | 19/76 (25%) ICU | 14.8 ± 1.3 ICU | 13.2 ± 1.4 | 19/76 (25%) |
| | | Oxepa | | 27.9 ± 2.1 hospital | | |
| | | Stand EN | | 31.1 ± 2.4 hospital | | |
| Singer et al,[81] 2006 | ARDS and ALI (n = 100) | Oxepa | 14/46 (30%) at 28 d[b] | 13.5 ± 11.8 ICU | 12.1 ± 11.3 | NR |
| | | Stand EN | 26/49 (53%) at 28 d | 15.6 ± 11.8 ICU | 14.7 ± 12.0 | |
| Pontes-Arruda et al,[82] 2006 | Severe sepsis ICU (n = 165) | Oxepa | 26/83 (31%) at 28 d[b] | 17.2 ± 4.9 ICU[b] | 14.6 ± 4.3[b] | 32/83 (39%)[b] |
| | | Stand EN | 38/82 (46%) at 28 d | 23.4 ± 3.5 ICU | 22.2 ± 5.1 | 66/82 (80%) |

*Abbreviations:* LOS, length of stay; NR, not reported.
[a] Oxepa, Abbott Nutrition, Columbus, OH, USA.
[b] $P < .05$.

*Data from* McClave SA, Martindale RG, Vanek VW, et al. Guidelines for the provision and assessment of nutrition support therapy in the adult critically ill patient: Society of Critical Care Medicine (SCCM) and American Society for Parenteral and Enteral Nutrition (A.S.P.E.N.). JPEN J Parenter Enteral Nutr 2009;33:277–316; and Kien CL, Young VR, Rohrbaugh DK, et al. Increased rates of whole body protein synthesis and breakdown in children recovering from burns. Ann Surg 1978;187:383–91.

immune-enhancing nutrients was associated with preservation of lean body mass.[93] A consensus panel from a recent conference on immune-enhancing enteral therapy recommended the use of IEDs in the following 2 groups of patients: (1) severely malnourished patients (albumin levels <3.5 g/dL) undergoing upper GI tract surgery and patients with albumin levels less than 2.8 g/dL undergoing lower GI tract surgery and (2) patients with blunt or penetrating torso trauma with an injury severity score greater than 18, or an abdominal trauma index less than 20.[94]

## SUMMARY

Nutritional support of critically ill or injured patients has undergone significant advances in the last few decades. These advances are the direct result of the growing scientific progress and increased knowledge of the biology and biochemistry of key metabolic and nutrient changes induced by injury, sepsis, and other critical illnesses, both in adults and children. As this knowledge has increased, the science of nutritional support has become more disease based and disorder based. Depending on the individual patient's metabolic needs, key nutrients are replenished or added in larger amounts to supplement specific deficiencies or to prevent further deterioration and clinical consequences. However, choosing or constructing the ideal nutrient formulations for the various critically ill or injured patients is increasingly complex: the resultant specifically designed formulas, like manna from Heaven, will be expected to mitigate the body's metabolic response to injury, balance oxidative processes, and help regulate or moderate the immune system, which may be deranged because of the underlying disease, while additionally providing the balanced nutrients required for normal maintenance, structure, and function.

This is a daunting challenge, indeed, and much more sophisticated, labor-intensive, and judicious clinical investigation and care will be required to accomplish the desired accumulation of the unequivocal knowledge and data leading to optimal patient outcomes.

## REFERENCES

1. Ziegler T. Parenteral nutrition in the critically ill patient. N Engl J Med 2009;361: 1088–97.
2. Cuthbertson DP. Observations on the disturbance of metabolism produced by injury to the limbs. Q J Med 1932;1:233–46.
3. Hill AG, Hill GL. Metabolic response to severe injury. Br J Surg 1998;85:884–90.
4. Ingenblek Y, Berstein L. The stressful condition as a nutritional adaptive dichotomy. Nutrition 1999;15(4):305–20.
5. Azimuddin K, Latifi R, Ivatury R. Acute phase proteins in critically ill patients. In: Latifi R, Dudrick SJ, editors. The biology and practice of current nutritional support. 2nd edition. Georgetown (TX): Landes Bioscience; 2003. p. 63–71.
6. Kudlackova M, Andel M, Hajkova H, et al. Acute phase proteins and prognostic inflammatory and nutritional index (PINI) in moderately burned children aged up to three years. Burns 1990;16:53–6.
7. Boosalis MG, Ott L, Levine AS, et al. Relationship of visceral proteins to nutritional status in chronic and acute stress. Crit Care Med 1989;17:741–74.
8. Castell JV, Gomez-Lechon MJ, David M, et al. Acute-phase response of human hepatocytes: regulation of acute-phase protein synthesis by interleukin-6. Hepatology 1990;12:1179–86.
9. Issihiki H, Akira S, Sugita T, et al. Reciprocal expression of NF-IL6 and C/EBP in hepatocytes: possible involvement of NF-IL6 in acute phase protein gene expression. New Biol 1991;3(1):63–70.

10. Bankey PE, Mazuski JE, Ortiz M, et al. Hepatic acute phase protein synthesis is indirectly regulated by tumor necrosis factor. J Trauma 1990;30:1181–7.
11. Latifi R, Caushaj PE. Nutrition support in critically ill patients: current status and practice. J Clin Ligand Assay 1999;22:279–84.
12. Wilmore DW, Orcutt TW, Mason AD Jr, et al. Alterations in hypothalamic function following thermal injury. J Trauma 1975;15:697–703.
13. Birkhahn RH, Long CL, Fitkin D, et al. Effects of major skeletal trauma on whole body protein turnover in man measured by L-[1, 14C]-leucine. Surgery 1980;88:294–308.
14. Kien CL, Young VR, Rohrbaugh DK, et al. Increased rates of whole body protein synthesis and breakdown in children recovering from burns. Ann Surg 1978;187:383–91.
15. Levenson SM, Pulaski EJ, del Guercio LR. Metabolic changes associated with injury. In: Zimmerman LM, Levine R, editors. Physiological principles of surgery. 2nd edition. Philadelphia: WB Saunders; 1964. p. 5–7.
16. Young VR, Munro HN. N-methylhistidine (3-methylhistidine) and muscle protein turnover: an overview. Fed Proc 1978;37:2291–300.
17. Bilmazes C, Kien CL, Rohrbaugh DK, et al. Quantitative contributors by skeletal muscle to elevated rates of whole-body protein breakdown in burned children as measured by 3-methylhistidine output. Metabolism 1978;27:671–6.
18. Williamson DH, Farrell R, Kerr A, et al. Muscle protein catabolism after injury in man as measured by urinary excretion of 3-methylhistidine. Clin Sci Mol Med 1977;52:527–33.
19. Long CL, Schiller WR, Blakemore WS, et al. Muscle protein catabolism in the septic patient as measured by 3-methylhistidine excretion. Am J Clin Nutr 1977;30:1349–52.
20. Essen P, McNurlan MA, Gamrin L, et al. Tissue protein synthesis rates in critically ill patients. Crit Care Med 1998;26:92–100.
21. Latifi R, Dudrick SJ, editors. Surgical nutrition: strategies in critically ill. Austin (TX): Springer-Verlag/R.G.Landes; 1995.
22. Garber AJ, Karl IE, Kipnis DM. Alanine and glutamine synthesis and release from skeletal muscle. I: glycolysis and amino acid release. J Biol Chem 1976;251:826–35.
23. Souba WW, Wilmore DW. Postoperative alteration of arteriovenous exchange of amino acids across the gastrointestinal tract. Surgery 1983;94:342–50.
24. Souba WW, Klimberg VS, Plumley DA, et al. The role of glutamine in maintaining a healthy gut and supporting the metabolic response to injury and infection. J Surg Res 1990;48:383–91.
25. Fox AD, Kripke SA, Berman JM, et al. Dexamethasone administration induces increased glutaminase specific activity in the jejunum and colon. J Surg Res 1988;44:391.
26. Souba WW, Smith RJ, Wilmore DW. Effect of glucocorticoids on glutamine metabolism in visceral organs. Metabolism 1985;34:450–6.
27. Plumley DA, Souba WW, Hautamaki D, et al. Accelerated lung amino acid release in hyperdynamic septic surgical patients. Arch Surg 1990;125:57.
28. Austgen TR, Chen MK, Flynn TC, et al. The effects of endotoxin on the splanchnic metabolism of glutamine and related substrates. J Trauma 1991;6:742–51.
29. Austgen TR, Chen MK, Moore W, et al. Endotoxin and renal glutamine metabolism. Arch Surg 1991;126:23.
30. Souba WW, Smith RJ, Wilmore DW. Glutamine metabolism by the intestinal tract. JPEN J Parenter Enteral Nutr 1985;9:608–17.

31. Hwang TL, O'Dwyer ST, Smith RJ, et al. Preservation of small bowel mucosa using glutamine-enriched parenteral nutrition. Surg Forum 1986;38:56.

32. Zapata-Sirvent RL, Hnasbrough JF, Ohara MM, et al. Bacterial translocation of various diets including fiber-and glutamine enriched enteral formulas. Crit Care Med 1994;22:690–6.

33. Fox AD, Kripke SA, DePaula J, et al. Effect of a glutamine-supplemented enteral diet on methotrexate-induced enterocolitis. JPEN J Parenter Enteral Nutr 1988;12:325–31.

34. Klimberg VS, Souba WW, Dolson DJ, et al. Prophylactic glutamine protects the intestinal mucosa from radiation injury. Cancer 1990;66:62–8.

35. Li SJ, Nussbaum MS, McFadden DW, et al. Addition of L-glutamine to total parenteral nutrition and its effects on portal insulin and glucagon and the development of hepatic steatosis in rats. J Surg Res 1990;48:421–6.

36. Helton WS, Jacobs DO, Bonner-Weir S, et al. Effects of glutamine-enriched parenteral nutrition on the exocrine pancreas. JPEN J Parenter Enteral Nutr 1990;14:344–52.

37. Burke DJ, Alverdy JC, Aoys E, et al. Glutamine-supplemented total parenteral nutrition improves gut immune function. Arch Surg 1989;124:1396–9.

38. Hammarqvist F, Wernerman J, Ali R, et al. Addition of glutamine to total parenteral nutrition after elective abdominal surgery spares free glutamine in muscle, counteracts the fall in muscle protein synthesis, and improves nitrogen balance. Ann Surg 1989;209:455–61.

39. Stein TP, Yoshida S, Yamasaki K, et al. Amino acid requirements of critically ill patients. In: Latifi R, editor. Amino acids in critical care and cancer. Austin (TX): RG Landes Company; 1994. p. 9–25.

40. Barbul A. Arginine and immune function. Nutrition 1990;6:59–62.

41. Barbul A, Sisto DA, Wasserkrug HL, et al. Arginine stimulates lymphocyte immune response in healthy humans. Surgery 1981;90:244–51.

42. Stinnett J, Alexander JW, Watanabe C, et al. Plasma and skeletal muscle amino acids following severe burn injury in patients and experimental animals. Ann Surg 1982;195:75–89.

43. Xiao-jun C, Chih-chun Y, Wei-shia H, et al. Changes of serum amino acids in severely burned patients. Burns 1983;10:109–15.

44. Rose WC. Amino acid requirements of man. Fed Proc 1949;8(2):546–52.

45. Roth E, Funovics J, Muhlbacher F, et al. Metabolic disorders in severe abdominal sepsis: glutamine deficiency in skeletal muscle. Clin Nutr 1982;1(1):25–41.

46. Askanazi J, Carpentier YA, Michelsen CB, et al. Muscle and plasma amino acids following injury. Influence of intercurrent infection. Ann Surg 1980;192(1):78–85.

47. Ziegler TR, Ogden LG, Singleton KD, et al. Parenteral glutamine increases serum heat shock protein 70 in critically ill patients. Intensive Care Med 2005;31(8):1079–86.

48. Conejero R, Bonet A, Grau T, et al. Effect of a glutamine-enriched enteral diet on intestinal permeability and infectious morbidity at 28 days in critically ill patients with systemic inflammatory response syndrome: a randomized, single-blind, prospective, multicenter study. Nutrition 2002;18(9):716–21.

49. Garrel D, Patenaude J, Nedelec B, et al. Decreased mortality and infectious morbidity in adult burn patients given enteral glutamine supplements: a prospective, controlled, randomized clinical trial. Crit Care Med 2003;31(10):2444–9.

50. Houdijk AP, Rijnsburger ER, Jansen J, et al. Randomised trial of glutamine-enriched enteral nutrition on infectious morbidity in patients with multiple trauma. Lancet 1998;352(9130):772–6.

51. Hall JC, Dobb G, Hall J, et al. A prospective randomized trial of enteral glutamine in critical illness. Intensive Care Med 2003;29(10):1710–6.
52. Wischmeyer PE, Lynch J, Liedel J, et al. Glutamine administration reduces gram-negative bacteremia in severely burned patients: a prospective, randomized, double-blind trial versus isonitrogenous control. Crit Care Med 2001;29(11): 2075–80.
53. McClave SA, Martindale RG, Vanek VW, et al. Guidelines for the provision and assessment of nutrition support therapy in the adult critically ill patient: Society of Critical Care Medicine (SCCM) and American Society for Parenteral and Enteral Nutrition (A.S.P.E.N.). JPEN J Parenter Enteral Nutr 2009;33(3): 277–316.
54. Rose WC. The nutritive significance of the amino acids and certain related compounds. Science 1937;86(2231):298–300.
55. Davis SL. Plasma levels of prolactin, growth hormone and insulin in sheep following the infusion of arginine, leucine and phenylalanine. Endocrinology 1972;91(2):549–55.
56. Daly JM, Reynolds J, Thom A, et al. Immune and metabolic effects of arginine in the surgical patient. Ann Surg 1988;208(4):512–23.
57. Heyland DK, Novak F, Drover JW, et al. Should immunonutrition become routine in critically ill patients? A systematic review of the evidence. JAMA 2001;286(8): 944–53.
58. Bower RH, Cerra FB, Bershadsky B, et al. Early enteral administration of a formula (Impact) supplemented with arginine, nucleotides, and fish oil in intensive care unit patients: results of a multicenter, prospective, randomized, clinical trial. Crit Care Med 1995;23(3):436–49.
59. Bertolini G, Iapichino G, Radrizzani D, et al. Early enteral immunonutrition in patients with severe sepsis: results of an interim analysis of a randomized multi-centre clinical trial. Intensive Care Med 2003;29(5):834–40.
60. Zhou M, Martindale RG. Arginine in the critical care setting. J Nutr 2007;137(6 Suppl 2):1687S–92S.
61. Galban C, Montejo JC, Mesejo A, et al. An immune-enhancing enteral diet reduces mortality rate and episodes of bacteremia in septic intensive care unit patients. Crit Care Med 2000;28(3):643–8.
62. Kulkarni AD, Rudolph FB, Van Buren CT. The role of dietary sources of nucleo-tides in immune function: a review. J Nutr 1994;124(Suppl 8):1442S–6S.
63. Van Buren CT, Kulkarni AD, Fanslow WC, et al. Dietary nucleotides, a requirement for helper/inducer T lymphocytes. Transplantation 1985;40(6):694–7.
64. Beale RJ, Bryg DJ, Bihari DJ. Immunonutrition in the critically ill: a systematic review of clinical outcome. Crit Care Med 1999;27(12):2799–805.
65. Grimble GK, Westwood OM. Nucleotides as immunomodulators in clinical nutri-tion. Curr Opin Clin Nutr Metab Care 2001;4(1):57–64.
66. Heyland DK, Dhaliwal R, Suchner U, et al. Antioxidant nutrients: a systematic review of trace elements and vitamins in the critically ill patient. Intensive Care Med 2005;31(3):327–37.
67. Crimi E, Liguori A, Condorelli M, et al. The beneficial effects of antioxidant supple-mentation in enteral feeding in critically ill patients: a prospective, randomized, double-blind, placebo-controlled trial. Anesth Analg 2004;99(3):857–63.
68. Angstwurm MW, Engelmann L, Zimmermann T, et al. Selenium in Intensive Care (SIC): results of a prospective randomized, placebo-controlled, multiple-center study in patients with severe systemic inflammatory response syndrome, sepsis, and septic shock. Crit Care Med 2007;35(1):118–26.

69. Gennari R, Alexander JW, Eaves-Pyles T. Effect of different combinations of dietary additives on bacterial translocation and survival in gut-derived sepsis. JPEN J Parenter Enteral Nutr 1995;19(4):319–25.

70. Blackburn GL, Moldawer LL, Usui S, et al. Branched-chain amino acid administration and metabolism during starvation, injury, and infection. Surgery 1979; 86(2):307–15.

71. Yoshida S, Lanza-Jacoby S, Stein TP. Leucine and glutamine metabolism in septic rats. Biochem J 1991;276(Pt 2):405–9.

72. Freund HR, James JH, Fischer JE. Nitrogen-sparing mechanisms of singly administered branched-chain amino acids in the injured rat. Surgery 1981; 90(2):237–43.

73. García-de-Lorenzo A, Ortíz-Leyba C, Planas M, et al. Parenteral administration of different amounts of branch-chain amino acids in septic patients: clinical and metabolic aspects. Crit Care Med 1997;25(3):418–24.

74. Calder PC. Branched-chain amino acids and immunity. J Nutr 2006;136(Suppl 1): 288S–93S.

75. Ware LB, Matthay MA. The acute respiratory distress syndrome. N Engl J Med 2000;342(18):1334–49.

76. Mancuso P, Whelan J, DeMichele SJ, et al. Dietary fish oil and fish and borage oil suppress intrapulmonary proinflammatory eicosanoid biosynthesis and attenuate pulmonary neutrophil accumulation in endotoxic rats. Crit Care Med 1997;25(7): 1198–206.

77. Needleman P, Raz A, Minkes MS, et al. Triene prostaglandins: prostacyclin and thromboxane biosynthesis and unique biological properties. Proc Natl Acad Sci U S A 1979;76(2):944–8.

78. Lee TH, Menica-Huerta JM, Shih C, et al. Characterization and biologic properties of 5,12-dihydroxy derivatives of eicosapentaenoic acid, including leukotriene B5 and the double lipoxygenase product. J Biol Chem 1984;259(4):2383–9.

79. Gadek JE, DeMichele SJ, Karlstad MD, et al. Effect of enteral feeding with eicosapentaenoic acid, gamma-linolenic acid, and antioxidants in patients with acute respiratory distress syndrome. Enteral Nutrition in ARDS Study Group. Crit Care Med 1999;27(8):1409–20.

80. Pacht ER, DeMichele SJ, Nelson JL, et al. Enteral nutrition with eicosapentaenoic acid, gamma-linolenic acid, and antioxidants reduces alveolar inflammatory mediators and protein influx in patients with acute respiratory distress syndrome. Crit Care Med 2003;31(2):491–500.

81. Singer P, Theilla M, Fisher H, et al. Benefit of an enteral diet enriched with eicosapentaenoic acid and gamma-linolenic acid in ventilated patients with acute lung injury. Crit Care Med 2006;34(4):1033–8.

82. Pontes-Arruda A, Aragao AM, Albuquerque JD. Effects of enteral feeding with eicosapentaenoic acid, gamma-linolenic acid, and antioxidants in mechanically ventilated patients with severe sepsis and septic shock. Crit Care Med 2006; 34(9):2325–33.

83. Marik PE, Zaloga GP. Immunonutrition in critically ill patients: a systematic review and analysis of the literature. Intensive Care Med 2008;34(11):1980–90.

84. Martindale R, Miles J. Is immunonutrition ready for prime time? JPEN J Parenter Enteral Nutr 2003;18:489–96.

85. Braga M, Gianotti L, Nespoli L, et al. Nutritional approach in malnourished surgical patients: a prospective randomized study. Arch Surg 2002;137:174–80.

86. Seto Y, Fukuda T, Yamada K, et al. Celiac lymph nodes: distant or regional for thoracic esophageal carcinoma? Dis Esophagus 2008;21:704–7.

87. Fukuda T, Seto Y, Ymada K, et al. Can immune-enhancing nutrients reduce postoperative complications in patients undergoing esophageal surgery? Dis Esophagus 2008;21:708–11.
88. Giger U, Buchler M, Farhadi J, et al. Preoperative immunonutrition suppresses perioperative inflammatory response in patients with major abdominal surgery—a randomized controlled pilot study. Ann Surg Oncol 2007;14(10):2798–806.
89. Helminen H, Raitanen M, Kellosalo J. Immunonutrition in elective gastrointestinal surgery patients. Scand J Surg 2007;96:46–50.
90. Klek S, Kulig J, Sierzega M, et al. The impact of immuno stimulating nutrition on infectious complications after upper gastrointestinal surgery: a prospective, randomized, clinical trial. Ann Surg 2008;248(2):212–20.
91. Ryan A, Power D. Letters to the editor: immuno-nutrition in upper gastrointestinal surgery. Ann Surg 2009;249(6):1062–3.
92. Okamoto Y, Okano K, Izuishi K, et al. Attenuation of the systemic inflammatory response and infectious complications after gastrectomy with preoperative oral arginine and omega-3 fatty acids supplemented immunonutrition. World J Surg 2009;33:1815–21.
93. Ryan AM, Reynolds J, Healy L, et al. Enteral nutrition with Eicosapentaenoic Acid (EPA) preserves lean body mass following esophageal cancer surgery: results of a double-blinded randomized controlled trial. Ann Surg 2009;3(249):355–63.
94. Heys SD, Walker LG, Smith I, et al. Enteral nutrition supplementation with key nutrients in patients with critical illness and cancer. Meta-analysis of randomized controlled clinical trials. Ann Surg 1999;229:446–77, 93.

# Nutrition in Critical Care

Robert H. Bartlett, MD*, Ronald E. Dechert, PhD

**KEYWORDS**

• Nutrition • Critical care • Metabolic care

Critical care has evolved from a prolonged recovery room stay for cardiac surgery patients to a full medical and nursing specialty in the last 5 decades. The ability to feed patients who cannot eat has evolved from impossible to routine clinical practice in the last 4 decades. Nutrition in critically ill patients based on measurement of metabolism has evolved from a research activity to clinical practice in the last 3 decades. The authors of this article have participated in that evolution. We were there in the first intensive care units (ICUs), placed the first central lines, ran the first PEN (Parenteral and Enteral Nutrition) teams, and started ASPEN. We remember the first time we saw induced anabolism, the promise of continuous hemofiltration, and the first solution of amino acids. We did the research. We made the mistakes. We made some progress, and we brought thousands of critical care patients from cachexia to health.

Our prophets were Moore, Rhoads, and Elwyn. Our high priest has been Stan Dudrick. When Stan asked us to take a fresh look at what we do and have done, we had to agree.

Like so much of medicine and life, a fresh look reveals old facts in new packages. This article is as much a summary of how we got to 2010 as a speculation of where we will be in 2020. Because the authors have participated in this evolution, we have seen good ideas come and go and come again. This cycle results in progress but also in cynicism. Readers, please forgive us for the cynicism. It is meant to be instructive.

Before 1960 there were no ICUs and no parenteral nutrition; there was not much nutrition at all. Books were written about the physiology of starvation caused by gastric outlet obstruction or other problems. *Metabolic Care of the Surgical Patient* was published by Moore[1] in 1959. It remains the bible of fluid, electrolyte, and metabolic physiology in normal and injured people. In that book, he predicted that anabolism could be induced by feeding, but he did not know how to do it (**Fig. 1**).

Between 1960 and 1970, the first ICUs were established, primarily because the advent of cardiac surgery filled the recovery room, creating a problem for the next

The authors have no conflicts to disclose.

Department of Surgery, University of Michigan Hospitals, B560 MSRB II/SPC 5686, 1150 West Medical Center Drive, Ann Arbor, MI 48109, USA

* Corresponding author.

*E-mail address:* robbar@umich.edu

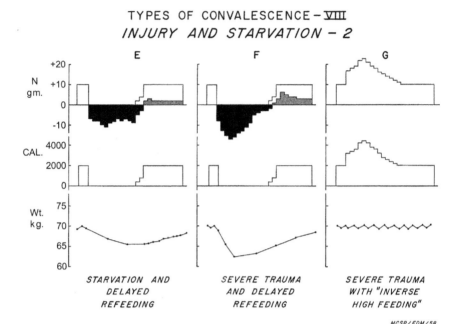

TYPES OF CONVALESCENCE – VIII

*INJURY AND STARVATION – 2*

*MCSP/FDM/58*

**Fig. 1.** Moore used balance diagrams to represent metabolism following injury or illness. He postulated that matching caloric and protein losses with feeding could prevent catabolism, but had no way to accomplish it. (*From* Moore FD. Metabolic care of the surgical patient. 1st edition. Philadelphia: WB Saunders; 1959:1011; with permission.)

day's patients. The back of the recovery room, and then some separate place in the hospital was set aside for these patients. People came from around the world to see a patient who had been intubated and ventilated overnight. Ventilated patients were the impetus, and soon there were nurses who learned how to manage the ventilator, and oxygen therapists who helped to service them. The same nurses and the residents responsible for the patients learned about continuous monitoring and interventions for shock. Myocardial infarction monitoring units were established and continuous electrophysiology was studied. Gastrostomies and small bowel tubes were occasionally used for feeding. Whole blood was used for blood loss and anemia. Bleeding stopped instantly when fresh, warm, whole blood was given. The cause of protein catabolism after illness or injury was believed to be endogenous cortisol.[1]

In the 1960s, the surgical laboratory at the University of Pennsylvania was an exciting place. A small group of surgical investigators discovered that very hyperosmolar solutions could be administered into rapidly flowing blood without causing thrombosis. This observation led to evaluation of concentrated glucose and peptide solutions for parenteral feeding. This evaluation resulted in the classic paper with the long title proving that parenteral nutrition was possible (**Fig. 2**).[2]

From 1970 to 1980, critical care evolved from simple ventilator management using simple ventilators to complex management and devices. Some of this was good (positive expiratory end pressure, humidification) and some was bad (inspiratory pressure of more than 40 cm H20, making patients accommodate to the ventilator). Endotracheal tubes designed for the operating room had little hard balloons that injured the trachea. Hemodialysis was used for acute renal failure when the blood urea nitrogen reached 200 to 300 mg/dl. We learned to recognize uremic frost and mouse breath.

# Can Intravenous Feeding as the Sole Means of Nutrition Support Growth in the Child and Restore Weight Loss in an Adult?

## An Affirmative Answer

STANLEY J. DUDRICK,* M.D., DOUGLAS W. WILMORE,† M.D., HARRY M. VARS,‡ PH.D., JONATHAN E. RHOADS,§ M.D.

*From the Department of Surgery and Harrison Department of Surgical Research, School of Medicine, University of Pennsylvania, the Veterans Administration Hospital and The Children's Hospital of Philadelphia, Philadelphia, Pennsylvania 19104*

**Fig. 2.** The classic paper from the surgical research laboratory at the University of Pennsylvania showing that total parenteral nutrition was possible. (*From* Dudrick SJ, Wilmore DW, Vars HM, et al. Can intravenous feeding as the sole means of nutrition support growth in the child and restore weight loss in an adult? an affirmative answer. Ann Surg 1969;169(6): 974–84; with permission.)

Separation of blood into components was efficient and made it possible to give only the component that was needed. We still stopped bleeding with fresh warm blood direct from the donor.

In that decade total parenteral nutrition (TPN) went from a curiosity in a few academic centers to routine practice. Placement of central lines, and apparatus to place lines, became standard practice.[3,4] Teams composed of pharmacists, nurses, doctors, and dieticians were established to prepare the formulas and monitor the practice.[5,6] Key research studies showed the interactive roles of energy and protein metabolism (**Fig. 3**).[7,8] The complications were frequent and serious: yeast infection, staphylococcus infection, hyperglycemia, and fatty liver, but the results were usually rewarding. If a little is good, a lot is not necessarily better. In time, we learned the metabolic and respiratory problems associated with 3000 or 4000 glucose calories a day.[9–11] A few research centers measured the metabolic rate, energy balance, and protein balance, bringing some clinical science to the bedside.[12–14] Diffuse solutions of polypeptides gave way to individual amino acids.[15,16] We learned from Norway that lipids could be given parenterally,[17] and that all of the required energy could be supplied by lipid emulsion rather than by glucose.[18]

The FreAmine story is worth recounting. The source of protein in the original TPN solutions was hydrolysate of proteins from cow blood or cow milk. These proteins were polypeptides that led to complications in some cases. In 1975, large quantities of pure amino acids became available, and the McGaw Laboratories Company made a solution of pure amino acids to replace the protein hydrolysates. They called the original solution FreAmine (FreAmine I, McGaw Laboratories, California; personal communication, 1975, RHB). The composition of amino acids in FreAmine is shown in **Fig. 4**. It included the known human essential amino acids and several others. It did not contain glutamine. The concentration of these amino acids was precise, down to 3 decimal places. We wondered why this specific mixture of amino acids was chosen, and visited the McGaw facility, which was close to our hospital. At the back of the building, we met the chemist who devised the formula for FreAmine. He explained that there were no definite data for normal human blood amino acid composition, so he copied the composition of amino acids in hen's egg albumin (hence, since 1976, TPN solutions have been a mixture of sugar and chicken soup). Because we

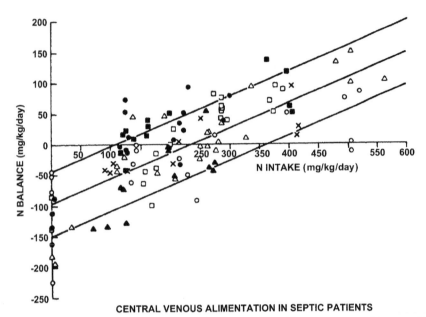

**Fig. 3.** Positive caloric balance (represented by diagonal lines) is necessary to achieve positive protein balance. (*From* Long CL, Crosby F, Geiger JW, et al. Parenteral nutrition in the septic patient: nitrogen balance, limiting plasma amino acids, and calorie to nitrogen ratios. Am J Clin Nutr 1976;29(4):380–91; with permission.)

| | Amino Acids, mg/100 ml | |
|---|---|---|
| | **8.5% Amino Acid, Crystalline** | **5% Amino Acid, Crystalline** |
| L-isoleucine | 590 | 360 |
| L-leucine | 770 | 470 |
| L-lysine acetate | 870 | 360 |
| L-methionine | 450 | 200 |
| L-phenylalanine | 480 | 220 |
| L-threonine | 340 | 260 |
| L-tryptophan | 130 | 80 |
| L-valine | 560 | 400 |
| L-tyrosine | . . . | 44 |
| L-alanine | 600 | 640 |
| L-arginine | 310 | 490 |
| L-glycine | 1,700 | 640 |
| L-proline | 950 | 430 |
| L-serine | 500 | 210 |
| L-histidine | 240 | 150 |
| L-cysteine | 20 | . . . |

**Fig. 4.** The composition of the first pure amino acid solution: FreAmine. FreAmine (McGaw) and a 5% amino acid solution from Abbot were used in this 1976 study. (*From* Gazzaniga AB, Day AT, Bartlett RH, et al. Endogenous caloric sources and nitrogen balance: regulation in postoperative patients. Arch Surg 1976;111:1357–61; with permission.)

were close to McGaw, we used some of the first FreAmine solutions. We noticed that all the patients hyperventilated on FreAmine, which was useful to prevent pulmonary complications, but was exhausting for the patients. It turned out that the amino acids were hydrolyzed with hydrochloric acid and were all the acidic chloride salts. McGaw solved this problem by adding acetate, producing the chloride and acetate salts of amino acids. When infused into patients, this caused metabolic alkalosis (because the acetate took up a hydrogen ion when it was metabolized). TPN infusion with acetate salts of pure amino acids has caused metabolic alkalosis in ICUs ever since. FreAmine with acetate was called FreAmine 2.[19]

In 1980 to 1990, critical care units became routine in major hospitals. Critical care was, and is, a nursing discipline, and the American Association of Critical Care Nurses (AACN) grew into prominence. Some physicians specialized in critical care in addition to their other practices. Societies and journals were established to serve the new specialty. The concept of accommodating the ventilator to the patient returned in many centers, and assist-control ventilators became available.[20,21] The phenomenon of stretch injury to the alveoli, long recognized in the laboratory,[22,23] found its way to clinical practice. The concept of resting the lung from ventilator injury with extracorporeal support by an extracorporeal membrane oxygenation (ECMO) became routine practice in neonatal respiratory failure.[24] Continuous hemofiltration, or continuous renal replacement therapy (CRRT), was invented in Germany[25] and brought to the United States in 1982.[26,27] In the ICUs, CRRT opened new possibilities for managing fluid overload, for removing any limits on nutrition, and for better management of renal failure.[26] Mixed venous oximetry became standard practice, resulting in better understanding of oxygen kinetics in critically ill patients.[28,29] Routine use of pulmonary artery catheters led to better understanding in the management of hemodynamics. Blood components rather than whole blood became essentially the only source of blood replacement. The cause of protein catabolism following illness and injury was shown to be hormonal, based primarily on a molecule named tumor necrosis factor[30] (probably the same molecule called cachectin by Clowes and colleagues[31] a decade later). Tumor necrosis factor was the first of the white cell–mediated molecules, which grew in numbers and became known by the collective name of cytokines.

Nutrition by central access with glucose, fat, and amino acid solutions became routine. The complications were largely controlled. The older generation, who believed that infection was a contraindication rather than an indication for feeding, gradually gave way. PEN teams, hospital manuals, and books on parenteral nutrition flowered, then wilted, as the technique became standard practice. ASPEN became a regular destination for critical care nutritionists. Because patients survived for weeks or months with no oral or enteral feeding, we learned about the importance of trace metals, essential amino and fatty acids, and esoteric vitamins.[32,33] Detailed measurement of metabolism, and planning of nutrition based on those measurements, became standard practice in many ICUs.[12,34] The value and timing of nutrition in critically ill patients was shown in these studies (**Fig. 5**).[35] Specialized TPN solutions were designed to treat chronic obstructive pulmonary disease,[36] renal failure,[37] and other specific abnormalities.[38] Hemofiltration, which was introduced in the 1980s, became standard practice for managing critically ill patients,[26] permitting feeding without limit, which had not been possible with intermittent dialysis.[39] The mortality for acute renal failure in critical care dropped from 90% to 50% when it became clear that starvation and intermittent hemodialysis were contributing to the mortality (**Fig. 6** CRRT).[40–42] The interest in, and provision of, nutrition in critical care became standard practice in pediatric and neonatal ICUs. New attention to enteral feeding revealed the dependence of the gut mucosa on glutamine.[43] Measuring nutrition status related to healing

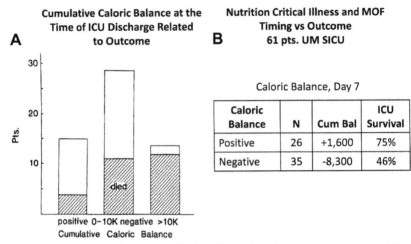

Fig. 5. In 1982, we showed that mortality in critically ill patients was associated with negative energy (and protein) balance during the ICU stay (*A*). In 1984, we showed that timing of nutrition in critically ill patients is important. Mortality was lower in patients who achieved positive caloric balance during the first week in the ICU (*B*). (*From* Bartlett RH, Dechert RE, Mault JR, et al. Measurement of metabolism in multiple organ failure. Surgery 1982;92(4):771–9; with permission; and Kresowik TF, Dechert RE, Mault JR, et al. Does nutritional support affect survival in critically ill patients? Surgical Forum 1984;35:108; with permission.)

and host defenses became standard practice in many ICUs. Measurements such as absolute lymphocyte count, triceps skin fold, and reaction to common skin test antigens were used. These studies showed that patients who had been starving (eg, because of esophageal cancer) had poor nutrition and major complications after operation. If patients were fed parenterally until these markers showed good nutrition status, the complications of operation were much less.[44] In the process of these studies, Meakins and Christou coined the term acquired immunologic deficiency syndrome (AIDS)[45] (**Fig. 7**).

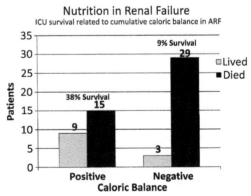

Fig. 6. Continuous hemofiltration facilitated unlimited feeding of energy sources and proteins, resulting in improved survival outcomes in acute renal failure. (*From* Bartlett RH, Mault JR, Dechert RE, et al. Continuous arteriovenous hemofiltration: improved survival in surgical acute renal failure? Surgery 1986;100(2):400–8; with permission.)

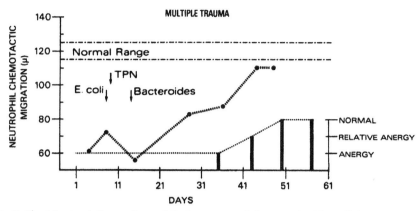

**Fig. 7.** The Montreal Group showed that anergy and decreased white cell function caused by acute illness are improved when adequate nutrition is supplied. (*From* Meakins JL, Pietsch JB, Bubenick O, et al. Delayed hypersensitivity: indicator of acquired failure of host defenses in sepsis and trauma. Ann Surg 1977;186(3):241–50; with permission.)

In 1990 to 2000, intensive care grew into a major specialty with residencies, boards, journals, and societies. Several scoring systems were introduced to predict mortality risk and outcome based on physiologic measurements.[46,47] Panels designed definitions for Acute Respiratory Distress Syndrome (ARDS),[48] sepsis,[49] and renal failure.[50] Algorithms for cardiac arrest, infection, and arrhythmias were proposed. The concept of closed ICUs arose, with both benefits and problems. The ICU syndrome became commonplace (intubation and ventilation, sedation because of intubation, paralysis because of the respiratory failure, nosocomial pneumonia, super-sized antibiotics because of the pneumonia, fluid overload, prolonged supine position, decubiti, renal failure, emergence of unusual organisms because of the antibiotics, cachexia and malnutrition, systemic sepsis, and often lingering demise). Three-dimensional imaging with computed tomography (CT) scans allowed percutaneous needle access to body cavities that had not been possible previously, which led to the concept of needle tissue diagnosis and percutaneous access to fluid collections for drainage for diagnosis and, in some cases, as treatment.[51] Echocardiography provided a direct look at the heart, and with some assumptions, the calculation of cardiac output and pressure gradients. The combination of hemodynamic monitoring and urgent treatment of shock based on that monitoring and reported by Rivers and Ahrens[52] led to improved results in acute treatment of shock. Although not commonly believed to be a major contributor to the advance of critical care medicine, external fixation of fractures has changed the management of patients with multiple injuries from weeks of bed care to early ambulation, which has had an impact throughout critical care.[53]

Enteral feeding became the new interest in ICU nutrition. Composition of enteral feeding was the subject of great discussion. Many patients had a tube in each nostril, one for feeding and one for gastric aspiration. Trophic feedings to prevent mucosal injury became routine **(Fig. 8)**.[54] The role of gastroesophageal reflux (with or without feeding) and pharyngeal organisms in the pathogenesis of nosocomial pneumonia was much discussed as a new phenomenon.[55] The concept of postpyloric feeding became an obsession, resulting in frequent trips to radiology. The timing of feeding was believed to be important, although the degree or magnitude of daily feeding remained controversial. Numerous studies reported a failure to meet daily caloric goals in patients in the ICU

**GUT INSULT**

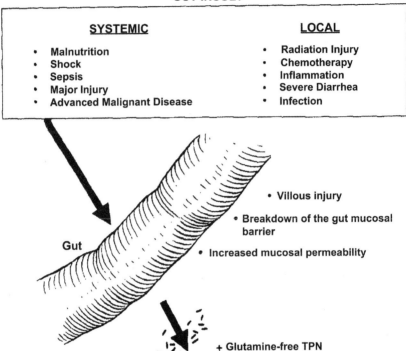

| SYSTEMIC | LOCAL |
|---|---|
| • Malnutrition | • Radiation Injury |
| • Shock | • Chemotherapy |
| • Sepsis | • Inflammation |
| • Major Injury | • Severe Diarrhea |
| • Advanced Malignant Disease | • Infection |

Gut

• Villous injury

• Breakdown of the gut mucosal barrier

• Increased mucosal permeability

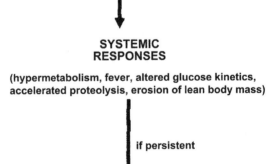

+ Glutamine-free TPN

migration of luminal bacteria and toxins into the mesenteric lymphatics and/or portal venous blood

**SYSTEMIC RESPONSES**

(hypermetabolism, fever, altered glucose kinetics, accelerated proteolysis, erosion of lean body mass)

if persistent

**M.S.O.F.**

**Fig. 8.** Maintenance of normal intestinal mucosa by small amounts of enteral glutamine (ie, evidence that lack of glutamine was largely responsible for small bowel atrophy during TPN). (*From* Souba WW, Klimberg VS, Plumley DA, et al. The role of glutamine in maintaining a healthy gut and supporting the metabolic response to injury and infection. J Surg Res 1990;48:383–91; with permission.)

because of our inability to maintain enteral support. Cyclic feeding began to receive practical support, in part because of the disruptions of enteral feeding commonly found in our ICU populations. Some proposed beginning feedings in the recovery room after an abdominal operation.[56] A variety of additives to parenteral nutrition were proposed to block hypermetabolism, enhance anabolism, and reduce central inflammation.

Between 2000 and 2010, critical care depended increasingly on mechanical artificial organs: ventilators, CRRT, ventricular assist devices (VADs), ECMO, and the most widely used artificial organ, the central line, representing the artificial gut. Damage by these mechanical devices was recognized, especially damage to the lung by over-zealous mechanical ventilation.[57] Evidence became the watchword, and some proposed that there was no evidence to support nutrition in sick patients.[58] As in any complex technology, attention to the details and a checklist to follow those details, proved valuable.

Tight glucose control with parenteral feeding was advocated by Van den Berghe[59] and others to minimize complications of parenteral nutrition. Later studies showed that the main advantage of tight glucose control was simply good nutrition.[60]

Nutrition in the most recent decade was focused on the right balance of enteral and parenteral feeding. Peripheral TPN was commonly used in ICUs, by infusing 5% amino acids and 10% sugar. The placement of central lines with fluoroscopic guidance became standard practice, resulting in many trips to radiology. The individual components of feeding mixtures and the amounts given were often guided by balance studies based on metabolic measurements,[12,13,18,34,35] recycling to Dr Moore's original predictions.[1]

The current status of critical care is that less is better (or too much was bad). Ventilation is based on spontaneous breathing with inspiratory pressure limited to 20 to 30 cm of water or less (remember the Engström ventilator with the 30-cm water column). Sedation is minimal and paralysis is out. Management is simplified by pulse oximetry and central venous oximetry. Fluid overload persists, but is easily managed by CRRT. The most potent antibiotics are reserved for culture-proven infection. Some of the less-is-better approach is questionable. Limiting transfusion and protein infusion makes for profound anemia[61] and low colloid osmotic pressure.[62]

The current status of nutrition in critical illness is to begin nutrition soon after the onset of acute injury or illness, with the goal of maintaining positive caloric and protein balance in the first week.[35] Recent guidelines were developed in a joint effort between the Society of Critical Care Medicine and the American Society for Parenteral and Enteral Nutrition, which acknowledges and supports the importance of nutritional monitoring and support in the care and recovery of critically ill populations.[63] The amount, route, and nature of feedings are based on measurements or revised estimates (using standardized predictive equations) of metabolism and the balance of proteins, fat, and carbohydrates. Enteral feeding is preferred as much as possible.

In the decade beginning in 2020, we expect that critical care will return to more physiologic-based measurement. Spontaneous breathing with pressure-limited ventilators will be the standard (remember the Bird Mark IV). The threshold for extracorporeal gas exchange will be low, eliminating ventilator-induced lung injury. There will be advances in extracorporeal life support (ECLS) and practices that allow ECLS without mechanical ventilation, thereby eliminating the potential for further induced lung injury. Continuous hemodynamic and oxygen kinetic monitoring will be combined, leading to care based on oxygen delivery and consumption rather than blood pressure (remember treating negative base excess). The threshold for mechanical support of perfusion will be low, eliminating overdose of toxic $\alpha$ agonists. An unlimited supply of safe fresh whole blood (initially from registered donors, then from factories of cultured liver and bone marrow) will replace blood components and return anemia to a physiologic condition rather than a goal. Routine administration of drugs that cause more harm than good when given to ICU patients will be eliminated (ranitidine, β blockers, heparin) and replaced with other routine drugs that do more harm than good (remember prophylactic digitalis?). Extracorporeal blood processing to treat sepsis will emerge, but, nonetheless, ICU patients will still die of sepsis.

We expect that nutrition in critical illness will also return to physiologic-based management. Caloric and protein balance measurements will be routine, and the amounts and composition of feedings will be based on maintaining positive protein (nitrogen) balance. Studies relating positive nitrogen balance to better outcomes will be met with positive results. Control of hypermetabolism with drugs and antimediators will be tried again, but draining the pus will still be the best solution to localized infection. Nutrition algorithms will still be "Enough, but not too much," and a new generation of outcome studies will claim that there is no evidence to support it. Immunomodulation by nutrition, and the use of nutraceutical products (remember growth hormone and Anabolin?) will be touted as the newest advances in efforts to treat critically ill patients, and only a few randomized controlled trials will be performed to test these hypotheses thoroughly. Overall, thousands of patients who would have died before Stan Dudrick will return to their happy, healthy lives. Thanks Stan!

## REFERENCES

1. Moore FD. Metabolic care of the surgical patient. 1st edition. Philadelphia: WB Saunders; 1959. p. 1011.
2. Dudrick SJ, Wilmore DW, Vars HM, et al. Can intravenous feeding as the sole means of nutrition support growth in the child and restore weight loss in an adult? An affirmative answer. Ann Surg 1969;169(6):974–84.
3. Parsa MH, Habif DV, Ferrer JM, et al. Intravenous hyperalimentation: indications, techniques and complications. Bull N Y Acad Med 1972;48(7):920–42.
4. Wilmore DW, Dudrick SJ. Safe long-term venous catheterization. Arch Surg 1969; 98:256–8.
5. Wesley JR, Khalidi N, Faubion WC, et al. Home parenteral nutrition: a hospital-based program with commercial logistic support. JPEN J Parenter Enteral Nutr 1984;8(5):585–8. 4b.
6. Shils ME. A program for total parenteral nutrition at home. Am J Clin Nutr 1975;28: 1429–35.
7. Kinney JM, Long CL, Gump FE, et al. Tissue composition of weight loss in surgical patients. I. Elective operation. Ann Surg 1968;168:459–74.
8. Duke JH Jr, Jorgenson SB, Broell JR, et al. Contribution of protein to caloric expenditure following surgery. Surgery 1970;68:168–74. 5b.
9. Rubecz I, Mestyan J. Energy metabolism and intravenous nutrition of premature infants. I. The response of oxygen consumption, respiratory quotient and substrate utilization to infusion of aminosol-glucose. Biol Neonate 1973;23(1):45–58.
10. Askanazi J, Carpenter YA, Elwyn DH, et al. Influence of total parenteral nutrition on fuel utilization in injury and sepsis. Ann Surg 1980;19(1):40–6.
11. Covelli HD, Black JW, Olsen MS, et al. Respiratory failure precipitated by high carbohydrate loads. Ann Intern Med 1981;95(5):579–81.
12. Bartlett RH, Allyn PA, Medley T, et al. Nutritional therapy based on positive caloric balance in burn patients. Arch Surg 1977;112(8):974–80.
13. Wilmore DW. Measurement of metabolism in critically ill patients. New York: Plenum; 1977.

14. Dechert RE, Wesley JR, Schafer LE, et al. A water-sealed indirect calorimeter for measurement of oxygen consumption ($VO_2$), carbon dioxide production ($Vco_2$), and energy expenditure in infants. JPEN J Parenter Enteral Nutr 1988;12(3):256–9.
15. Shohl AT, Blackfan KD. Intravenous administration of crystalline amino acids in infants. J Nutr 1940;20:305–16.
16. Wretlind A. Free amino acids in a dialyzed casein digest. Acta Physiology Scand 1947;13:45–54.
17. Shuberth O, Wretlind A. Intravenous infusion of fat emulsions, phosphatides and emulsifying agents. Acta Chir Scand 1961;278(Suppl):1–21.
18. Gazzaniga AB, Bartlett RH, Shobe JB. Nitrogen balance in patients receiving either fat or carbohydrate for total intravenous nutrition. Ann Surg 1975;182(2): 163–8.
19. Tweedle DE, Fitzpatrick GF, Brennan MF, et al. Intravenous amino acids as the sole nutritional substrate. Ann Surg 1977;186(1):60–73.
20. Krauss AN. Assisted ventilation: a critical review. Clin Perinatol 1980;7(1):61–74.
21. Davis H 2nd, Lefrak SS, Miller D, et al. Prolonged mechanically assisted ventilation. An analysis of outcome and charges. JAMA 1980;243(1):43–5.
22. Kolobow T, Pesenti A, Solca ME, et al. A new approach to the prevention and treatment of acute pulmonary insufficiency. Int J Artif Organs 1980;3(2):86–93.
23. Gattinoni L, Pesenti A, Caspani ML, et al. The role of total static lung compliance in the management of severe ARDS unresponsive to conventional treatment. Int Care Med 1984;10(3):121–6.
24. Bartlett RH, Andrews AF, Toomasian JM, et al. Extracorporeal membrane oxygenation for newborn respiratory failure: forty-five cases. Surgery 1982;92(2):425–33.
25. Kramer P, Schrader J, Bohnsack, et al. Continuous arteriovenous haemofiltration. A new kidney replacement therapy. Proc Eur Dial Transplant Assoc 1981;18:743–9.
26. Bartlett RH, Mault JR, Dechert RE, et al. Continuous arteriovenous hemofiltration: improved survival in surgical acute renal failure? Surgery 1986;100(2):400–8.
27. Golper TA. Continuous arteriovenous hemofiltration in acute renal failure. Am J kidney Dis 1985;6(6):373–86.
28. Baele PL, McMichan JC, Marsh HM, et al. Continuous monitoring of mixed venous oxygen saturation in critically ill patients. Anesth Analg 1982;61(6):513–7.
29. Orlando R 3rd. Continuous mixed venous oximetry in critically ill surgical patients. 'High-tech' cost-effectiveness. Arch Surg 1986;121(4):470–1.
30. Old LJ. Tumor necrosis factor. Clin Bull 1976;6(3):118–20.
31. Clowes GH Jr, George BC, Villee CA Jr, et al. Muscle proteolysis induced by a circulating peptide in patients with sepsis or trauma. N Engl J Med 1983; 308(10):545–52.
32. Rhoads JE, Steiger E, Dudrick SJ, et al. Intravenous hyperalimentation. Med Clin North Am 1970;54(3):577–89.
33. Dudrick SJ, Rhoads JE. Total intravenous feeding. Sci Am 1972;226(5):73–80.
34. Bartlett RH, Dechert RE, Mault JR, et al. Measurement of metabolism in multiple organ failure. Surgery 1982;92(4):771–9.
35. Kresowik TF, Dechert RE, Mault JR, et al. Does nutritional support affect survival in critically ill patients? Surgical Forum 1984;35(108).
36. Pulmocare: Abbott Laboratories Inc; 2007.
37. Renalcal: Nestle Nutrition; 2011.
38. TraumaCal: Novartis Nutrition; 2011.
39. Mault JR, Kresowik TF, Dechert RE, et al. Continuous arteriovenous hemofiltration: the answer to starvation in acute renal failure? Trans Am Soc Artif Intern Organs 1984;30:203–6.

40. Mault JR, Bartlett RH, Dechert RE, et al. Starvation: a major contribution to mortality in acute renal failure? Trans Am Soc Artif Intern Organs 1983;29:390–5.

41. Mault JR, Dechert RE, Lees P, et al. Continuous arteriovenous filtration: an effective treatment for surgical acute renal failure. Surgery 1987;101(4):478–84.

42. Swartz RD, Messana JM, Orzol S, et al. Comparing continuous hemofiltration with hemodialysis in patients with severe acute renal failure. Am J Kidney Dis 1999; 34(3):424–32.

43. Bragg LE, Thompson JS, Rikkers LF. Influence of nutrient delivery on gut structure and function. Nutrition 1991;7(4):237–43.

44. Meakins JL, Pietsch JB, Bubenick O, et al. Delayed hypersensitivity: indicator of acquired failure of host defenses in sepsis and trauma. Ann Surg 1977;186(3): 241–50.

45. Centers for Disease Control. Update on acquired immune deficiency syndrome (AIDS) - United States. MMWR Morb Mortal Wkly Rep 1982;31(37):507–8, 513–4.

46. Knaus WA, Draper EA, Wagner DP, et al. APACHE II: a severity of disease classification system. Crit Care Med 1985;13(10):818–29.

47. Vincent JL, de Mendonca A, Cantraine F, et al. Use of the SOFA score to assess the incidence of organ dysfunction/failure in intensive care units: results of a multicenter, prospective study. Working group on "sepsis-related problems" of the European Society of Intensive Care Medicine. Crit Care Med 1988;26(11): 1793–800.

48. Bernard GR, Artigas A, Brigham KL, et al. The American-European Consensus Conference on ARDS. Definitions, mechanisms, relevant outcomes, and clinical trial coordination. Am J Respir Crit Care Med 1994;149:818–24.

49. Moreno R, Vincent JL, Matos R, et al. The use of maximum SOFA score to quantify organ dysfunction/failure in intensive care. Results of a prospective, multicentre study. Working Group on Sepsis related Problems of ESICM. Int Care Med 1999;25(7):686–96.

50. Bock HA. Pathogenesis of acute renal failure: new aspects. Contrib Nephrol 1998;124:43–55.

51. vanSonnenberg E, D'Agostino HB, Casola G, et al. Lung abscess: CT-guided drainage. Radiology 1991;178(2):347–51.

52. Rivers EP, Ahrens T. Improving outcomes for severe sepsis and septic shock: tools for early identification of at-risk patients and treatment protocol implementation. Crit Care Clin 2008;24(Suppl 3):S1–47.

53. Hammer R. A new device for external fixation. Acta Orthop Scand 1988;59(6): 708–11.

54. Morlion BJ, Stehle P, Wachtler P, et al. Total parenteral nutrition with glutamine dipeptide after major abdominal surgery: a randomized, double-blind, controlled study. Ann Surg 1998;227(2):302–8.

55. Brownlee IA, Aseeri A, Ward C, et al. From gastric aspiration to airway inflammation. Monaldi Arch Chest Dis 2010;73(2):54–63.

56. Marik PE, Zaloga GP. Early enteral nutrition in acutely ill patients: a systematic review. Crit Care Med 2001;29(12):2264–70.

57. Rosenberg AL, Dechert RE, Park PK, et al. Review of a large clinical series: association of cumulative fluid balance on outcome in acute lung injury: a retrospective review of the ARDSnet tidal volume study cohort. J Intensive Care Med 2009; 24(1):35–46.

58. Koretz RL. Nutritional supplementation in the ICU. How critical is nutrition for the critically ill? Am J Respir Crit Care Med 1995;151:570–3.

59. Van den Berghe G, Wouters P, Weekers F, et al. Intensive insulin therapy in critically ill patients. N Engl J Med 2001;345(19):1359–67.

60. Haga KK, McClymont KL, Clarke S, et al. The effect of tight glycaemic control, during and after cardiac surgery, on patient mortality and morbidity: a systematic review and meta-analysis. J Cardiothorac Surg 2011;6:3.

61. Prewitt RM, McCarthy J, Wood LD. Treatment of acute low pressure pulmonary edema in dogs: relative effects of hydrostatic and oncotic pressure, nitroprusside, and positive end-expiratory pressure. J Clin Invest 1981;67(2):409–18.

62. Ohqvist G, Settergren G, Bergstrom K, et al. Plasma colloid osmotic pressure during open-heart surgery using non-colloid or colloid priming solution in the extracorporeal circuit. Scan J Thorac Cardiovasc Surg 1981;15(3):251–5.

63. McClave SA, Martindale RG, Vane VW, et al. Guidelines for the provision and assessment of nutrition support therapy in the adult critically ill patient: Society of Critical Care Medicine (SCCM) and American Society for Parenteral and Enteral Nutrition (A.S.P.E.N) JPEN 2009;33:277–316.

# What, How, and How Much Should Patients with Burns be Fed?

Felicia N. Williams, MD[a], Ludwik K. Branski, MD[a],
Marc G. Jeschke, MD, PhD[b], David N. Herndon, MD[a],*

**KEYWORDS**

- Hypermetabolic response • Burn injury • Trauma • Nutrition

Severe burn injury represents a significant problem worldwide. More than 1 million burn injuries occur annually in the United States. Although most of these burn injuries are minor, approximately 10% of patients with burns require admission to a hospital or major burn center for appropriate treatment every year.[1] Recent reports revealed a 50% decline in burn-related deaths and hospital admissions in the United States over the last 20 years, mainly because of effective prevention strategies, decreasing the number and severity of burns.[2,3] Advances in therapeutic strategies, including advances in resuscitation, wound coverage, better support of hypermetabolic response to injury, more appropriate infection control, and improved treatment of inhalation injury, have further improved the clinical outcome of this unique patient population over the past years. However, severe burns remain a devastating injury affecting nearly every organ system and leading to significant morbidity and mortality.[4]

## METABOLIC CHANGES AFTER SEVERE BURN INJURY

Severe burns covering more than 40% total body surface area (TBSA) are typically followed by a period of stress, inflammation, and hypermetabolism, characterized by a hyperdynamic circulatory response with increased body temperature, glycolysis, proteolysis, lipolysis, and futile substrate cycling.[5–7] These responses are present in

There are no financial ties between any of the authors and any corporate entity or product mentioned in this manuscript.

Supported by SHC Grant #8660, SHC Grant # 8490, SHC Grant # 8640, SHC Grant # 8760, SHC Grant # 9145, NIH Training Grant #2T32GM0825611, NIH Center Grant #1P50GM60338-01, NIH Grant #5RO1GM56687-03, NIH R01-GM56687, NIH Grant # R01-HD049471, NIDDR H133A020102, NIDDR H133A70019, NIGMS U54/GM62119, American Surgical Association.

[a] Department of Surgery, Shriners Hospital for Children and University of Texas Medical Branch, 815 Market Street, Galveston, TX 77550, USA

[b] Ross Tilley Burn Centre, Sunnybrook Health Sciences Centre, and Department of Surgery, Division of Plastic Surgery, University of Toronto, 2075 Bayview Avenue, Toronto, ON M4N 3M5, Canada

* Corresponding author.

*E-mail address:* dherndon@utmb.edu

all trauma, surgical, or critically ill patients, but the severity, length, and magnitude are unique for patients with burns.[4,8] Marked and sustained increases in catecholamine, glucocorticoid, glucagons, and dopamine secretion are believed to initiate the cascade of events leading to the acute hypermetabolic response with its ensuing catabolic state.[5,9–16] The response is characterized by supraphysiologic metabolic rates, constitutive muscle and bone catabolism, growth retardation, insulin resistance, and increased risk for infection.[5–7,17,18] If untreated, physiologic exhaustion ensues, and the insult becomes fatal.[19–22] This period is characterized by profoundly accelerated glycolysis, lipolysis, proteolysis, insulin resistance, liver dysfunction, and decreases of lean body mass (LBM) and total body mass.[23–29] A 10% loss of total body mass leads to immune dysfunction; 20% leads to decreased wound healing; 30% leads to severe infections; and a 40% loss leads to death.[30] Severely burned, catabolic patients can lose up to 25% of total body mass after acute severe burn injury.[25]

The cause of this complex response is not well understood. However, it is hypothesized that interleukin 1 (IL-1) and IL-6, platelet-activating factor, tumor necrosis factor (TNF), endotoxin, neutrophil-adherence complexes, reactive oxygen species, nitric oxide, and coagulation as well as complement cascades have also been implicated in regulating this response to burn injury.[31] Once these cascades are initiated, their mediators and by-products seem to stimulate the persistent and increased metabolic rate associated with altered glucose metabolism seen after severe burn injury.[32] The primary mediators of this response after severe burn injury are catecholamines, corticosteroids, and inflammatory cytokines.[33] There is a 10-fold to 50-fold increase of plasma catecholamines and corticosteroid levels that lasts up to 12 months after burn injury.[34,35] Inflammatory cytokine levels, serum hormones, acute proteins, and constitutive proteins are altered immediately after burn injury and remain abnormal throughout the acute hospitalization up to 2 months after burn injury compared with normal levels.[34]

Several studies have indicated that these metabolic phenomena after burn injury occur in a timely manner, suggesting 2 distinct patterns of metabolic regulation after injury.[36] The first phase occurs within the first 48 hours of injury and has classically been called the ebb phase,[36,37] characterized by decreases in cardiac output, oxygen consumption, and metabolic rate as well as impaired glucose tolerance associated with its hyperglycemic state. These metabolic variables gradually increase within the first 5 days after injury to a plateau phase (called the flow phase), characteristically associated with hyperdynamic circulation and the hypermetabolic state mentioned earlier.

Multiorgan dysfunction is the hallmark of the acute phase response after burn injury.[8] Immediately after burn injury, patients may have low cardiac values characteristic of early shock.[38] However, by 4 days after burn injury, at the onset of shock, they have cardiac outputs greater than 150% compared with nonburned, healthy volunteers.[34] Heart rates of our patients approach 160% compared with nonburned, healthy patients.[28] After burn injury, patients have increased cardiac work that lasts well into the rehabilitation phase.[4,39] Myocardial oxygen consumption values far surpass values of marathon runners and are sustained well into the rehabilitation phase.[39,40] Profound hepatomegaly occurs after burn injury. The liver increases its size by 225% by 2 weeks after burn injury and remains increased at discharge by 200%.[34]

Insulin release during this period was found to be twice that of controls in response to glucose load,[41,42] and plasma glucose levels are markedly increased, indicating the development of an insulin resistance.[42,43] Current understanding has been that these metabolic alterations resolve soon after complete wound closure. However, recent studies found that the hypermetabolic response to burn injury may last for more than 12 months after the initial event.[5,9,16,44] We found in a recent study that sustained hypermetabolic alterations after burn injury, indicated by persistent increases of total urine cortisol levels, serum cytokines, catecholamines, and basal energy require-ments, were accompanied by impaired glucose metabolism and insulin sensitivity that persisted for up to 3 years after the initial burn injury.[45]

Glucose metabolism in severely burned patients is dramatically deranged. To provide glucose, a major fuel source to vital organs, release of the stress mediators mentioned earlier opposes the anabolic actions of insulin.[46] By enhancing adipose tissue lipolysis[47] and skeletal muscle proteolysis,[48] they increase gluconeogenic substrates, including glycerol, alanine, and lactate, thus augmenting hepatic glucose production in burned patients.[49–51] In healthy individuals glucose metabolism is tightly regulated, and under normal circumstances, a postprandial increase in blood glucose concentration stimulates release of insulin from pancreatic β cells. Insulin mediates peripheral glucose uptake into skeletal muscle and adipose tissue and suppresses hepatic gluconeogenesis, thereby maintaining blood glucose homeostasis.[49,50] However, in severe burns metabolic alterations can cause signifi-cant changes in energy substrate metabolism. Hyperglycemia fails to suppress hepatic glucose release during this time,[52] and the suppressive effect of insulin on hepatic glucose release is attenuated, significantly contributing to posttrauma hyperglycemia.[53] Catecholamine-mediated enhancement of hepatic glycogenolysis, as well as direct sympathetic stimulation of glycogen breakdown, can further aggra-vate the hyperglycemia in response to stress.[49] Catecholamines have also been shown to impair glucose disposal via alterations of the insulin signaling pathway and glucose transporter type 4 translocation in muscle and adipose tissue, resulting in peripheral insulin resistance.[50,54] Researchers have shown an impaired activation of insulin receptor substrate 1 at its tyrosine binding site and an inhibition of AKT in muscle biopsies of children at 7 days after burn injury.[53] There is a link among impaired liver and muscle mitochondrial oxidative function, altered rates of lipolysis, and impaired insulin signaling after burn injury, attenuating the suppressive actions of insulin both on hepatic glucose production and on the stimulation of muscle glucose uptake.[42,47,52,53] Another counterregulatory hormone of interest during stress of the critically ill is glucagon. Glucagon, like epinephrine, leads to increased glucose production through both gluconeogenesis and glycogenolysis.[55] The action of glucagon alone is not maintained over time; however, its action on gluconeogenesis is sustained in an additive manner by the presence of epinephrine, cortisol, and growth hormone.[46,55] Similarly, epinephrine and glucagon have an additive effect on glycogenolysis.[55] Proinflammatory cytokines contribute indirectly to postburn hyperglycemia by enhancing the release of the aforementioned stress hormones.[56–58] Other groups showed that inflammatory cytokines, including TNF, IL-6 and monocyte chemotactic protein 1 also act via direct effects on the insulin signal transduction pathway through modification of signaling properties of insulin receptor substrates, contributing to postburn hyperglycemia via liver and skeletal muscle insulin resistance.[59–61] Alterations in metabolic pathways as well as proin-flammatory cytokines, such as TNF, have also been implicated in significantly contributing to lean muscle protein breakdown, both during the acute and convales-cent phases in response to burn injury.[62,63] In contrast to starvation, in which lipolysis and ketosis provide energy and protect muscle reserves, burn injury considerably reduces the ability of the body to use fat as an energy source.

Skeletal muscle is thus the major source of fuel in the burned patient, which leads to marked wasting of LBM within days after injury.[4,64] This muscle breakdown has been shown with whole-body and cross-leg nitrogen balance studies in which pronounced negative nitrogen balances persisted for 6 and 9 months after injury.[65] Because skeletal muscle has been shown to be responsible for up to 80% of whole-body insulin-stimulated glucose uptake, decreases in muscle mass may significantly contribute to this persistent insulin resistance after burn injury.[66] The correlation between hyperglycemia and muscle protein catabolism has also been supported by Flakoll and colleagues,[67] who used an isotopic leucine tracer as an index of whole-body protein flux in normal volunteers. These investigators showed a significant increase in proteolysis rates occurring without any alteration in either leucine oxidation or nonoxidative disposal (an estimate of protein synthesis), suggesting that hyperglycemia induced increased protein breakdown. Flakoll and colleagues[67] further reported that increases of plasma glucose levels resulted in a marked stimulation of whole-body proteolysis during hyperinsulinemia. Net loss of protein leads to loss of LBM, and severe muscle wasting leads to decreased strength and failure to rehabilitate fully. The resultant muscle weakness was further shown to prolong mechanical ventilatory requirements, and delay mobilization in protein-malnourished patients, thus markedly contributing to the incidence of mortality in these patients.[68] This loss of protein is directly related to increases in metabolic rate and may persist up to 9 months after critical burn injury, often resulting in significantly negative whole-body and cross-leg nitrogen balances. Severely burned patients have a nitrogen loss of 20 to 25 $g/m^2$ TBSA/d, and if unattended, lethal cachexia becomes imminent in less than 30 days. Persistent protein catabolism may also account for the delay in growth frequently observed in our pediatric patient population for up to 2 years after burn injury.[17]

Perturbations, such as sepsis, increase metabolic rates and protein catabolism up to 40% compared with patients with like-size burns who do not develop sepsis.[5,69] A vicious cycle ensues, because patients who are catabolic are more susceptible to sepsis because of changes in immune function and immune response. The emergence of multiresistant organisms has led to increases in sepsis-related infections and death overall.[70–72] Inflammatory cells, in response to burn wounds and burn wound infections, metabolize glucose anaerobically to pyruvate and lactate.[73] These compounds are returned to the liver for gluconeogenesis, which produces recycled energy for use by leukocytes and fibroblasts in the burn wound.[74,75]

In past years, therapeutic approaches have therefore focused mainly on reversing the hypermetabolic response, with its ensuing catabolic state after burn injury, using many different strategies.

### Nutritional Support of the Severely Burned Patient

The hypermetabolic response for a severely burned patient surpasses that in any other disease state.[14] Determinants of successful initial burn treatment include early aggressive resuscitation (including nutrition), control of infection, and early closure of the burn wound. Aggressive, early enteral feeding improves outcomes in the burned patient by mitigating the degree and extent of catabolism.[76,77] Attempting to overcompensate by providing excess calories and/or protein is ineffective and likely to increase such complications as hyperglycemia, $CO_2$ retention, and azotemia.[64] Thus, the primary goal of nutritional support in patients with burns is to satisfy acute, burn-specific requirements, and not to overfeed.

Patients with 40% TBSA treated with vigorous oral alimentation alone can lose a quarter of their preadmission weight by 3 weeks after injury.[25] Attempts to feed severely burned patients orally failed because of altered mental status, inhalation injuries that compromised pulmonary function, gastrointestinal dysfunction, and/or feeding intolerance.[25] The amount of nutrition necessary to provide adequate support and prevent severe catabolism was intolerable for these patients. Inanition proved fatal as severely burned victims succumbed to severe systemic infections and respiratory failure.[25,78] Thus, the primary goal of nutritional support is to address the ever-evolving metabolic needs in severely burned patients. Nutrition should be tailored to promote wound healing, to increase resistance to infection, and to prevent persistent loss of muscle protein. During the acute hospitalization of severely burned patients, attempts to optimize nutrition are countered by immobility and evolving catabolic responses to injury; attempts to achieve a positive nitrogen balance are repeatedly thwarted.

Total parenteral nutrition (TPN) for the nutrition and rehabilitation of severely burned patients surfaced in the 1970s.[79,80] TPN allows for the provision of elemental components that do not require digestion or a functioning alimentary tract. Dextrose is the main calorie source in TPN, and protein is supplied as crystalline amino acid solutions. Lipid emulsions can comprise a significant proportion of the calories in TPN. Use of TPN has now been largely replaced by enteral nutrition (EN) in patients with burns.

Adults can maintain body weight after severe burn injury only with aggressive, continuous nutrition of 25 kcal per kilogram body weight per day plus 40 kcal per percent TBSA burn per day.[81,82] Children require 1800 kcal per square meter of body surface plus 2200 kcal per square meter of burn area per day to maintain body weight.[83] The mechanism by which patients are fed affects outcomes. Research shows that parenteral nutrition alone or even in combination with EN could lead to overfeeding, liver failure, impaired immune response, and increased mortality by 3-fold.[84–86] EN reduces translocation bacteremia and sepsis, maintains gut motility, and preserves first-pass nutrient delivery to the liver.[76] For these patients, parenteral nutrition should be reserved primarily for those who have enteral feeding intolerance or prolonged ileus.

### Timing of Nutrition

Advances in burn care have altered the magnitude of the postburn hypermetabolic response, but not the nature of the response.[64] A major determinant of outcome for patients with severe burns is time to treatment. Any delays in resuscitation lead to poorer outcomes.[87] In the acute phase, in the unfed patient, there is significant gut mucosal damage and increased bacterial translocation, which collectively lead to decreased nutrient absorption.[88,89] Therefore, optimal nutritional support for the severely burned patient is best accomplished by early initiation of EN. Moreover, multiple studies report that early institution of enteral feeding can significantly modulate the hypermetabolic response to severe burns.[76,77] Laboratory studies showed significant decreases in metabolic rates by 2 weeks after burn injury in animals fed enterally and continuously by 2 hours after burn injury compared with animals fed 3 days after burn injury, indicating the benefits of early initiation.[76] Significant modulation of catecholamine levels and support of gut mucosal integrity have been shown with early EN.[90] In human studies, early continuous EN delivered calculated caloric requirements (resting energy expenditure) by postburn day 3, nearly prevented the hypermetabolic response, and significantly decreased circulating levels of catecholamines, cortisol, and glucagon.[90,91] Early enteral feeding preserved gut mucosal integrity, motility, and intestinal blood flow.[76] Intestinal hypoperfusion or ileus, secondary to delays in resuscitation, can be reversed by reperfusion or adequate resuscitation. Postburn ileus spares the small bowel and primarily affects the stomach and colon.[92] Patients can be safely fed enterally in the duodenum or jejunum 6 hours after severe burn injury, whether or not they have total gastroduodenal function.[93] Nasojejunal or nasoduodenal feeding should be initiated as soon as possible to facilitate the full resuscitation of the severely burned patient.

### The Nutritional Requirements

Caloric requirements can be accurately determined by measuring resting energy expenditures with bedside carts.[94,95] Preservation of LBM should be a nutritional goal for severe burn victims, because a major consequence of the hypermetabolic response is severe total body catabolism. Appropriate nutrient delivery can be accomplished by feeding 1.2 to 1.4 times the measured resting energy expenditures (in kilocalories per square meter per day). Goran and colleagues[94] found that by feeding patients 1.2 times the measured resting energy expenditures, body weight may be maintained, but with a loss of 10% of LBM. Although others found an increase in body weight by feeding 1.4 times the resting energy expenditure, the gains were in fat deposition, not LBM.[95,96]

The major energy source for patients with burns should be carbohydrates, which serve as fuel for wound healing, provide glucose for metabolic pathways, and spare the amino acids needed for catabolic patients with burns. It is estimated that critically ill, burned patients have caloric requirements that exceed the body's ability to use glucose, which is approximately 7 g/kg/d (2240 kcal for an 80-kg man).[97] Providing a limited amount of dietary fat reduced requirements for carbohydrates and can improve glucose tolerance significantly.

The hypermetabolic, catabolic response to severe burns suppresses lipolysis and limits the extent to which lipids can be used for energy. Thus, fat should comprise no more than about 30% of nonprotein calories, or about 1 g/kg/d of intravenous lipids in TPN.[98] Thirty percent may be overwhelming in burned patients. In an animal model, immune function was further compromised with diets containing more than even 15% lipids, advocating the use of low-fat diets in severely burned patients.[99,100] The composition of administered fat is more important than the quantity. Most common lipid sources contain ω-6 free fatty acids (ω-6 FFAs) such as linoleic acid, which are metabolized through synthesis of arachidonic acid, a precursor of proinflammatory cytokines such as prostaglandin $E_2$. ω-3 FFAs are metabolized without provoking proinflammatory compounds. Diets high in ω-3 FFAs have been associated with an improved inflammatory response, improved outcomes, and reduced incidences of hyperglycemia.[101,102]

Proteolysis is another hallmark of the hypermetabolic response after severe burn injury. Protein catabolism in patients with burns can exceed 150 g/d, or almost half a pound of skeletal muscle.[64] Increased protein catabolism leads to decreased wound healing, immunoincompetence, and loss of LBM.[64] There is some evidence that increased protein replacement for severely burned patients may be beneficial.[103,104] Healthy individuals require 1 g per kilogram body weight per day of protein intake.[105,106] However, based on in vivo kinetics studies measuring oxidation rates of essential and nonessential amino acids, patients with burns have 50% higher use rates than healthy individuals in the fasting state.[103,104,107] Thus, patients with burns require a minimum of 1.5 to 2 g per kilogram body weight per day protein intake.[16,64,108] However, any higher amount of supplementation in burned children leads to increased urea production without improvements in LBM or muscle protein synthesis.[109]

Amino acids have a key role in recovery after injury. Alanine and glutamine (GLU) are important transport amino acids, created in skeletal muscle to supply energy to the liver and to aid in wound healing.[110] GLU serves as a primary fuel for enterocytes and lymphocytes, and aids in maintaining small bowel integrity, preserving gut-associated immune function, and limiting intestinal permeability after acute injury.[111,112] GLU is rapidly depleted from both serum and muscle after severe burn injury, limiting visceral protein synthesis, and underscoring the importance of GLU replacement after severe burn injury.[110,113] When GLU was given at 25 g/kg/d, severely burned patients had a decrease in incidence of infections, improved visceral protein levels, decreased length of stay, and reduced mortality.[114–116] Replacement of branched-chain amino acids led to improvements in nitrogen balance, but had no effect on survival.[117]

Vitamins and other micronutrients are also profoundly affected by the hypermetabolic-catabolic response after burn injury (**Table 1**).[118–121] Decreased levels of vitamins A, C, and D, iron, zinc, and selenium have been implicated in decreased wound healing and immune dysfunction after severe burn injury.[118,122] Vitamin A replacement is important for wound healing and epithelial growth.[120,123] Vitamin C is paramount for synthesis and the cross-linking of collagen after burn injury, and patients with burns often require up to 20 times the recommended daily allowance.[120,122] Vitamin D is essential in the prevention of further bone catabolism after burn injury.[122] Iron is an important cofactor in oxygen-carrying proteins.[64] Zinc supplementation contributes to improvements in wound healing, DNA replication, and lymphocyte function.[124] Selenium replacement improves cell-mediated immunity.[125] Collectively, replacement of these micronutrients has contributed to the improvement in morbidity of severely burned patients.

Milk, traditionally an isocaloric isoprotein, but high-fat diet, consisting of 44% fat, 42% carbohydrate, and 14% protein, became standard of care for the pediatric burned patient.[126,127] Although it was well tolerated, fat did not serve as the optimal energy source for these patients. There was continued protein degradation, and LBM gains paled compared with high-carbohydrate diets, consisting of 3% fat, 15% protein, and 82% carbohydrate.[127] The high-carbohydrate diet increased protein synthesis, increased effective endogenous insulin production, and improved LBM. Increased endogenous insulin levels, stimulated by high-carbohydrate delivery, may have contributed to improved muscle protein synthesis.[127] Parenteral formulas, which are traditionally 70% dextrose, 15% amino acids, and 20% lipids, can be manipulated and adjusted to meet patients' caloric needs. However, TPN is associated with increased proinflammatory cytokines, increased pulmonary dysfunction, and increased mortality.[84,85,128,129] Thus, all TPN formulas containing fat emulsions should be reserved for patients that cannot tolerate EN.

### Overfeeding

The overfeeding of severely burned patients can lead to major complications. Overfeeding with carbohydrates results in increased respiratory quotients, increased fat synthesis, and increased $CO_2$ elimination. Ventilated patients become more difficult to manage and to wean from support.[130] Excess carbohydrate or fat can also lead to fat deposition in the liver.[131] Excess protein replacement leads to increases in blood urea nitrogen, which could lead to acute renal failure, increased propensity to sepsis, and death.[131] Overfeeding can lead to hyperglycemia, which is already present in up to 90% of all critically ill patients, leading to increased morbidity and mortality.[132] This iatrogenic hyperglycemia is even harder to treat because both endogenous and exogenous insulin effects are often countered by the surge of catabolic hormones.[33,133] These complications are not specific to parenteral or enteral feeding, but are manifestations of attempts to overcompensate for the losses suffered by severely burned patients.

Positive changes in body weight are among the best predictors of overall nutritional status. Significant weight loss, particularly rapid and unplanned, is a predictor of mortality.[134] However, resuscitation and maintenance fluid increases may mask ongoing loss of LBM so that patients can suffer significant inanition and still weigh more than they did at the time of admission. In addition, fluid shifts associated with infections, ventilator support, hypoproteinemia, and increases in aldosterone and antidiuretic hormone lead to wide fluctuations in weight that have little to do with

**Table 1**
Summary of the main effects of various pharmacologic interventions to alter the hypermetabolic response to burn injury

| Drug | Inflammatory Response | Stress Hormones | Body Composition | Net Protein Balance | Insulin Resistance | Hyperdynamic Circulation |
|---|---|---|---|---|---|---|
| rhGH | Improved | No difference | Improved | No difference | Hyperglycemia | No difference |
| IGF-1 | Improved | No difference | Improved | Improved | Improved | No difference |
| Oxandrolone | Improved | No difference | Improved | Improved | No difference | No difference |
| Insulin | Improved | No difference | Improved | Improved | Improved | No difference |
| Propranolol | Improved | Improved | Improved | Improved | Improved | Improved |
| Oxandrolone + propranolol | Improved (preliminary) | Improved (preliminary) | Improved (preliminary) | Improved (preliminary) | Improved (preliminary) | Improved (preliminary) |

Data from [23,28,30,53,121,138,141,143,149,150,152,153,156,158,185–200], and From Williams FN, Herndon DN, Jeschke MG. The hypermetabolic response to burn injury and interventions to modify this response. Clin Plast Surg 2009;36(4):591; with permission.

nutritional status.[135] Judicious monitoring of long-term trends is paramount in the clinical management of severely burned patients.

Determination of nitrogen balance, serum proteins, and abnormalities of immune function also aids the assessment of nutritional supplementation after burn injury.[122,136,137] Although no single laboratory test is fully reliable in nutritional monitoring, regular metabolic assessment is paramount in the ever-evolving physiologic response after burn injury.

### The Hormonal Response in Severe Burns

Increased levels of catecholamines, cortisol, and glucagon perpetuate the profound changes in metabolic rates, growth, and physiology observed in patients with burns. Anabolic agents such as recombinant human growth hormone (rhGH), insulin, insulin-like growth factor (IGF-1), and IGF-binding protein 3 (IGFBP-3) in combination with testosterone and oxandrolone have been shown to abate postburn metabolism. To counter increased levels of catecholamines, the adrenergic antagonist propranolol has been used with profound results. Other glucose modulators, besides insulin, have also been shown to attenuate postburn metabolic derangements. The use of anabolic or anticatabolic agents in severely burned children, in addition to standard of care, has led to significant decreases in protein catabolism.

## PHARMACOLOGIC MODALITIES
### rhGH

Intramuscular administration of rhGH at doses of 0.2 mg/kg as a daily injection during the acute burn phase favorably influenced the hepatic acute phase response,[138,139] increased serum concentrations of its secondary mediator IGF-I,[140] improved muscle protein kinetics, maintained muscular growth,[141,142] decreased donor site healing time by 1.5 days,[143] improved resting energy expenditure, and attenuated hyperdynamic circulation.[144] These beneficial effects of rhGH are mediated by IGF-1, and patients receiving treatment showed 100% increases in serum IGF-I and IGFBP-3 relative to healthy individuals.[145,146] However, in a prospective, multicenter, double-blind, randomized, placebo-controlled trial involving 247 patients and 285 critically ill nonburned patients, Takala and colleagues[146] found that high doses of rhGH (0.10 ± 0.02 mg/kg body weight) were associated with increased morbidity and mortality. Others showed growth hormone treatment to be associated with hyperglycemia and insulin resistance.[147,148] However, neither short-term nor long-term administration of rhGH was associated with an increase in mortality in severely burned children.[144,149]

### IGF

IGF-I mediates the effects of growth hormone. The infusion of equimolar doses of recombinant human IGF-1 and IGFBP-3 to burned patients has been shown to be effective in improving protein metabolism in catabolic pediatric patients and adults with significantly less hypoglycemia than rhGH alone.[150,151] It attenuates muscle catabolism and improves gut mucosal integrity in children with severe burns.[151] Immune function is effectively improved by attenuation of the type 1 and type 2 hepatic acute phase responses, increased serum concentrations of constitutive proteins, and vulnerary modulation of the use of body protein resulting from hypercatabolism.[151–154] However, studies by Langouche and van den Berghe[155] indicate that the use of IGF-1 alone is not effective in nonburned critically ill patients.

## Oxandrolone

Treatment with anabolic agents such as oxandrolone, a testosterone analogue that possesses only 5% of its virilizing androgenic effects, improves muscle protein catabolism via enhanced protein synthesis efficiency,[156] reduces weight loss, and increases donor site wound healing.[157] In a large prospective, double-blind, randomized, single-center study, oxandrolone given at a dose of 0.1 mg/kg every 12 hours shortened length of acute hospital stay, maintained LBM, and improved body composition and hepatic protein synthesis.[158] These effects were independent of age.[159] Long-term treatment with this oral anabolic during rehabilitation in the outpatient setting is more favorably regarded by pediatric patients than parenteral anabolic agents. Oxandrolone use in children successfully abates the effects of burn-associated hypermetabolism on body tissues and significantly improves body mass over time, increasing LBM at 6, 9, and 12 months after burn injury, and bone mineral content by 12 months after injury compared with unburned controls.[160] Patients treated with oxandrolone experience few complications relative to those treated with rhGH. However, although anabolic agents can increase LBM, exercise is essential to developing strength.[161]

## Propranolol

β-Adrenergic blockade with propranolol probably represents the most efficacious anticatabolic therapy in the treatment of burns.[8] Long-term use of propranolol during acute care in patients with burns, at a dose titrated to reduce heart rate by 15% to 20%, was noted to diminish cardiac work.[39] It also reduced fatty infiltration of the liver, which typically occurs in these patients as the result of enhanced peripheral lipolysis and altered substrate disposition. Reduction of hepatic fat results from decreased peripheral lipolysis and reduced palmitate delivery and uptake by the liver,[162,163] resulting in smaller livers and avoiding the hepatomegaly that frequently adversely affects diaphragmatic function. Stable isotope serial body composition studies showed that administration of propranolol reduces skeletal muscle wasting and increases LBM after burn injury.[28,164] The underlying mechanism of action of propranolol is still unclear; however, its effects seem to occur as a result of increased protein synthesis in the presence of persistent protein breakdown and reduced peripheral lipolysis.[165] Recent data suggest that administration of propranolol at 4 mg/kg body weight every 24 hours also markedly decreased the amount of insulin necessary to reduce increased blood glucose levels after burn injury.[40] Propranolol may thus constitute a promising approach to overcoming postburn insulin resistance.

## ATTENUATION OF HYPERGLYCEMIA AFTER BURN INJURY
### Insulin

Insulin probably represents one of the most extensively studied therapeutic agents, and novel therapeutic applications are continually being explored. Insulin decreases blood glucose levels by mediating increased peripheral glucose uptake by skeletal muscle and adipose tissue, and suppressing hepatic gluconeogenesis. It also increases DNA replication and protein synthesis via control of amino acid uptake, increases fatty acid synthesis and decreases proteiolysis.[166] The latter action makes insulin particularly attractive for the treatment of hyperglycemia in severely burned patients because insulin given during acute hospitalization has been shown to improve muscle protein synthesis, accelerate donor site healing, and attenuate LBM loss and the acute phase response.[121,167–173] In addition to its anabolic actions, insulin was shown to exert totally unexpected antiinflammatory effects, potentially neutralizing the proinflammatory actions of glucose.[170,171,174] These results suggest a dual benefit of insulin administration: reduction of proinflammatory effects of glucose by restoration of euglycemia, and a possible additional insulin-mediated antiinflammatory effect.[175] Van den Berghe and colleagues[132] confirmed the beneficial effects of insulin in a recent large milestone study. Insulin administered to maintain glucose at levels less than 110 mg/dL decreased mortality, incidence of infections, sepsis, and sepsis-associated multiorgan failure in critically ill surgical patients. Intensive insulin therapy also significantly reduces newly acquired kidney injury, accelerating weaning from mechanical ventilation and accelerating discharge from the intensive care unit (ICU) and the hospital.[176] The ideal target blood glucose range for the severely burned patient has not been identified unequivocally, and several groups are undertaking clinical trials to define ideal blood glucose levels for the treatment of patients in the ICU and burned patients: a study by Finney and colleagues[177] suggests maintaining blood glucose levels of 140 mg/dL and less, whereas the Surviving Sepsis Campaign recommends maintenance of blood glucose levels less than 150 mg/dL.[178] However, maintaining a continuous hyperinsulinemic, euglycemic clamp in patients with burns is particularly difficult because these patients are being continuously fed large caloric loads via enteral feeding tubes. Because patients with burns require weekly operations and daily dressing changes, EN occasionally needs to be stopped, which may lead to disruption of gastrointestinal motility and increased risk of hypoglycemia.[4]

### Metformin

Metformin (Glucophage), a biguanide, has recently been suggested as an alternative means to correct hyperglycemia in severely injured patients.[179] By inhibiting gluconeogenesis and augmenting peripheral insulin sensitivity, metformin directly counters the 2 main metabolic processes that underlie injury-induced hyperglycemia.[180–182] In addition, metformin has only rarely been associated with hypoglycemic events, thus possibly minimizing this concern, which is associated with the use of exogenous insulin.[183] In a small randomized study reported by Gore and colleagues,[179] metformin reduced plasma glucose concentration, decreased endogenous glucose production, and accelerated glucose clearance in severely burned patients. A follow-up study evaluating the effects of metformin on muscle protein synthesis confirmed these observations and showed an increased fractional synthetic rate of muscle protein and improvement in net muscle protein balance in metformin-treated patients.[182] Thus, metformin, analogous to insulin, may have efficacy in critically injured patients as both an antihyperglycemic and a muscle protein anabolic agent. On the other hand, despite the advantages and potential therapeutic uses, treatment with metformin, or other biguanides, has been associated with lactic acidosis.[183,184] To avoid metformin-associated lactic acidosis, the use of this medication is contraindicated in certain diseases or illnesses in which there is a potential for impaired lactate elimination (hepatic or renal failure) or tissue hypoxia, and it should be used with caution in patients with acute burns.

### Novel Therapeutic Options

Other ongoing trials, with the goal of decreasing postburn hyperglycemia, include the use of glucagonlike peptide 1 and peroxisome proliferator-activated receptor $\gamma$ (PPAR-$\gamma$) agonists (eg, pioglitazone, thioglitazones) or the combination of various antidiabetic drugs. PPAR-$\gamma$ agonists, such as fenofibrate, have been shown to improve insulin sensitivity in patients with diabetes. Cree and colleagues[53] found in a recent double-blind, prospective, placebo-controlled, randomized trial that fenofibrate treatment significantly decreased plasma glucose concentrations by improving insulin sensitivity and mitochondrial glucose oxidation. Fenofibrate also led to significantly increased tyrosine phosphorylation of the insulin receptor and IRS-1 in muscle tissue after a hyperinsulinemic-euglycemic clamp when compared with placebo-treated patients, indicating improved insulin receptor signaling.[53]

## SUMMARY

Severely burned patients have profound nutritional requirements secondary to the prolonged postburn hypermetabolic, hypercatabolic response. Enteral nutritional support should be initiated early to optimize total burn care and decrease long-term morbidity. Neither nonpharmacologic nor pharmacologic strategies are sufficient to abate completely the catabolic response to severe burn injury. All therapeutic strategies have contributed to some extent to the improvements in morbidity and mortality (see **Table 1**). Early EN has contributed to the significant decline in LBM loss of severely catabolic patients.[34,44] Modulation of the hypermetabolic response is paramount in the optimal restoration of structure and function of severely burned patients and remains an elusive completely fulfilled goal despite the significant advances made in this area in the past few decades.

## REFERENCES

1. Nguyen TT, Gilpin DA, Meyer NA, et al. Current treatment of severely burned patients. Ann Surg 1996;223(1):14–25.
2. Brigham PA, McLoughlin E. Burn incidence and medical care use in the United States: estimates, trends, and data sources. J Burn Care Rehabil 1996;17(2):95–107.
3. Wolf S. Critical care in the severely burned: organ support and management of complications. In: Herndon DN, editor. Total burn care. 3rd edition. London: Saunders Elsevier; 2007. p. 454–76.
4. Herndon DN, Tompkins RG. Support of the metabolic response to burn injury. Lancet 2004;363(9424):1895–902.
5. Hart DW, Wolf SE, Mlcak R, et al. Persistence of muscle catabolism after severe burn. Surgery 2000;128(2):312–9.
6. Reiss E, Pearson E, Artz CP. The metabolic response to burns. J Clin Invest 1956;35(1):62–77.
7. Yu YM, Tompkins RG, Ryan CM, et al. The metabolic basis of the increase in energy expenditure in severely burned patients. JPEN J Parenter Enteral Nutr 1999;23(3):160–8.
8. Williams FN, Jeschke MG, Chinkes DL, et al. Modulation of the hypermetabolic response to trauma: temperature, nutrition, and drugs. J Am Coll Surg 2009;208(4):489–502.
9. Mlcak RP, Jeschke MG, Barrow RE, et al. The influence of age and gender on resting energy expenditure in severely burned children. Ann Surg 2006;244(1):121–30.
10. Przkora R, Barrow RE, Jeschke MG, et al. Body composition changes with time in pediatric burn patients. J Trauma 2006;60(5):968–71.
11. Dolecek R. Endocrine changes after burn trauma–a review. Keio J Med 1989;38(3):262–76.
12. Jeffries MK, Vance ML. Growth hormone and cortisol secretion in patients with burn injury. J Burn Care Rehabil 1992;13(4):391–5.
13. Klein GL, Bi LX, Sherrard DJ, et al. Evidence supporting a role of glucocorticoids in short-term bone loss in burned children. Osteoporos Int 2004;15(6):468–74.

14. Goodall M, Stone C, Haynes BW Jr. Urinary output of adrenaline and noradrenaline in severe thermal burns. Ann Surg 1957;145(4):479–87.
15. Coombes EJ, Batstone GF. Urine cortisol levels after burn injury. Burns Incl Therm Inj 1982;8(5):333–7.
16. Norbury WB, Herndon DN. Modulation of the hypermetabolic response after burn injury. In: Herndon DN, editor. Total burn care. 3rd edition. New York: Saunders Elsevier; 2007. p. 420–33.
17. Rutan RL, Herndon DN. Growth delay in postburn pediatric patients. Arch Surg 1990;125(3):392–5.
18. Wilmore DW, Mason AD Jr, Pruitt BA Jr. Insulin response to glucose in hypermetabolic burn patients. Ann Surg 1976;183(3):314–20.
19. Goldstein DS, Kopin IJ. Evolution of concepts of stress. Stress 2007;10(2): 109–20.
20. Selye H. Stress and the general adaptation syndrome. Br Med J 1950;1(4667): 1383–92.
21. Selye H. An extra-adrenal action of adrenotropic hormone. Nature 1951; 168(4265):149–50.
22. Selye H, Fortier C. Adaptive reaction to stress. Psychosom Med 1950;12(3): 149–57.
23. Herndon D. Mediators of metabolism. J Trauma 1981;21:701–5.
24. Lee JO, Herndon DN. Modulation of the post-burn hypermetabolic state. Nestle Nutr Workshop Ser Clin Perform Programme 2003;8:39–49 [discussion: 49–56].
25. Newsome TW, Mason AD Jr, Pruitt BA Jr. Weight loss following thermal injury. Ann Surg 1973;178(2):215–7.
26. Barrow RE, Hawkins HK, Aarsland A, et al. Identification of factors contributing to hepatomegaly in severely burned children. Shock 2005;24(6):523–8.
27. Barrow RE, Wolfe RR, Dasu MR, et al. The use of beta-adrenergic blockade in preventing trauma-induced hepatomegaly. Ann Surg 2006;243(1):115–20.
28. Herndon DN, Hart DW, Wolf SE, et al. Reversal of catabolism by beta-blockade after severe burns. N Engl J Med 2001;345(17):1223–9.
29. Wolfe RR, Herndon DN, Peters EJ, et al. Regulation of lipolysis in severely burned children. Ann Surg 1987;206(2):214–21.
30. Chang DW, DeSanti L, Demling RH. Anticatabolic and anabolic strategies in critical illness: a review of current treatment modalities. Shock 1998;10(3):155–60.
31. Sheridan RL. A great constitutional disturbance. N Engl J Med 2001;345(17): 1271–2.
32. Pereira C, Murphy K, Jeschke M, et al. Post burn muscle wasting and the effects of treatments. Int J Biochem Cell Biol 2005;37(10):1948–61.
33. Wilmore DW, Long JM, Mason AD Jr, et al. Catecholamines: mediator of the hypermetabolic response to thermal injury. Ann Surg 1974;180(4):653–69.
34. Jeschke MG, Chinkes DL, Finnerty CC, et al. Pathophysiologic response to severe burn injury. Ann Surg 2008;248(3):387–401.
35. Wilmore DW, Aulick LH. Metabolic changes in burned patients. Surg Clin North Am 1978;58(6):1173–87.
36. Wolfe RR. Review: acute versus chronic response to burn injury. Circ Shock 1981;8(1):105–15.
37. Cuthbertson DP, Angeles Valero Zanuy MA, Leon Sanz ML. Post-shock metabolic response. 1942. Nutr Hosp 2001;16(5):175–82.
38. Cuthbertson D. Post-shock metabolic response. Lancet 1942;(1):433–6.
39. Baron PW, Barrow RE, Pierre EJ, et al. Prolonged use of propranolol safely decreases cardiac work in burned children. J Burn Care Rehabil 1997;18(3):223–7.

40. Williams FN, Herndon DN, Kulp GA, et al. Propranolol decreases cardiac work in a dose-dependent manner in severely burned children. Surgery 2011;149(2): 231–9.

41. Galster AD, Bier DM, Cryer PE, et al. Plasma palmitate turnover in subjects with thermal injury. J Trauma 1984;24(11):938–45.

42. Cree MG, Aarsland A, Herndon DN, et al. Role of fat metabolism in burn trauma-induced skeletal muscle insulin resistance. Crit Care Med 2007;35(Suppl 9): S476–83.

43. Childs C, Heath DF, Little RA, et al. Glucose metabolism in children during the first day after burn injury. Arch Emerg Med 1990;7(3):135–47.

44. Jeschke MG, Mlcak RP, Finnerty CC, et al. Burn size determines the inflammatory and hypermetabolic response. Crit Care 2007;11(4):R90.

45. Gauglitz GG, Herndon DN, Kulp GA, et al. Abnormal insulin sensitivity persists up to three years in pediatric patients post-burn. J Clin Endocrinol Metab 2009; 94(5):1656–64.

46. Khani S, Tayek JA. Cortisol increases gluconeogenesis in humans: its role in the metabolic syndrome. Clin Sci (Lond) 2001;101(6):739–47.

47. Wolfe RR, Herndon DN, Jahoor F, et al. Effect of severe burn injury on substrate cycling by glucose and fatty acids. N Engl J Med 1987;317(7):403–8.

48. Gore DC, Jahoor F, Wolfe RR, et al. Acute response of human muscle protein to catabolic hormones. Ann Surg 1993;218(5):679–84.

49. Robinson LE, van Soeren MH. Insulin resistance and hyperglycemia in critical illness: role of insulin in glycemic control. AACN Clin Issues 2004;15(1):45–62.

50. Gearhart MM, Parbhoo SK. Hyperglycemia in the critically ill patient. AACN Clin Issues 2006;17(1):50–5.

51. Carlson GL. Insulin resistance and glucose-induced thermogenesis in critical illness. Proc Nutr Soc 2001;60(3):381–8.

52. Wolfe RR, Durkot MJ, Allsop JR, et al. Glucose metabolism in severely burned patients. Metabolism 1979;28(10):1031–9.

53. Cree MG, Zwetsloot JJ, Herndon DN, et al. Insulin sensitivity and mitochondrial function are improved in children with burn injury during a randomized controlled trial of fenofibrate. Ann Surg 2007;245(2):214–21.

54. Hunt DG, Ivy JL. Epinephrine inhibits insulin-stimulated muscle glucose transport. J Appl Physiol 2002;93(5):1638–43.

55. Gustavson SM, Chu CA, Nishizawa M, et al. Interaction of glucagon and epinephrine in the control of hepatic glucose production in the conscious dog. Am J Physiol Endocrinol Metab 2003;284(4):E695–707.

56. Mastorakos G, Chrousos GP, Weber JS. Recombinant interleukin-6 activates the hypothalamic-pituitary-adrenal axis in humans. J Clin Endocrinol Metab 1993; 77(6):1690–4.

57. Lang CH, Dobrescu C, Bagby GJ. Tumor necrosis factor impairs insulin action on peripheral glucose disposal and hepatic glucose output. Endocrinology 1992;130(1):43–52.

58. Akita S, Akino K, Ren SG, et al. Elevated circulating leukemia inhibitory factor in patients with extensive burns. J Burn Care Res 2006;27(2):221–5.

59. Fan J, Li YH, Wojnar MM, et al. Endotoxin-induced alterations in insulin-stimulated phosphorylation of insulin receptor, IRS-1, and MAP kinase in skeletal muscle. Shock 1996;6(3):164–70.

60. del Aguila LF, Claffey KP, Kirwan JP. TNF-alpha impairs insulin signaling and insulin stimulation of glucose uptake in C2C12 muscle cells. Am J Physiol 1999;276(5 Pt 1):E849–55.

61. Sell H, Dietze-Schroeder D, Kaiser U, et al. Monocyte chemotactic protein-1 is a potential player in the negative cross-talk between adipose tissue and skeletal muscle. Endocrinology 2006;147(5):2458–67.
62. Baracos V, Rodemann HP, Dinarello CA, et al. Stimulation of muscle protein degradation and prostaglandin E2 release by leukocytic pyrogen (interleukin-1). A mechanism for the increased degradation of muscle proteins during fever. N Engl J Med 1983;308(10):553–8.
63. Jahoor F, Desai M, Herndon DN, et al. Dynamics of the protein metabolic response to burn injury. Metabolism 1988;37(4):330–7.
64. Saffle JR, Graves C. Nutritional support of the burned patient. In: Herndon DN, editor. Total burn care. 3rd edition. London: Saunders Elsevier; 2007. p. 398–419.
65. Hart DW, Wolf SE, Chinkes DL, et al. Determinants of skeletal muscle catabolism after severe burn. Ann Surg 2000;232(4):455–65.
66. DeFronzo RA, Jacot E, Jequier E, et al. The effect of insulin on the disposal of intravenous glucose. Results from indirect calorimetry and hepatic and femoral venous catheterization. Diabetes 1981;30(12):1000–7.
67. Flakoll PJ, Hill JO, Abumrad NN. Acute hyperglycemia enhances proteolysis in normal man. Am J Physiol 1993;265(5 Pt 1):E715–21.
68. Arora NS, Rochester DF. Respiratory muscle strength and maximal voluntary ventilation in undernourished patients. Am Rev Respir Dis 1982;126(1):5–8.
69. Greenhalgh DG, Saffle JR, Holmes JH, et al. American Burn Association consensus conference to define sepsis and infection in burns. J Burn Care Res 2007;28(6):776–90.
70. Murray CK, Loo FL, Hospenthal DR, et al. Incidence of systemic fungal infection and related mortality following severe burns. Burns 2008;34(8):1108–12.
71. Pruitt BA Jr, McManus AT, Kim SH, et al. Burn wound infections: current status. World J Surg 1998;22(2):135–45.
72. Williams FN, Herndon DN, Hawkins HK, et al. The leading causes of death after burn injury in a single pediatric burn center. Crit Care 2009;13(6):R183.
73. Im MJ, Hoopes JE. Energy metabolism in healing skin wounds. J Surg Res 1970;10(10):459–64.
74. Falcone PA, Caldwell MD. Wound metabolism. Clin Plast Surg 1990;17(3):443–56.
75. Wilmore DW, Aulick LH, Mason AD, et al. Influence of the burn wound on local and systemic responses to injury. Ann Surg 1977;186(4):444–58.
76. Mochizuki H, Trocki O, Dominioni L, et al. Mechanism of prevention of postburn hypermetabolism and catabolism by early enteral feeding. Ann Surg 1984; 200(3):297–310.
77. Dominioni L, Trocki O, Fang CH, et al. Enteral feeding in burn hypermetabolism: nutritional and metabolic effects of different levels of calorie and protein intake. JPEN J Parenter Enteral Nutr 1985;9(3):269–79.
78. Wilmore DW. Nutrition and metabolism following thermal injury. Clin Plast Surg 1974;1(4):603–19.
79. Ireton-Jones CS, Gottschlich MM. The evolution of nutrition support in burns. J Burn Care Rehabil 1993;14(2 Pt 2):272–80.
80. Popp MB, Law EJ, MacMillian BG. Parenteral nutrition in the burned child: a study of twenty-six patients. Ann Surg 1974;179(2):219–25.
81. Curreri PW, Richmond D, Marvin J, et al. Dietary requirements of patients with major burns. J Am Diet Assoc 1974;65(4):415–7.
82. Wilmore DW, Curreri PW, Spitzer KW, et al. Supranormal dietary intake in thermally injured hypermetabolic patients. Surg Gynecol Obstet 1971;132(5): 881–6.

83. Hildreth MA, Herndon DN, Desai MH, et al. Reassessing caloric requirements in pediatric burn patients. J Burn Care Rehabil 1988;9(6):616–8.

84. Herndon DN, Barrow RE, Stein M, et al. Increased mortality with intravenous supplemental feeding in severely burned patients. J Burn Care Rehabil 1989; 10(4):309–13.

85. Herndon DN, Stein MD, Rutan TC, et al. Failure of TPN supplementation to improve liver function, immunity, and mortality in thermally injured patients. J Trauma 1987;27(2):195–204.

86. Jeejeebhoy KN. Total parenteral nutrition: potion or poison? Am J Clin Nutr 2001; 74(2):160–3.

87. Wolf SE, Rose JK, Desai MH, et al. Mortality determinants in massive pediatric burns. An analysis of 103 children with > or = 80% TBSA burns (> or = 70% full-thickness). Ann Surg 1997;225(5):554–65 [discussion: 565–9].

88. Deitch EA. Intestinal permeability is increased in burn patients shortly after injury. Surgery 1990;107(4):411–6.

89. van Elburg RM, Uil JJ, de Monchy JG, et al. Intestinal permeability in pediatric gastroenterology. Scand J Gastroenterol Suppl 1992;194:19–24.

90. Mochizuki H, Trocki O, Dominioni L, et al. Reduction of postburn hypermetabolism by early enteral feeding. Curr Surg 1985;42(2):121–5.

91. McDonald WS, Sharp CW Jr, Deitch EA. Immediate enteral feeding in burn patients is safe and effective. Ann Surg 1991;213(2):177–83.

92. Tinckler LF. Surgery and intestinal motility. Br J Surg 1965;52:140–50.

93. Moss G. Maintenance of gastrointestinal function after bowel surgery and immediate enteral full nutrition. II. Clinical experience, with objective demonstration of intestinal absorption and motility. JPEN J Parenter Enteral Nutr 1981;5(3): 215–20.

94. Goran MI, Peters EJ, Herndon DN, et al. Total energy expenditure in burned children using the doubly labeled water technique. Am J Physiol 1990;259(4 Pt 1): E576–85.

95. Gore DC, Rutan RL, Hildreth M, et al. Comparison of resting energy expenditures and caloric intake in children with severe burns. J Burn Care Rehabil 1990;11(5):400–4.

96. Hart DW, Wolf SE, Herndon DN, et al. Energy expenditure and caloric balance after burn: increased feeding leads to fat rather than lean mass accretion. Ann Surg 2002;235(1):152–61.

97. Wolfe RR, Allsop JR, Burke JF. Glucose metabolism in man: responses to intravenous glucose infusion. Metabolism 1979;28(3):210–20.

98. Demling RH, Seigne P. Metabolic management of patients with severe burns. World J Surg 2000;24(6):673–80.

99. Mochizuki H, Trocki O, Dominioni L, et al. Optimal lipid content for enteral diets following thermal injury. JPEN J Parenter Enteral Nutr 1984;8(6):638–46.

100. Garrel DR, Razi M, Lariviere F, et al. Improved clinical status and length of care with low-fat nutrition support in burn patients. JPEN J Parenter Enteral Nutr 1995;19(6):482–91.

101. Alexander JW, Saito H, Trocki O, et al. The importance of lipid type in the diet after burn injury. Ann Surg 1986;204(1):1–8.

102. Huschak G, Zur Nieden K, Hoell T, et al. Olive oil based nutrition in multiple trauma patients: a pilot study. Intensive Care Med 2005;31(9):1202–8.

103. Wolfe RR, Goodenough RD, Burke JF, et al. Response of protein and urea kinetics in burn patients to different levels of protein intake. Ann Surg 1983; 197(2):163–71.

104. Yu YM, Young VR, Castillo L, et al. Plasma arginine and leucine kinetics and urea production rates in burn patients. Metabolism 1995;44(5):659–66.
105. Melville S, McNurlan MA, McHardy KC, et al. The role of degradation in the acute control of protein balance in adult man: failure of feeding to stimulate protein synthesis as assessed by L-[1-13C]leucin infusion. Metabolism 1989; 38(3):248–55.
106. Hoerr RA, Matthews DE, Bier DM, et al. Effects of protein restriction and acute refeeding on leucine and lysine kinetics in young men. Am J Physiol 1993;264(4 Pt 1):E567–75.
107. Yu YM, Ryan CM, Burke JF, et al. Relations among arginine, citrulline, ornithine, and leucine kinetics in adult burn patients. Am J Clin Nutr 1995;62(5): 960–8.
108. Matthews DE, Marano MA, Campbell RG. Splanchnic bed utilization of leucine and phenylalanine in humans. Am J Physiol 1993;264(1 Pt 1):E109–18.
109. Patterson BW, Nguyen T, Pierre E, et al. Urea and protein metabolism in burned children: effect of dietary protein intake. Metabolism 1997;46(5):573–8.
110. Soeters PB, van de Poll MC, van Gemert WG, et al. Amino acid adequacy in pathophysiological states. J Nutr 2004;134(Suppl 6):1575S–82S.
111. De-Souza DA, Greene LJ. Intestinal permeability and systemic infections in critically ill patients: effect of glutamine. Crit Care Med 2005;33(5):1125–35.
112. Souba WW. Glutamine: a key substrate for the splanchnic bed. Annu Rev Nutr 1991;11:285–308.
113. Gore DC, Jahoor F. Glutamine kinetics in burn patients. Comparison with hormonally induced stress in volunteers. Arch Surg 1994;129(12):1318–23.
114. Garrel D. The effect of supplemental enteral glutamine on plasma levels, gut function, and outcome in severe burns. JPEN J Parenter Enteral Nutr 2004; 28(2):123 [author reply: 123].
115. Wischmeyer PE, Lynch J, Liedel J, et al. Glutamine administration reduces Gram-negative bacteremia in severely burned patients: a prospective, randomized, double-blind trial versus isonitrogenous control. Crit Care Med 2001; 29(11):2075–80.
116. Zhou YP, Jiang ZM, Sun YH, et al. The effect of supplemental enteral glutamine on plasma levels, gut function, and outcome in severe burns: a randomized, double-blind, controlled clinical trial. JPEN J Parenter Enteral Nutr 2003;27(4): 241–5.
117. Cerra FB, Mazuski JE, Chute E, et al. Branched chain metabolic support. A prospective, randomized, double-blind trial in surgical stress. Ann Surg 1984; 199(3):286–91.
118. Gamliel Z, DeBiasse MA, Demling RH. Essential microminerals and their response to burn injury. J Burn Care Rehabil 1996;17(3):264–72.
119. Dietary Reference Intakes: The Essential Guide to Nutrient Requirements. Otten JJ, Pitzi-Hellwig J, Meyers LD, editors. Washington, DC: National Academic Press 2006.
120. Mayes T, Gottschlich MM, Warden GD. Clinical nutrition protocols for continuous quality improvements in the outcomes of patients with burns. J Burn Care Rehabil 1997;18(4):365–8 [discussion: 364].
121. Ferrando AA, Chinkes DL, Wolf SE, et al. A submaximal dose of insulin promotes net skeletal muscle protein synthesis in patients with severe burns. Ann Surg 1999;229(1):11–8.
122. Gottschlich MM, Mayes T, Khoury J, et al. Hypovitaminosis D in acutely injured pediatric burn patients. J Am Diet Assoc 2004;104(6):931–41 [quiz: 1031].

123. Rock CL, Dechert RE, Khilnani R, et al. Carotenoids and antioxidant vitamins in patients after burn injury. J Burn Care Rehabil 1997;18(3):269–78 [discussion: 268].

124. Selmanpakoglu AN, Cetin C, Sayal A, et al. Trace element (Al, Se, Zn, Cu) levels in serum, urine and tissues of burn patients. Burns 1994;20(2):99–103.

125. Hunt DR, Lane HW, Beesinger D, et al. Selenium depletion in burn patients. JPEN J Parenter Enteral Nutr 1984;8(6):695–9.

126. Lee J. The pediatric burned patient. In: Herndon DN, editor. Total burn care. 3rd edition. Philadelphia: Saunders Elsevier; 2007. p. 485–93.

127. Hart DW, Wolf SE, Zhang XJ, et al. Efficacy of a high-carbohydrate diet in catabolic illness. Crit Care Med 2001;29(7):1318–24.

128. Battistella FD, Widergren JT, Anderson JT, et al. A prospective, randomized trial of intravenous fat emulsion administration in trauma victims requiring total parenteral nutrition. J Trauma 1997;43(1):52–8 [discussion: 58–60].

129. Fong YM, Marano MA, Barber A, et al. Total parenteral nutrition and bowel rest modify the metabolic response to endotoxin in humans. Ann Surg 1989;210(4): 449–56 [discussion: 456–7].

130. Askanazi J, Rosenbaum SH, Hyman AI, et al. Respiratory changes induced by the large glucose loads of total parenteral nutrition. JAMA 1980;243(14): 1444–7.

131. Klein CJ, Stanek GS, Wiles CE 3rd. Overfeeding macronutrients to critically ill adults: metabolic complications. J Am Diet Assoc 1998;98(7):795–806.

132. van den Berghe G, Wouters P, Weekers F, et al. Intensive insulin therapy in the critically ill patients. N Engl J Med 2001;345(19):1359–67.

133. Turina M, Fry DE, Polk HC Jr. Acute hyperglycemia and the innate immune system: clinical, cellular, and molecular aspects. Crit Care Med 2005;33(7):1624–33.

134. Shopbell J, Hopkins B, Shronts E. Nutrition screening and assessment. In: Gottschlich MM, editor. A case-based core curriculum. Silver Spring (MD): Society of Parenteral and Enteral Nutrition; 2001.

135. Zdolsek HJ, Lindahl OA, Angquist KA, et al. Non-invasive assessment of intercompartmental fluid shifts in burn victims. Burns 1998;24(3):233–40.

136. Graves C, Saffle J, Morris S. Comparison of urine urea nitrogen collection times in critically ill patients. Nutr Clin Pract 2005;20(2):271–5.

137. Rettmer RL, Williamson JC, Labbe RF, et al. Laboratory monitoring of nutritional status in burn patients. Clin Chem 1992;38(3):334–7.

138. Jeschke MG, Herndon DN, Wolf SE, et al. Recombinant human growth hormone alters acute phase reactant proteins, cytokine expression, and liver morphology in burned rats. J Surg Res 1999;83(2):122–9.

139. Wu X, Herndon DN, Wolf SE. Growth hormone down-regulation of Interleukin-1beta and Interleukin-6 induced acute phase protein gene expression is associated with increased gene expression of suppressor of cytokine signal-3. Shock 2003;19(4):314–20.

140. Jeschke MG, Chrysopoulo MT, Herndon DN, et al. Increased expression of insulin-like growth factor-I in serum and liver after recombinant human growth hormone administration in thermally injured rats. J Surg Res 1999;85(1):171–7.

141. Aili Low JF, Barrow RE, Mittendorfer B, et al. The effect of short-term growth hormone treatment on growth and energy expenditure in burned children. Burns 2001;27(5):447–52.

142. Hart DW, Herndon DN, Klein G, et al. Attenuation of posttraumatic muscle catabolism and osteopenia by long-term growth hormone therapy. Ann Surg 2001; 233(6):827–34.

143. Herndon DN, Barrow RE, Kunkel KR, et al. Effects of recombinant human growth hormone on donor-site healing in severely burned children. Ann Surg 1990; 212(4):424–9 [discussion: 430–1].

144. Branski LK, Herndon DN, Barrow RE, et al. Randomized controlled trial to determine the efficacy of long-term growth hormone treatment in severely burned children. Ann Surg 2009;250(4):514–23.

145. Klein GL, Wolf SE, Langman CB, et al. Effects of therapy with recombinant human growth hormone on insulin-like growth factor system components and serum levels of biochemical markers of bone formation in children after severe burn injury. J Clin Endocrinol Metab 1998;83(1):21–4.

146. Takala J, Ruokonen E, Webster NR, et al. Increased mortality associated with growth hormone treatment in critically ill adults. N Engl J Med 1999;341(11):785–92.

147. Demling RH. Comparison of the anabolic effects and complications of human growth hormone and the testosterone analog, oxandrolone, after severe burn injury. Burns 1999;25(3):215–21.

148. Gore DC, Honeycutt D, Jahoor F, et al. Effect of exogenous growth hormone on glucose utilization in burn patients. J Surg Res 1991;51(6):518–23.

149. Ramirez RJ, Wolf SE, Barrow RE, et al. Growth hormone treatment in pediatric burns: a safe therapeutic approach. Ann Surg 1998;228(4):439–48.

150. Moller S, Jensen M, Svensson P, et al. Insulin-like growth factor 1 (IGF-1) in burn patients. Burns 1991;17(4):279–81.

151. Herndon DN, Ramzy PI, DebRoy MA, et al. Muscle protein catabolism after severe burn: effects of IGF-1/IGFBP-3 treatment. Ann Surg 1999;229(5): 713–20 [discussion: 720–2].

152. Spies M, Wolf SE, Barrow RE, et al. Modulation of types I and II acute phase reactants with insulin-like growth factor-1/binding protein-3 complex in severely burned children. Crit Care Med 2002;30(1):83–8.

153. Jeschke MG, Herndon DN, Barrow RE. Insulin-like growth factor I in combination with insulin-like growth factor binding protein 3 affects the hepatic acute phase response and hepatic morphology in thermally injured rats. Ann Surg 2000; 231(3):408–16.

154. Cioffi WG, Gore DC, Rue LW 3rd, et al. Insulin-like growth factor-1 lowers protein oxidation in patients with thermal injury. Ann Surg 1994;220(3):310–6 [discussion: 316–9].

155. Langouche L, Van den Berghe G. Glucose metabolism and insulin therapy. Crit Care Clin 2006;22(1):119–29, vii.

156. Hart DW, Wolf SE, Ramzy PI, et al. Anabolic effects of oxandrolone after severe burn. Ann Surg 2001;233(4):556–64.

157. Demling RH, Orgill DP. The anticatabolic and wound healing effects of the testosterone analog oxandrolone after severe burn injury. J Crit Care 2000;15(1):12–7.

158. Jeschke MG, Finnerty CC, Suman OE, et al. The effect of oxandrolone on the endocrinologic, inflammatory, and hypermetabolic responses during the acute phase postburn. Ann Surg 2007;246(3):351–60 [discussion: 360–2].

159. Demling RH, DeSanti L. The rate of restoration of body weight after burn injury, using the anabolic agent oxandrolone, is not age dependent. Burns 2001;27(1): 46–51.

160. Murphy KD, Thomas S, Mlcak RP, et al. Effects of long-term oxandrolone administration in severely burned children. Surgery 2004;136(2):219–24.

161. Suman OE, Thomas SJ, Wilkins JP, et al. Effect of exogenous growth hormone and exercise on lean mass and muscle function in children with burns. J Appl Physiol 2003;94(6):2273–81.

162. Barret JP, Jeschke MG, Herndon DN. Fatty infiltration of the liver in severely burned pediatric patients: autopsy findings and clinical implications. J Trauma 2001;51(4):736–9.

163. Aarsland A, Chinkes D, Wolfe RR, et al. Beta-blockade lowers peripheral lipolysis in burn patients receiving growth hormone. Rate of hepatic very low density lipoprotein triglyceride secretion remains unchanged. Ann Surg 1996;223(6):777–87 [discussion: 787–9].

164. Gore DC, Honeycutt D, Jahoor F, et al. Propranolol diminishes extremity blood flow in burned patients. Ann Surg 1991;213(6):568–74.

165. Pereira CT, Jeschke MG, Herndon DN. Beta-blockade in burns. Novartis Found Symp 2007;280:238–51.

166. Pidcoke HF, Wade CE, Wolf SE. Insulin and the burned patient. Crit Care Med 2007;35(Suppl 9):S524–30.

167. Pierre EJ, Barrow RE, Hawkins HK, et al. Effects of insulin on wound healing. J Trauma 1998;44(2):342–5.

168. Thomas SJ, Morimoto K, Herndon DN, et al. The effect of prolonged euglycemic hyperinsulinemia on lean body mass after severe burn. Surgery 2002;132(2):341–7.

169. Zhang XJ, Chinkes DL, Wolf SE, et al. Insulin but not growth hormone stimulates protein anabolism in skin would and muscle. Am J Physiol 1999;276(4 Pt 1):E712–20.

170. Jeschke MG, Klein D, Herndon DN. Insulin treatment improves the systemic inflammatory reaction to severe trauma. Ann Surg 2004;239(4):553–60.

171. Jeschke MG, Klein D, Bolder U, et al. Insulin attenuates the systemic inflammatory response in endotoxemic rats. Endocrinology 2004;145(9):4084–93.

172. Jeschke MG, Rensing H, Klein D, et al. Insulin prevents liver damage and preserves liver function in lipopolysaccharide-induced endotoxemic rats. J Hepatol 2005;42(6):870–9.

173. Klein D, Schubert T, Horch RE, et al. Insulin treatment improves hepatic morphology and function through modulation of hepatic signals after severe trauma. Ann Surg 2004;240(2):340–9.

174. Gauglitz GG, Toliver-Kinsky TE, Williams FN, et al. Insulin increases resistance to burn wound infection-associated sepsis. Crit Care Med 2010;38(1):202–8.

175. Dandona P, Chaudhuri A, Mohanty P, et al. Anti-inflammatory effects of insulin. Curr Opin Clin Nutr Metab Care 2007;10(4):511–7.

176. Van den Berghe G, Wilmer A, Hermans G, et al. Intensive insulin therapy in the medical ICU. N Engl J Med 2006;354(5):449–61.

177. Finney SJ, Zekveld C, Elia A, et al. Glucose control and mortality in critically ill patients. JAMA 2003;290(15):2041–7.

178. Dellinger RP, Levy MM, Carlet JM, et al. Surviving Sepsis Campaign: international guidelines for management of severe sepsis and septic shock: 2008. Crit Care Med 2008;36(1):296–327.

179. Gore DC, Wolf SE, Herndon DN, et al. Metformin blunts stress-induced hyperglycemia after thermal injury. J Trauma 2003;54(3):555–61.

180. DeFronzo RA, Goodman AM. Efficacy of metformin in patients with non-insulin-dependent diabetes mellitus. The Multicenter Metformin Study Group. N Engl J Med 1995;333(9):541–9.

181. Stumvoll M, Nurjhan N, Perriello G, et al. Metabolic effects of metformin in non-insulin-dependent diabetes mellitus. N Engl J Med 1995;333(9):550–4.

182. Gore DC, Herndon DN, Wolfe RR. Comparison of peripheral metabolic effects of insulin and metformin following severe burn injury. J Trauma 2005;59(2):316–23.

183. Bailey CJ, Turner RC. Metformin. N Engl J Med 1996;334(9):574–9.
184. Luft D, Schmulling RM, Eggstein M. Lactic acidosis in biguanide-treated diabetics: a review of 330 cases. Diabetologia 1978;14(2):75–87.
185. Heszele MFC, Price SR. Insulin-like growth factor I: the yin and yang of muscle atrophy. Endocrinology 2004;145(11):4803–5.
186. Barret JP, Dziewulski P, Jeschke MG, et al. Effects of recombinant human growth hormone on the development of burn scarring. Plast Reconstr Surg 1999;104(3): 726–9.
187. Takagi K, Suzuki F, Barrow RE, et al. Recombinant human growth hormone modulates Th1 and Th2 cytokine response in burned mice. Ann Surg 1998; 228(1):106–11.
188. Takagi K, Suzuki F, Barrow RE, et al. Growth hormone improves immune function and survival in burned mice infected with Herpes simplex virus type? J Surg Res 1997;69(1):166–70.
189. Low JFA, Herndon DN, Barrow RE. Effect of growth hormone on growth delay in burned children: a 3-year follow-up study. Lancet 1999;354(9192):1789.
190. Demling RH, DeSanti L. Oxandrolone, an anabolic steroid, significantly increases the rate of weight gain in the recovery phase after major burns. J Trauma 1997;43(1):47–51.
191. Aarsland A, Chinkes DL, Sakurai Y, et al. Insulin therapy in burn patients does not contribute to hepatic triglyceride production. J Clin Invest 1998;101(10): 2233–9.
192. Minnich A, Tian N, Byan L, et al. A potent PPAR alpha agonist stimulates mitochondrial fatty acid beta-oxidation in liver and skeletal muscle. Am J Physiol Endocrinol Metab 2001;280(2):E270–9.
193. Schnabel D, Grasemann C, Staab D, et al. A multicenter, randomized, double-blind, placebo-controlled trial to evaluate the metabolic and respiratory effects of growth hormone in children with cystic fibrosis. Pediatrics 2007;119(6): E1230–8.
194. Herndon DN, Barrow RE, Rutan TC, et al. Effect of propranolol administration on hemodynamic and metabolic responses of burned pediatric patients. Ann Surg 1988;208(4):484–92.
195. Engelhardt D, Dorr G, Jaspers C, et al. Ketoconazole blocks cortisol secretion in man by inhibition of adrenal 11-beta-hydroxylase. Klin Wochenschr 1985; 63(13):607–12.
196. Engelhardt D, Mann K, Hormann R, et al. Ketoconazole inhibits cortisol secretion of an adrenal adenoma in vivo and in vitro. Klin Wochenschr 1983;61(7): 373–5.
197. Loose DS, Stover EP, Feldman D. Ketoconazole binds to glucocorticoid receptors and exhibits glucocorticoid antagonist activity in cultured cells. J Clin Invest 1983;72(1):404–8.
198. Hart DW, Wolf SE, Chinkes DL, et al. Beta-blockade and growth hormone after burn. Ann Surg 2002;236(4):450–7.
199. Jeschke MG, Finnerty CC, Kulp GA, et al. Combination of recombinant human growth hormone and propranolol decreases hypermetabolism and inflammation in severely burned children. Pediatr Crit Care Med 2008;9(2):209–16.
200. Debroy MA, Wolf SE, Zhang XJ, et al. Anabolic effects of insulin-like growth factor in combination with insulin-like growth factor binding protein-3 in severely burned adults. J Trauma 1999;47(5):904–10.

# Nutrition Management of Patients with Malignancies of the Head and Neck

James Paul O'Neill, MD, MRCSI, MBA, MMSc, ORL-HNS*,
Ashok R. Shaha, MD

**KEYWORDS**

- Head and neck cancer • Nutrition • Surgery • Chemotherapy
- Radiotherapy

Cancers of the head and neck are a complex group of genetic-based diseases derived from alterations, which include activation of proto-oncogenes and inactivation of tumor suppressor genes. A higher incidence is observed in men than in women, and significant tobacco and alcohol use are major risk factors. Other behavioral risk factors include betel nut chewing and the ever-defining risk imposed by human papilloma virus infection. Despite the major importance of the tumor burden for these patients, the pattern and progression of nutritional deterioration is highly influenced by anatomic location of the tumor and stage of the disease. In 1932 malnutrition was observed as being a poor prognostic indicator of cancer therapy in terms of mortality and morbidity.[1] Today we know malnutrition to be a multifactorial medical and social problem, which clearly has a negative impact on patients' prognosis.

Cancer cachexia can be caused by diminished oral intake and by catabolic factors secreted by the tumor, such as interleukins, interferon-gamma, and tumor necrosis factor, amongst others. Immunosuppression is related to the immunosuppressive capacity and effects of the tumor and surgical intervention. Head and neck cancers account for approximately 3% to 5% of all cancers in the United States. A multidisciplinary management approach involves experienced individuals trained in head and neck cancer surgery, microvascular reconstructive surgery, maxillofacial prosthodontics, oculoplastic surgery, nutrition, and speech and swallowing therapy. Nutrition is a key factor in patients' preoperative and postoperative course. Treatment strategies,

No financial disclosures.
Department of Head and Neck Surgery, Memorial Sloan Kettering Cancer Center, 1275 York Avenue, New York, NY 10065, USA
* Corresponding author.
*E-mail address:* Oneillj1@mskcc.org

Surg Clin N Am 91 (2011) 631–639
doi:10.1016/j.suc.2011.02.005
0039-6109/11/$ – see front matter. Published by Elsevier Inc.

whether comprised of surgical excision, radiotherapy, or a combined approach often result in a temporary or permanent nutritional burden. Furthermore, the etiologic risk factors involved have, in themselves, an impact upon the nutritional status of these patients. It is well recognized that malnutrition is reported in up to 50% of patients presenting with a head and neck malignancy and that adequate nutrition support improves therapeutic tolerance, chemotherapeutic response, immunologic function, and decreases wound and flap morbidity.[2]

## HEAD AND NECK CANCER

To understand the nutritional importance and impact in head and neck cancers we must first appreciate the variety of malignancies within this region, their presenting features, and the treatment modalities employed. All cancers are staged in accordance with the American Joint Committee for Cancer.[3] The predominant pathologic histology is squamous cell carcinoma (SCC). More than two-thirds of SCC of the head and neck region are locally advanced at the time of initial diagnosis. Advances in radiotherapy (RT) have been associated with the multidisciplinary approach to treatment, including the conformal applications of new strategies, such as intensity modulated radiation therapy and proton beam and its association with targeted chemotherapeutic agents. Radiation therapy, despite its success in the head and neck, also has a myriad of associated morbidities, such as xerostomia, mucositis, dysgeusia, odynophagia, dysphagia, osteoradionecrosis, tissue fibrosis, stricture formation, and so forth. These morbidities have immediate and long-term implications for patients' nutritional status and quality of life.

In the last 2 decades clinical research strategies have focused on the addition of chemotherapy (CT) to the armamentarium used against head and neck cancer. Traditional CT has been considered a standard therapy for patients who initially present with systemic metastatic disease, who develop recurrence, or who have persistent disease after local therapy. CT can be considered a standard component, along with RT, for nasopharyngeal carcinomas, oropharyngeal and laryngopharyngeal cancers, and most unresectable tumors. Treatment paradigms include various forms of curative combined modality therapies, including concurrent chemoradiation (CRT), induction chemotherapy followed by irradiation, and sequential therapy (induction chemotherapy followed by concurrent chemoradiation).

The oral cavity extends from the skin-vermillion junction of the lips to the hard and soft palate above and to the line of the circumvallate papillae below. The oral cavity can be further divided into the mucosal lip, buccal mucosa, upper and lower alveolar ridges, hard palate, and floor of the mouth. About 36,540 new cases (25,420 in men and 11,120 in women) of oral cavity and oropharyngeal cancer will present in Americans in 2010.[4] More than 95% of patients with oral cavity cancer have a history of smoking, drinking alcohol, or both, and the synergistic effect of their combination has been well established. More than 60 carcinogens are found in mainstream cigarette smoke and the majority of these are also found in passive smoke. To evaluate the effects of smoking, 40 current and 40 age- and gender-matched never smokers underwent buccal biopsies and it was observed that smoking altered the expression of numerous genes. Increases were found in genes involved in xenobiotic metabolism, oxidant stress, eicosanoid synthesis, nicotine signaling, and cell adhesion. In addition to being a major etiologic factor in carcinogenesis, smoking alters the activity of chemopreventive agents, promotes the clearance of selected targeted anticancer therapies, reduces the efficacy of cancer treatment, and increases the risk of a second primary.[5]

Oral cavity tumors are seen predominantly in patients aged older than 50 years. Early, curable lesions are rarely symptomatic; thus, improvement in survival requires early detection by screening. Treatment is accomplished with surgery, RT, or both. The overall 5-year survival rate (all sites and stages combined) is greater than 50%. Oral and oropharyngeal cancers are increasingly seen in younger patients but its suspected relationship to human papillomavirus infection remains unclear.

The pharynx is subdivided into the nasopharynx, which extends from the posterior choanae to the free border of the soft palate; the oropharynx extending from the superior plane of the soft palate to the superior level of the hyoid bone (or floor of the vallecula); and the hypopharynx, which extends from the level of the hyoid bone to the lower border of the cricoid cartilage. An estimated 2850 cases of hypopharyngeal cancer are diagnosed each year, about 2250 in men and 600 in women. Every anatomic site may be further broken down to anatomic subdivisions and current therapeutic modalities include concurrent CRT with surgery and reconstruction for salvage. Pharyngeal tumors, in particular oropharynx and hypopharynx, frequently present with progressive dysphagia and odynophagia. Subsites, such as the tongue base, can have an insidious nature to them and can mask considerably advanced tumors before overt presentation.

The larynx is subdivided into the supraglottis, glottis, and subglottis regions. Approximately 12,720 new cases of laryngeal cancer (10,110 in men and 2610 in women) are expected in 2010. Furthermore, 3600 people (2870 men and 730 women) will die of their disease. The supraglottis is composed of the lingual and laryngeal aspects of the epiglottis, which is further divided into its suprahyoid and infrahyoid epiglottic components; the arytenoids; aryepiglottic folds; and finally the false cords or ventricular bands. The inferior limit of the supraglottis is the line between the lateral margin of the ventricle and the superior surface of the vocal cord. During embryologic development the supraglottic structures are derived from the buccopharyngeal anlage of the third and fourth branchial arches. In contrast, the glottic and subglottic structures develop from the tracheobronchial anlage of the fifth and sixth branchial arches. The glottic region consists of the superior and inferior surfaces of the vocal cords, including the anterior and posterior commissures. The subglottic region is between the lower boundaries of the glottis and in the lower margin of the cricoid cartilage. Of the nearly 13,000 new cases of laryngeal cancer diagnosed annually in the United States, 30% to 40% of these tumors are thought to arise in the supraglottis. Like other head and neck cancers, there is a higher incidence in men than in women, and significant tobacco and alcohol use are major risk factors for the development of supraglottic squamous cell carcinoma. The vast majority (95%) of these tumors are squamous cell carcinoma and greater than 25% of these patients have disseminated nodal metastases upon presentation. Glottic cancers rarely metastasize to the regional lymphatics secondary to the poor lymphatic drainage in this area. Treatment usually consists of some combination of surgery, CT, and RT. Indications for radiation therapy vary with tumor characteristics and location. RT or surgery can cure small tumors (T1–T2) in any location. The choice of treatment is usually made based on the functional aspects and potential complications of the two modalities. For example, T1 and T2 N0 tumors of the larynx can be treated with RT with 90% cure rates for T1 tumors and 70% cure rates for T2 tumors.

Larynx preservation is often chosen for these smaller tumors because voice preservation obviously improves quality of life. The goal of any intervention is complete treatment of the primary tumor and any draining lymphatics at risk for occult metastatic spread. Combined therapy (surgery and RT) is usually recommended for advanced (T3–T4) lesions. An expanding body of literature also supports chemotherapy with

RT for advanced disease. Two-thirds of patients present with locoregional advanced disease and of these, approximately 50% are cured despite the frequent use of both treatment modalities.

The major salivary glands include the parotid, submandibular, and sublingual glands. The benign histology varies wherein pleomorphic adenoma and Warthin tumors (papillary cystadenoma lymphomatosum) are the most common variants of benign disease. Approximately 20% to 25% of all parotid tumors are malignant, an incidence which rises to 40% to 45% for the submandibular gland and to 50% to 81% for sublingual and minor salivary glands. Malignant disease consists mostly of the mucoepidermoid variant followed by adenoid cystic cancer. They occur at a rate of about 2 cases per 100,000 people per year in the United States. Patients with advanced stage, high-grade tumor, positive surgical margins, perineural invasion, and lymph node metastasis usually receive postoperative RT. Adjuvant radiation to the primary bed site maximizes the curative potential. RT also adds a considerable survival advantage in advanced disease. Five-year survival of 19% was reported at Memorial Sloan Kettering Cancer Center for stage III and IV salivary gland tumors, which was increased to 49% with surgery and adjuvant RT. Furthermore, local control improved from 40% to 69% over a 5-year period.[6]

### Assessment of Nutritional Deficiency

Defining malnutrition is not in itself an easy task. A recent study attempting to reveal the elements defining malnutrition could not find uniform agreement in an expert panel. Deficiencies of energy or protein and decrease in fat-free mass were most often mentioned to be particularly important in defining malnutrition as were involuntary weight loss, body mass index (BMI), and decreased or no nutritional intake. Opinions on cutoff points regarding these elements differed strongly amongst their expert panelists.[7]

Body weight and BMI have been the traditional outcome measures of dietetic analysis. Actual body weight is used for nonobese patients and ideal body weight is used for obese patients. This practice allows for estimation of lean body mass and is calculated based upon gender and height. If one uses actual body weight to estimate dietary needs in an obese patient, this practice may result in over feeding. During the malignant process dietary requirements can vary depending upon the nutritional status at presentation, the necessity for nutritional maintenance or repletion preoperatively, and whether patients are in a catabolic state in the postoperative period. The average patient requires 30 to 35 kcal/Kg maintenance and 40 to 45 kcal/Kg for repletion or during catabolic periods, which converts to about 2000 to 2500 kcal/d for maintenance and 3000 to 4000 kcal/d for repletion. Estimations of nutritional loss can be calculated using several methods. Percent ideal body weight is computed as the midpoint of the weight range for a given height and frame size. The percentage of ideal body weights of 80% to 90%, 70% to 79%, and less than 69% can be interpreted as mild malnutrition, moderate malnutrition, and severe malnutrition, respectively. Percent weight loss during the past 6 months is calculated by dividing the difference between usual weight (ie, the body weight 6 months before presentation) and the actual current weight.[8]

A modified nutritional index may be calculated as another assessment based on albumin, percentage ideal body weight, and total lymphocyte count. An index value less than 1.31, which is the mean of the reference group, was considered to be a deviation from a normal nutritional status.[9] Blood albumin levels have also been used to valuate nutrition status. Under stable conditions values between 27 and 35 g/L reflect mild depletion; between 21 and 27 g/L, moderate depletion; and less than 21 g/L, severe depletion.[8]

Subjective global assessment (SGA) has proved to be a good nutritional assessment and prognostic indicator in several clinical situations. SGA is considered a gold standard method for validating new nutritional assessment and screening methods. This assessment is based on components of the medical history, changes in weight, dietary intake and functional capacity, gastrointestinal symptoms with nutritional impact, and metabolic stress of disease. It also includes a physical examination identifying the loss of subcutaneous fat, muscle wasting, and ankle/sacral swelling.[10] The scored patient generated subjective global assessment is a quick, valid, and reliable nutrition assessment tool that enables malnourished hospital patients with cancer to be identified and triaged for nutrition support and enhances the clinical applicability of the SGA assessment.[11]

### Malnutrition, Morbidity, and Mortality

In a report of 64 patients undergoing major surgery for advanced head and neck cancer and studied prospectively with logistic regression to link nutritional parameters to postoperative complications, malnutrition levels between 20% and 67% were documented. A weight loss of more than10% preoperatively was identified as the greatest risk for postoperative complications.[12] A follow-up study related the combination of male gender, preoperative weight loss of more than 5%, and major postoperative morbidities to early death in patients with advanced head and neck cancer.[13]

The question arises whether we should consider preoperative or postoperative nutritional supplementation and if so with what feeding regimens. A study of 47 patients with oral and laryngeal cancers allocated into 2 groups, one group who received an enteral diet (for a mean 22-day period) supplemented with arginine and fiber and a second group who received an isocaloric iso-nitrogenous enteral formula. Fistulae were less frequently encountered in the enriched-nutrition group with 0% in group 1, compared with 20.8% in group 2. Additionally, there was a significant reduction in length of postoperative stay in group 1, of 22.8 days, compared with group 2, which was 31.2 days.[14] However, time periods appear to play an important role as a previous study giving a similar arginine enriched diet, failed to support the hypothesis that preoperative feeding (9 days), either with or without arginine supplementation, improved clinical outcome, immune function, or nutritional status compared with ad libitum oral food intake.[15]

On the other hand, nutrition has a definite impact upon patients undergoing radiation therapy. RT toxicities depend upon anatomic location, tumor histology, total radiation dose, fractionation, irradiated area volume, and injury repair mechanisms associated with radiation high turnover cellular damage.

Quality of life (QoL) is a multidimensional construct. It is a subjective analysis of functional status, psychosocial wellbeing, health and disease perception, and therapeutic symptom scores. A study of 125 patients with a variety of cancers, undergoing RT, had nutritional status evaluated using SGA. They also had QoL evaluated using a standardized instrument for use as a measure of health outcome and Quality of Life Questionnaire (QLQ)-C30.[16,17] The investigators evaluated their patients QoL, nutritional status, and nutrient intake at the beginning and end of RT. They also evaluated the hypothetical advantages of nutritional counseling and symptoms associated with a reduced QoL and nutritional intake. The patients with head and neck cancer, among others in the patient pool, were categorized as high risk. They showed that RT-induced symptoms affecting nutrient intake, such as mucositis, xerostomia, dysphagia, nausea and vomiting, became evident only in patients categorized as high risk. Interestingly, nutritional intake within this high-risk group improved with nutritional counseling and QoL improved with increased nutritional intake.[18]

A subsequent study added that oral nutritional dietary supplementation does not seem to be as effective as proper nutritional assessment, compliance monitoring, and dietary counseling.[19]

### Modalities of Nutritional Support

Techniques of nutritional supplementation require an individual approach to patients, bearing in mind the cancer location, gastrointestinal (GI) functionality, feeding access, patient motivation, modality of therapy, and anticipated duration of therapy.[20] There are 2 main routes of nutritional support, enteral and parenteral nutrition. Enteral nutrition may be provided by nasogastric tube placement, surgical gastrostomy, percutaneous or endoscopically guided gastrostomy tube (PEG). Parenteral nutrition is administered via total parenteral nutrition (TPN). Patients with head and neck cancer usually have functional GI tracts, the preferred mode of nutritional support is enteral feeding. The authors do not advocate early PEG tube insertion in their patients despite difficulties maintaining adequate nutrition during the latter half of chemoradiation protocols, even for primary oropharyngeal cancers, as patients with PEG tubes inserted early in their treatment frequently forget how to swallow, and esophageal stricture formation often becomes a major morbid sequelae. This opinion does not necessarily have full support within the literature.

In a study of 45 patients with oropharyngeal cancer, 74% had PEG tubes inserted. This early nutritional intervention, according to the investigators, is feasible and efficient in preventing dehydration in patients with oropharyngeal cancer and may improve quality of life by decreasing the frequency of hospital admissions.[21] A retrospective review study concluded that prophylactic feeding gastrostomy tubes (GT) significantly reduce the incidence of severe weight loss and hospitalization for dehydration during RT when placed before onset of RT.[22]

Thus, the question arises as to consider just how safe are feeding tubes? A meta-analysis of 5752 patients following radiologic, endoscopic, and surgical gastrostomy for all types of pathology was conducted in 1995. The investigators concluded that radiologically inserted gastrostomy tubes (RIG) were slightly more successful than percutaneous endoscopic gastrostomy (99.2% vs 95.7%) and also safer, with lower rates of major complications (5.9% vs 9.4%). Patients within the study with a cancer diagnosis amounted to only 24% to 29% of the patient population. They reported a procedure-related fatality rate of 0.3% for RIG and 0.53% for PEG.[23] A prospective multi-institution study, systematic review, and meta-analysis of 172 patients specifically with head and neck disease compared PEG tube insertion with radiologically inserted gastrostomy tubes. Within the series, mortality rates were noted at 1.0% for PEG and 3.9% for RIG, higher than the previous meta-analysis in 1995. Major complication rates for PEG and RIG were 3.3% versus 15.6%, respectively. Patients with head and neck cancer are significantly more likely to experience major morbidity and mortality than patients without cancer. Past medical history, medical morbidities, oncological treatment course, and staging are all essential considerations.[24]

A study of 120 patients with stage III/IV head and neck cancer were retrospectively evaluated for the benefits and morbidities of prophylactic gastrostomy tube insertion. They initially reported gastrostomy tube insertion to be highly effective at reducing weight loss and requirements for intravenous hydration, however, among those who did not receive a gastrostomy tube, the weight loss that ensued was largely temporary and correctable, requiring no change in treatment compliance and no added hospital admissions.

Among the problems encountered for the patients with gastrostomy tube insertion was that a high percentage of patients who received prophylactic GT were still dependent on enteral feedings at 6 months and 1 year after treatment. It was also noted these patients had a higher incidence of esophageal stricture.[25] This observation is confirmed with psychological, physiologic studies and further retrospective reviews. A series from 1989 to 2002 of 222 patients receiving chemoradiation for head and neck squamous cell cancer reported esophageal strictures in 21% of these patients. The female sex, radiation fractionation twice daily, and a hypopharyngeal primary site were identified as significant predictive factors for stricture formation.[26] Earlier in the literature these results demonstrated that prophylactic gastrostomy tube placement was associated with a significantly increased need for esophageal dilatation in comparison with prophylactic nasogastric tube placement.[27]

Esophageal stricture dilatation in the post chemoradiation head and neck cancer candidate is an extremely dangerous procedure associated with major morbidities and mortality. As a result of recent reports, the authors do not think that a prophylactic gastrostomy tube is necessary for these patients. The authors are willing to accept the associated transient weight loss and nutritional deficits to offset the ominous prospect of an esophageal stricture formation and its hazardous remedy.

In a study randomizing 81 subjects to nasogastric enteral feeding or total parenteral nutrition in pharyngeal and laryngeal postoperative patients, the investigators found that each method had advantages and disadvantages. TPN was more expensive by $11.81 per day; however, nasogastric enteral feeding was not without its complications, with aspiration pneumonias developing in 9.8% of the subjects.[28] An earlier study in patients with gastrointestinal cancers compared 159 subjects assigned to enteral nutrition with 158 subjects assigned to parenteral nutrition.[29] It is obvious that rigid, conscientious adherence to established guidelines, principles, and practices of nutritional support is likely to result in improved outcomes for patients with head and neck cancer regardless of the feeding techniques used, provided that the feedings are administered with skill and competence.

## SUMMARY

Patients with head and neck cancer require multidisciplinary patient management, including proper assessment of nutritional status, attention to dietary requirements, counseling, and compliance maintenance. In the authors' approach to nutrition, they appreciate the necessity of nutritional management, but remain cognizant of the potential impact of nutritional support on the multimodality treatment algorithms of head and neck malignant disease. There remains a deficit within the literature of nutritional research specifically involving patients with head and neck cancer. This patient group requires further research investigations, including nutritional carcinogenesis, identification of populations at risk, nutrient supplementation, and alteration of dietary habits to determine definitively the impact of nutritional support on head and neck cancer treatment outcomes.

## REFERENCES

1. Warren S. The immediate cause of death in cancer. Am J Med Sci 1932;184:610–5.
2. Williams EF, Meguid MM. Nutritional concepts and considerations in head and neck surgery. Head Neck 1989;11(5):393–9.
3. American joint committee on cancer. 7th edition. New York (NY): Springer; 2010.
4. American Cancer Society. Cancer Facts & Figures 2010. Atlanta (GA): American Cancer Society; 2010.
5. Boyle JO, Gumus ZH, Choksi VL, et al. Effects of cigarette smoke on the human oral mucosal transcriptome. Cancer Prev Res 2010;3(3):266–78.

6. Armstrong JG, Harrison LB, Spiro RH, et al. Malignant tumors of major salivary gland origin. A matched pair analysis of the role of combined surgery and postoperative radiotherapy. Arch Otolaryngol 1990;116:290–3.

7. Meijers JM, van Bokhorst-de van der Schueren MA, Schols JM. Defining malnutrition, mission or mission impossible? Nutrition 2010;26(4):432–40.

8. Gottschlich MM, Matarese LE, Shronts EP. Nutrition support dietetics core curriculum. 2nd edition. Silversprings (MD): American Society for Parenteral and Enteral Nutrition; 1993.

9. Von Meyenfeldt MF, Meijerink WJ, Rouflart MM, et al. Perioperative nutritional support: a randomised clinical trial. Clin Nutr 1992;11:180–6.

10. Detsky AS, McLaughlin JR, Baker JP, et al. What is subjective global assessment of nutritional status? JPEN J Parenter Enteral Nutr 1987;11:8–13.

11. Bauer J, Capra S, Ferguson M. Use of the scored Patient-Generated Subjective Global Assessment (PG-SGA) as a nutrition assessment tool in patients with cancer. Eur J Clin Nutr 2002;56:779–85.

12. van Bokhorst-de van der Schueren MA, van Leeuwen PA, Sauerwein HP, et al. Assessment of malnutrition parameters in head and neck cancer and their relation to postoperative complications. Head Neck 1997;19(5):419–25.

13. van Bokhorst-de van der Schuer, van Leeuwen PA, Kuik DJ, et al. The impact of nutritional status on the prognoses of patients with advanced head and neck cancer. Cancer 1999;86(3):519–27.

14. De Luis DA, Aller R, Izaola O, et al. Post surgery enteral nutrition in head and neck cancer patients. Eur J Clin Nutr 2002;56:1126–9.

15. van Bokhorst-De Van Der Schueren MA, Quak JJ, von Blomberg-van der Flier BM, et al. Effect of perioperative nutrition, with and without arginine supplementation, on nutritional status, immune function, postoperative morbidity, and survival in severely malnourished head and neck cancer patients. Am J Clin Nutr 2001;73(2):323–32.

16. Brooks R. EuroQol: the current state of play. Health Policy 1990;37:53–72.

17. Aaronson NK, Ahmedzai S, Bergman B, et al. The European Organisation for research and Treatment of Cancer QLQ-C30: A quality of life instrument for use in International clinical trials in oncology. J Natl Cancer Inst 1993;85:365–76.

18. Ravasco P, Monteiro-Grillo I, Ermelinda Camilo M. Does nutrition influence quality of life in cancer patients undergoing radiotherapy? Radiother Oncol 2003;67:213–20.

19. Ravasco P, Monteiro-Grillo I, Marques Vidal P, et al. Impact of nutrition on outcome: a prospective randomized controlled trial in patients with head and neck cancer undergoing radiotherapy. Head Neck 2005;27:659–68.

20. Snyderman C. Nutrition and head and neck cancer. Curr Oncol Rep 2003;5:158–63.

21. Piquet MA, Ozsahin M, Larpin I, et al. Early nutritional interventional in oropharyngeal cancer patients undergoing radiotherapy. Support Care Cancer 2002;10(6):502–4.

22. Beaver ME, Matheny KE, Roberts DB. Predictors of weight loss during radiation therapy. Otolaryngol Head Neck Surg 2001;125(6):645–8.

23. Wollman B, D'Agostino HB, Walus-Wigle JR, et al. Radiologic, endoscopic, and surgical gastrostomy: an institutional evaluation and meta-analysis of the literature. Radiology 1995;197:699–704.

24. Grant D, Bradley P, Pothier D. Complications following gastrostomy tube insertion in patients with head and neck cancer: a prospective multi-institution study, systematic review and meta-analysis. Clin Otolaryngol 2009;34(2):103–12.

25. Chen A, Li B, Lau DH. Evaluating the role of prophylactic gastrostomy tube placement prior to definitive chemoradiotherapy for head and neck cancer. Int J Radiat Oncol Biol Phys 2010;78(4):1026–32.
26. Lee WT, Akst LM, Adelstein DJ, et al. Risk factors for hypopharyngeal/upper esophageal stricture formation after concurrent chemoradiation. Head Neck 2006;28:808–12.
27. Mekhail TM, Adelstein DJ, Rybicki LA, et al. Enteral nutrition during the treatment of head and neck carcinoma. Cancer 2001;91:1785–90.
28. Ryu J, Nam B, Jung Y. Clinical outcomes comparing parenteral and nasogastric tube nutrition after laryngeal and pharyngeal cancer surgery. Dysphagia 2009; 24(4):378–86.
29. Bozzetti F, Braga M, Gianotti L, et al. Postoperative enteral versus parenteral nutrition in malnourished patients with gastrointestinal cancer: a randomized multicenter trial. Lancet 2001;358:1487–92.

# Nutritional Support: We have Failed in Our Ability to Support Patients with Sepsis and Cancer

Josef E. Fischer, MD

**KEYWORDS**

• Sepsis • Cancer • Cachexia • Proteolysis

I first met Dr Stanley Dudrick 43 years ago. The circumstances were interesting. Dr Ronald Abel was a bright, irascible, promising intern at the Massachusetts General Hospital (MGH) who, in July of 1966, started his first rotation on the pediatric surgical service, having recently graduated from the University of Pennsylvania School Medical. I was a freshly minted third-year resident serving as chief resident on the pediatric surgical service under the redoubtable Dr Hardy Hendren. The rotation was memorable for several reasons, not the least of which was Dr Abel's description to me of a young resident at the University of Pennsylvania, who had enabled puppies to grow normally without eating. I was incredulous but believing. As we discussed this with Dr William Abbott, a fellow intern who had spent 3 years away and was now a second-year resident, we decided we would invite Dr Stanley Dudrick to come to Boston and give a talk in the Bigelow Amphitheater at MGH. I do not recall ever asking anybody for permission; that was the way things were at that time at the MGH; as long as one did not hurt anybody, one could do pretty much anything one wanted, and that was one of the great things about being a resident at that institution. With his true generosity, which he has always had, Stanley Dudrick came to the MGH and gave an exciting talk. Dr Stanley Dudrick then stayed an additional 2 days, taught us how to put in subclavian central venous lines, the composition of the nutritional solution, and how to prepare it with an interested pharmacist who volunteered his services and would make the solutions up after hours. We did not know precisely the proper components and dosages of the total parenteral nutrition (TPN) and were initially giving too much glucose and probably too much volume; the patients looked like

---

The author has nothing to disclose.

Harvard Medical School, Renaissance Park, 1135 Tremont Street, Suite 511-512, Boston, MA 02120, USA

*E-mail address:* jfische1@bidmc.harvard.edu

Surg Clin N Am 91 (2011) 641–651

doi:10.1016/j.suc.2011.02.001

0039-6109/11/$ – see front matter © 2011 Elsevier Inc. All rights reserved.

surgical.theclinics.com

beached whales, but we were able to sustain them and not do too much damage. In 1969, with all of us still residents, I was asked to organize what was to be the Hyper-alimentation Unit at the MGH, again, with the help of Ron Abel and Bill Abbot. Later, John Ryan joined us, as did Rita Colley, our first TPN nurse.

In the early 1970s, we rapidly accumulated up to 70 patients at any given time on the TPN service, which was spread throughout the hospital. I was running the service as a young staff person with several fellows, many of whom have gone on to great success in world surgery. Despite the success that we had at supporting most surgical malnourished patients, we never could understand, nor could we achieve, the ability to support patients with sepsis and patients with cancer nutritionally, and that remains true to this day.

## THE EVOLUTION OF TPN

We have learned much since that time. We have decreased the glucose load. We have a much better understanding of an appropriate calorie/nitrogen ratio. The use of a lipid supplement is still controversial as to whether it is used to prevent fatty acid deficiency or whether lipid should constitute a substantial percentage of calories in some clinical situations. Solutions with modified amino acid profiles are in use in special situations, such as renal and/or hepatic failure, and more recently in immuno-modulation, particularly in enteral feeding with the addition of arginine, nucleic acids, perhaps glutamine, and certainly fish oil. Yet, for patients who are most in need, those who are cachectic with cancer and those in whom proteolysis is running amuck with severe sepsis, we have made little progress in ameliorating their catabolism with nutrition support.

## METABOLIC BACKGROUND

To understand the difficulty in supporting such patients, it is necessary to review some of the metabolic pathways in normal nutritional support. The fate of carbohydrate administered to patients or animals is bimodal. It either increases ATP production by glycolysis or, under certain hormonal stimuli, ends up as glycogen for energy storage. Although glycolysis is universal, the brain requires glucose, as do red cells (it is thought that it takes 5 days to switch from glucose to ketone bodies to support the brain; the red cells never switch over); gluconeogenesis occurs largely in the liver and to a lesser extent in the kidney. There is a negative feedback system, so that when intracellular ATP is high, glycolysis is damped. The synthesis of ATP results from the reaction of phosphoenolpyruvate plus ADP to form pyruvate and ATP.

Other sources of fuel include long-chain fatty acids and acetyl coenzyme A, which is a product of long-chain fatty acids. These are also important fuels for ATP production and can normally decrease glycolysis but only when ATP levels are sufficiently high.

## THE HORMONAL ENVIRONMENT

Glucagon is released in response to low blood sugar. It inhibits glycolysis and stimu-lates gluconeogenesis. Glucagon binds to hepatocytes and increases adenyl cyclase, which in turn increases ATP and then increases or activates phosphofructokinase 2 and fructose bisphosphate 2, decreasing fructose and 2,6-bisphosphate. This, in turn, decreases glycolysis and increases gluconeogenesis largely from protein. Insulin, alter-natively, decreases glycolysis, decreases gluconeogenesis, and increases glycogen synthesis in its role as a storage hormone.

## MEDIATORS, CYTOKINES, AND HORMONES

**Fig. 1** illustrates the role of mediators, cytokines, glucocorticoids, counter-regulatory hormones, and possibly myostatins in sepsis. The mechanisms involved include transcription factors and nuclear cofactors, which cooperate in gene regulation involving atrogin-1 and MuRF1, which also participate in stimulating calpain and muscle proteolysis, resulting in the final product in sepsis and cancer, which is muscle wasting. This particular Gordian knot of hormones and various other mediators and stimuli has been difficult to unravel over the past four decades.

Is it possible that the basic problem with the inability to support patients with sepsis and cancer metabolically is due to the following metabolic mechanisms which follow.

## A HYPOTHESIS

1. Ineffective glycolysis results in the insufficient generation of ATP.
2. Whereas normally, administering fat for nutritional support obviates glycolysis, in these two situations, sepsis and cancer, the switch that shuts off glycolysis does not seem to work.
3. The continued need for gluconeogenesis may well be a membrane problem in which there are
   a. Insufficient transport mechanisms
   b. Disordered submembrane space
   c. A pathologic increase in processes that depends on cytoskeletal substructure
4. The cell is not a bag. It has an internal structure. The cell is surrounded by a cell membrane. The cell membrane has subcompartments and/or excrescences arising from the membrane, which provide order to the interior of the cell, a cytoskeletal structure. Various biochemical reactions that organize the cell may proceed better if there is a spatial relationship between the two enzymatic or metabolic processes because they are adherent to the cell membrane. Thus, if there is an aberrant pathophysiologic mechanism and two mechanisms attached to the cell membrane are adjacent to the cytoskeletal structure, these pathologic processes may be increased by the proximity of these adjacent enzymatic processes.

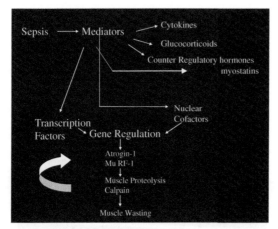

**Fig. 1.** Some of the factors involved in muscle breakdown and muscle wasting. Probably ubiquination involving NF-κB and non–NF-κB pathways is involved.

5. Are there any cytoskeletally spatially related processes that might explain some of the phenomena seen in sepsis and cancer?

## AEROBIC GLYCOLYSIS

Aerobic glycolysis[1] is a process involving sodium-potassium ATPase that takes place in an area adjacent to the cell membrane that produces lactate. Lactate is usually an end product. In addition, the failure to process lactate further via the metabolic cycle into the Krebs cycle means that the process of aerobic glycolysis results in only 8 ATPs produced per molecule of glucose rather than at least the 32 ATPs if the process continues through the Cori cycle. Aerobic glycolysis is stimulated by epinephrine and produces lactate. In the past, the appearance of lactate has led to the conclusion that anaerobic glycolysis is taking place because it has normally been supposed that if lactate is the final end product, the oxidation was incomplete and was producing lactate as an anaerobic end product. This is not necessarily the case. The process of aerobic glycolysis does produce lactate, but it does not produce it in an anaerobic environment. The reason that this process of aerobic glycolysis takes place is the proximity of stored glycogen, which fuels this system, and sodium-potassium ATPase, which is spatially related on, or close to, the cell membrane. Aerobic glycolysis stimulated by epinephrine and the release of glycogen in the presence of sodium-potassium ATPase yield a final end product of 8 ATPs per molecule of glucose.[1]

In the liver, this likely produces an energy shortage. To keep this engine running, increased gluconeogenesis results, in which the glucose produced gets to certain sites in the cell and to glycogen, and those sites are different from the sites normal circulating glucose gets to in the liver. This indicates a lack of membrane transport for circulating glucose in the first place, which is well known, and in the second place, it suggests that the mechanisms by which circulating glucose is synthesized glycogen are somewhat deficient, either because of spatial problems, or more likely, enzymatic or transport problems. The question then is, in the face of aerobic glycolysis, could this intracellular glycogen store attached to the cytoskeleton be the reason why gluconeogenesis continues in patients who are septic or have cancer? If the hypothesis is correct, and lactate is the final product, lactate conceivably might be recirculated to glucose in the liver and form glycogen, which then results in aerobic glycolysis once again (**Fig. 2**). This conceivably could be a fatal, futile cycle.

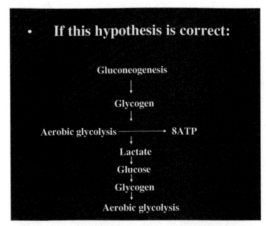

**Fig. 2.** A brief outline of a futile cycle, which may also contribute to mortality.

## WHAT DOES HYPERLACTATEMIA MEAN?

Traditionally, high blood lactate has been associated with hypotension, hypoperfusion, and hypoxia. For generations, students and residents have been taught that increased serum lactate means hypoperfusion and/or hypoxia, and sometimes it does, particularly with dead bowel, and blood lactate is a common test that most residents use when patients are hypotensive and septic to determine if there is a problem with perfusion or if there is something that is nonviable, such as bowel. The clinical corollary of this teaching is that even if blood pressure, pulse, urine output, and $Po_2$ are normal, as in burns, 2 weeks after the burn, resuscitation has not been completed. This is potentially dangerous, because continued resuscitation with high volume of fluids may be injurious. Recent studies have raised questions, however, concerning the origins and significance of lactate with respect to an association with hypoxia and hypoperfusion. If this theory is correct, resuscitation in the face of normal blood pressure, pulse, urine output, and $Po_2$ may be harmful.

From 1967 to 1969, Sir Miles Irving[2] demonstrated that after $\alpha$ and $\beta$ sympathetic blockade in hemorrhaged dogs, with a combination of phenoxybenzamine, an $\alpha$-blocker, and propranolol, a $\beta$-blocker, both plasma catecholamines and hyperlactatemia were reduced. This was reported in the Hunterian lecture delivered on October 24, 1967, at the University of Sydney in New South Wales, Australia.[2] More recently, our laboratory has shown that the production of lactate in vitro from extensor digitorum longus muscle, in shocked, burned, or septic rats, was decreased when ouabain was used to block the activities of sodium-potassium ATPase.[3] This was known previously, but our laboratory went on to show that the regulatory cascade controlling glycogen breakdown was often dependent on adenyl cyclase, stimulated by epinephrine, and mediated by the activation of phosphorylase $b$ kinase to phosphorylase $b$, to glycogen plus inorganic phosphate, and finally to glucose 6-phosphate. Furthermore, stimulation of lactate production in extensor digitorum longus either by epinephrine or amylin could be inhibited by ouabain (**Fig. 3**). In their article, James and colleagues[3,4] proposed the following hypothesis:

1. Within cells, oxidative and glycolytic energy conduction can proceed in separate compartments.
2. Most lactate production occurs in muscle, usually from glycogen.
3. Most lactate production is linked to aerobic glycolysis, which is linked in turn to sodium-potassium ATPase.
4. Epinephrine and insulin (insulin to a lesser extent) stimulates sodium-potassium ATPase to maintain membrane polarity and muscle contraction.

This then supposed that dependence of the sodium-potassium pump function on glycolysis is likely associated with a degree of compartmentalization. In vascular smooth muscle, Paul and coworkers suggested an association of glycolytic enzymes and sodium-potassium ATPase or calcium ATPase at the plasma membrane (**Fig. 4**).[5,6] This could be proved, or at least supported, by the alternative effects of epinephrine and ouabain on glycogen and lactate production (**Fig. 5**). They measured glycogen remaining versus lactate production, as expressed in glucose equivalents, after incubation of extensor digitorum longus in vitro in the presence or absence of either epinephrine or ouabain. An increase of lactate resulted in the decrease of glycogen (see **Fig. 5**). When epinephrine and ouabain were both added to the bath, however, the lactate production was largely blocked, whereas glycogen concentrations were maintained.

These results was in keeping with the hypothesis put forth by Thomas and coworkers[7] that a metabolic control analysis was involved in glycolytic flux control

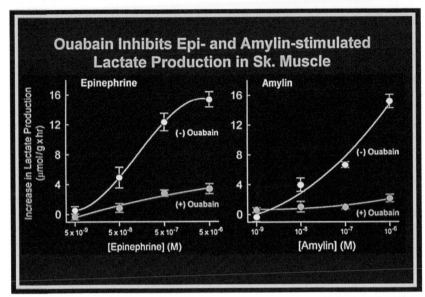

**Fig. 3.** Production of lactate in in vitro incubated skeletal muscle. Epinephrine and amylin separately stimulate lactate production, which may be blocked by ouabain, suggesting that sodium-potassium ATPase is involved.

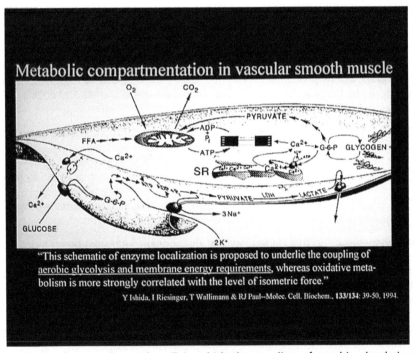

**Fig. 4.** A vascular smooth muscle cell in which the coupling of aerobic glycolysis and membrane energy requirements are pictured. Glycogen is proposed as a source of energy for sodium potassium ATPase and lactate is the final product. Proximity to the cell membrane is important. (*From* Ishida Y, Riesinger I, Wallimann T, et al. Compartmentation of ATP synthesis and utilization in smooth muscle: roles of aerobic glycolysis and creatine kinase. Mol Cell Biochem 1994;133–4:39–50; with permission.)

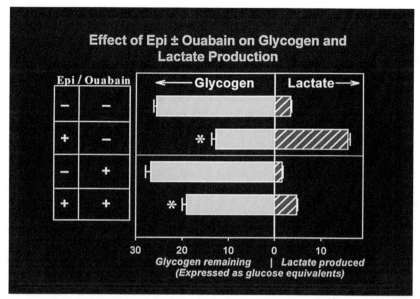

**Fig. 5.** Linkage of small stored glycogen and production of lactate. When ouabain is added, glycogen remains intact for the most part and lactate production is diminished. This indicates that sodium-potassium ATPase stimulated by epinephrine is at least partially responsible for lactate production.

and glycolytic-metabolite-concentration regulation. Thus, perhaps metabolic control analysis predicts the stimulation of sodium-potassium ATPase, which also stimulates glycolysis.

It is possible to explain these effects by an increase in the plasma concentration of insulin. In medical school we all have been taught to believe that insulin entry into the cell is blocked by a deficiency of transport across the cell membrane, perhaps involving glucose 6-phosphate. What if the actions of insulin were differentially blocked in some areas, however, such as glucose use by glycolysis, but not blocked in other areas, such as glycogen storage? In that sense, the differential effects of insulin might conceivably participate in the disorder in glucose metabolism, which is characteristic in sepsis and probably in cancer.

Finally, epinephrine was viewed traditionally as stimulating two entirely different processes: increasing glycogen phosphorylase, thereby increasing lactate production, and separately increasing sodium-potassium ATPase activity, thus increasing ion pumping membrane hyperphosphorylation. What Fischer and colleagues[4] suggested initially was that these two processes were linked because of their mutual proximity to each other at the cell membrane.[6]

## PROTEOLYSIS IN SEPSIS AND CANCER

Under normal circumstances in muscle protein, muscle synthesis and degradation are matched, and little, if any, net breakdown or synthesis of muscle occurs unless exercise and increased caloric or protein intake occur. In cachexia, however, brought on by a variety of stimuli, including sepsis and cancer, muscle breakdown far exceeds muscle synthesis. There has been a flurry of research in the area of muscle wasting in several conditions, including sepsis, burns, cancer, AIDS, renal failure, and starvation, to attempt to understand this process.

Currently, muscle wasting is believed to always be bad. In either acute sepsis or cancer, however, muscle wasting conceivably could be beneficial. Muscle wasting is thought of as deleterious because it results in chronic muscle weakness, delayed ambulation, increased risk for thromboembolic complications, prolonged stays in ICUs, and prolonged need for ventilatory support as well as delays in rehabilitation and in returning to work. Yet, the ability to support patients in ICUs is less than 60 years old. In early historic times, for example, if one were mauled by a saber-toothed tiger, survival depended not only on getting back to the cave but also perhaps on how much glucose and acute-phase protein were produced by gluconeogenesis. If positive immunologic effects could be produced, that might determine survival. It is only recently, with the advent of excellent nutritional support in ICUs, that we have begun to think of muscle wasting as all bad. In the past 30 years, however, we have begun to understand what some of the critical points are in muscle wasting: the mediators, signaling pathways, molecular regulation, gene transcription, and proteolytic pathways all mesh.

In the early 1990s, Dr Avram Hershko and Aaron Ciechanover[8] identified the ubiquitin and proteasome energy-requiring system for proteolysis. Both later received a Nobel prize for this important work. Yet, the breakdown of the myofibrils that was required for muscle breakdown to take place required calpain, a finding further elucidated in the late 1990s and in the early twenty-first century.[9] Muscle wasting is associated with increased transcription of several genes in the ubiquitin proteasome pathways, including the atrogenes, atrogin-1/MAFbx and MuRF1. The regulation of this pathway is by transcription factors C/EBPβ and FOX01/3a; nuclear cofactors, which are important, include P300, PGC-1α, and PGC-1β. The mechanism of stimulation to entering the nucleus involves the breakdown of blocking protein, such as IκB, nuclear factor (NF)-κB, and others, but its further delineation is beyond the scope of this review.

## MYOSTATIN

More recently, myostatins have achieved some notoriety. Myostatin is a member of transforming growth factor β family, which is heavily conserved. It was first described in 1997 by McPherron and colleagues,[10] although it may have been previously described in 1987 in Duchenne muscular dystrophy.[11] Natural and activating mutations of the myostatin gene in cattle are associated in Belgian Blue cattle in double-muscling of these heavily muscled cattle.[12–14] Glucocorticoid-induced skeletal muscle atrophy is associated with upregulation of the myostatin gene expression and is blocked by the steroid blocker RU-486. Dexamethasone treatment continued for 10 days, however, results in normal intramuscular concentration of myostatin. At least one mechanism of the ubiquitin proteolytic system is an NF-κB–independent and FOXO1-dependent mechanism activated by increased ubiquitin-associated genes, atrogin-1, MuRF1, and E214k.[15]

The significance is that inactivation of myostatin leads to muscle growth; the injection of RNA antisense nucleotides increased muscle growth in both normal and cancer cachectic mice.[16] Myostatin circulates in adult mice as a propeptide, which maintains it with a C-terminal dimer in a latent inactive state. Acidosis cleaves the shielding protein, as do metalloproteinases (which are implicated in cancer). Furthermore, injection of a mutant propeptide resistant to cleavage by BMP-1/TLD causes a significant increase in muscle mass when injected into adult mice. Although myostatin has been implicated in cachexia associated with AIDS and associated with liver cirrhosis, preliminary investigations in sepsis have failed to reveal increases in myostatins. Finally, oral glutamine in rats partially prevents muscle atrophy induced by dexamethasone; myostatin expression is also inhibited.

## THE FAT/GLUCOSE SWITCH

In sepsis, if fat is given, gluconeogenosis and proteolysis do not cease to occur. Recently, Cao and coworkers[17] identified the C16:1n7-palmitoleate, which strongly stimulates insulin action in the muscle and in liver as well. They called this molecule a lipokine. The mechanism of action of this lipokine involves specific fatty acid–binding protein, which binds to intracellular fatty acids and conveys them into their ultimate cellular destination (**Fig. 6**). As Olefsky[18] stated in his editorial concerning Cao's article,

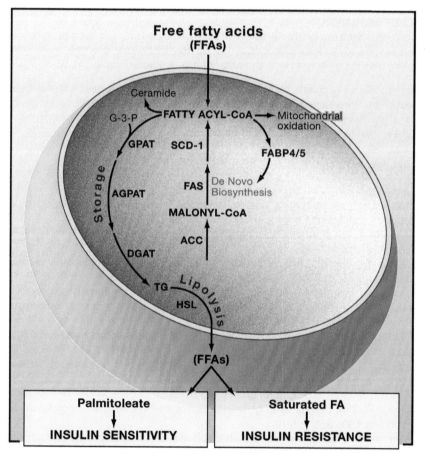

**Fig. 6.** A graphic presentation of the mechanisms involved in lipokine, the newest factor described, which may have profound effects on insulin sensitivity and some of its effects on the fate of various fatty acids. If the existence of leporines is confirmed, it may turn out that metabolic diseases, such as diabetes or sepsis, may be diseases of lipokines in which glucose metabolism disturbances are only secondary. (*From* Olefsky SN. Fat talks, liver and muscle listen. Cell 2008;134:914–6; with permission.)

metabolic diseases, such as diabetes or sepsis, may be diseases of lipokines or a fat metabolism in which the glucose metabolism is only secondary. This may be a fruitful area of investigation for further elucidation in the metabolism of sepsis and cancer.

## SUMMARY

I have attempted to address what I think remains the single most important problem in nutritional support. Using new discoveries and new cofactors, I have provided a hypothesis as to why it has been impossible to support septic and cancer cachectic patients optimally. The metabolic background of the inability to support patients with sepsis and cancer, among other catabolic states, may involve, in part, the following areas:

1. Aerobic glycolysis
2. Proteolysis, possibly secondary to myostatin, which is cleaved in the circulation by acidosis and possibly mediated by non–NF-κB ubiquination mediated in turn by FOX01 and atrogin
3. Lipokine, which may increase sensitivity in muscle and liver to insulin despite insulin resistance and increase glycogen synthesis from lactate and glucose, thereby facilitating aerobic glycolysis and a resultant futile, inefficient cycle.

This hypothesis suggests that at least one form of therapy, the injection of antisense nucleotides to decrease activity of myostatins, may enable the amelioration of some forms of cachexia associated with sepsis and cancer. Proving or disproving this hypothesis will be difficult but should be possible.

## REFERENCES

1. James JH, Fang CH, Schrantz SJ, et al. Linkage of aerobic glycolysis to sodium-potassium transport in rat skeletal muscle. Implications for increased muscle lactate production in sepsis. J Clin Invest 1996;98:2388–97.
2. Irving MH. The sympatho adrenal factor in hemorrhagic shock. Ann R Coll Surg Engl 1968;42:367–86.
3. James JH, Luchette FA, McCarter FD, et al. Lactate is an inreliable indicator of tissue hypoxia in injury or sepsis. Lancet 1999;354:505–8.
4. James JH, Wagner KR, King JK, et al. Stimulation of both aerobic glycolysis and Na(+)-K(+)-ATPase activity in skeletal muscle by epinephrine or amylin. Am J Physiol 1999;277:E176–86.
5. Paul RJ, Bauer M, Pease W. Vascular smooth muscle: aerobic glycolysis linked to sodium and potassium transport processes. Science 1979;206:1414–6.
6. Lynch RM, Paul RS. Compartmentation of glycolytic and glycogenlytic metabolism in vascular smooth muscle. Science 1983;222:1344–6.
7. Thomas S, Fell DS. A control analysis exploration of the role of ATP utilisation in glycolitic -flux control and glycolitic-metabolite-concentration regulation. EurJ Biochem 1998;258:958–67.
8. Hershko A, Ciechanover A. The ubiquitin system for protein degradation. Annu Rev Biochem 1992;61:761–807.
9. Williams AB, deCourten-Myers GM, Fischer JE, et al. Sepsis stimulates release of myofilaments in skeletal muscle by a calcium-dependent mechanism. FASEB J 1999;13:1435–43.
10. McPherron AC, Lawler AM, Lee SJ. Regulation of skeletal muscle mass in mice by a new TGF-1 super family member. Nature 1997;387:83–90.

11. Parsons SA, Millay DP, Sargent MA, et al. Age dependent effect of myostatin block on disease severity in a murine model of limb girdle muscular dystrophy. Am J Pathol 2006;168:1975–85.
12. Grobet L, Martin LJ, Pocelet D, et al. A deletion of the bovine myostatin gene causes the double muscled phenotype in cattle. Nat Genet 1997;17:71–4.
13. McPherron AC, Lee SJ. Double muscling in cattle due to mutations in the myostatin gene. Proc Natl Acad Sci U S A 1997;94:12451–7.
14. Kambadur R, Sharma M, Smith TP, et al. Mutations in myostatin (GDF8) in double-muscled Belgian blue and piedmontese cattle. Genome Res 1997;7:910–6.
15. McFarlane C, Plummer E, Thomas M, et al. Myostatin induces cachexia by activating the ubiquitous proteoylic system through an NF-KB independent FOX01-dependent mechanism. J Cell Physiol 2006;209:501–14.
16. Liu CM, Yang Z, Liu CW, et al. Myostatin antisense RNA-mediated muscle growth in normal and cancer cachexia mice. Gene Ther 2008;15:155–60.
17. Cao H, Gerhold K, Mayers JR, et al. Identification of a lipokine, a lipid hormone linking adipose tissue to systemic metabolism. Cell 2008;134(6):933–44.
18. Olefsky SN. Fat talks, liver and muscle listen. Cell 2008;134:914–6.

# Cachexia, Malnutrition, the Refeeding Syndrome, and Lessons from Goldilocks

J. Alexander Palesty, MD[a,b], Stanley J. Dudrick, MD[b,c],*

**KEYWORDS**

- Cachexia • Malnutrition • Nutritional support
- Refeeding syndrome

Although the explosion of interest in clinical nutrition became manifest more than two decades ago, the keen attention to nutrition and its practical applications to clinical situations continues at an unprecedented rate in the arenas of basic research, clinical investigation, and technologic development. Recognition of the importance of nutritional care has allowed patients with even the most advanced and/or complicated diseases to survive major physiologic insults with minimal morbidity and mortality. The advent of total parenteral nutrition (TPN), followed by the extraordinary progress in parenteral and enteral feedings and their currently widespread availability, in addition to the improved understanding of cellular biomechanics and biochemistry, has allowed clinicians to combat starvation and malnutrition with much more zeal and effectiveness because of their ability to deliver diets formulated and designed not only for general nutritional support but also specifically for the treatment of special patient problems and deficiencies.

Cachexia, in particular the cachexia of cancer, is one of the areas in which recent advances in clinical nutrition have had a profound impact on patient care. It is appreciated widely by clinicians that significant malnutrition accompanies malignant

The authors have nothing to disclose.

[a] Department of Surgery, University of Connecticut School of Medicine, 263 Farmington Avenue, Farmington, CT 06030, USA
[b] Department of Surgery, Saint Mary's Hospital, 56 Franklin Street, Waterbury, CT 06706, USA
[c] Department of Surgery, Yale University School of Medicine, 333 Cedar Street, New Haven, CT 06510, USA
* Corresponding author. Department of Surgery, Saint Mary's Hospital, 56 Franklin Street, Waterbury, CT 06706.
*E-mail address:* sdudrick@stmh.org

processes in approximately 50% of patients and eventually leads to severe wasting, which accounts for approximately 30% of cancer-related deaths overall.[1,2] The body wasting known as cancer cachexia is a complex syndrome characterized by progressive tissue depletion and decreased nutrient intake that is manifested clinically as inexplicable, recalcitrant anorexia and inexorable host weight loss. Decreased nutritional intake, increased metabolic expenditure, and dysfunctional metabolic processes, including hormonal and cytokine-related abnormalities, all seem to play roles in the development of cancer cachexia.[1,3] Although this condition of advanced protein-calorie malnutrition, sometimes described as the cancer anorexia-cachexia syndrome, is not entirely understood, it seems to be multifactorial, is a major cause of morbidity and mortality in cancer patients, and ultimately leads to death.

Therapeutic nutritional interventions to correct or reverse cachexia have met with little success, and, despite tremendous efforts throughout the decades, the exact nature of the mediators responsible for cancer cachexia remain elusive. The pathogenesis of cancer cachexia seems related to proinflammatory cytokines, alterations in the neuroendocrine axis, and tumor-derived catabolic factors. Despite trials of conventional and/or aggressive nutritional support by myriad feeding techniques, patients with cancer cachexia have failed to gain consistent significant benefits in terms of weight gain, functional ability, quality of life, or survival. Additionally, attempts to ameliorate the abnormal clinical and metabolic features of cancer cachexia with a variety of pharmacologic agents have met with only rare and limited success.

A thorough understanding of the basic metabolic derangements and the effects of the available nutritional supportive measures can assist in reducing the morbidity and mortality of malnourished and/or starving patients. It is the responsibility of health care providers to sick patients to maintain optimal organ and system integrity to allow cells to perform their individual specialized functions to their maximal capacity, thereby restoring and maintaining patients' homeostasis and nutritional health. Herein, a detailed overview of the cachexia of cancer and review of two of the sentinel articles on malnutrition, starvation, and refeeding and the lessons gleaned therefrom provide clinicians, both novice and expert, with efficacious and thought-provoking knowledge of the still rapidly evolving and vital discipline of nutritional care of malnourished patients.[4,5] An additional goal is to caution and familiarize practitioners of nutritional support regarding some of the consequences associated with attempting to re-establish the delicate physiologic balance of metabolic and nutritional homeostasis too rapidly and/or excessively.

## CACHEXIA AND CANCER

Cachexia results from the inexorable and recalcitrant progression of nutritional deterioration, which occurs in approximately 50% of patients with malignant disorders and in approximately 80% of patients with cancers involving the upper gastrointestinal tract. It is among the most debilitating and life-threatening aspects of cancer and results in body mass wasting that accounts for up to 30% of cancer-related deaths.[2] Clinically, the cancer-cachexia syndrome is characterized primarily by anorexia, early satiety, wasting, weight loss, weakness, fatigue, poor mental and physical performance, decreased capacity for wound healing, impaired immunologic function, and a compromised quality of life, none of which is resolved by forced nutrient intake.[1,2] Diminished nutritional intake, increased metabolic expenditure, and disordered or malfunctioning metabolic processes, including hormonal and cytokine-related abnormalities, all seem to play roles in the development of cancer cachexia.[2,3] Although this condition of advanced protein-calorie malnutrition, frequently referred to as the cancer anorexia-cachexia syndrome, is not entirely understood, it seems to be multifactorial, is a major cause of morbidity and mortality in cancer patients, and ultimately leads to death.[3,6]

The origin of the word, *cachexia*, is both descriptive and incriminating. It is derived from the Greek words, *kakos* (meaning bad) and *hexis* (meaning condition, habit, or state of being).[1,3] Cancer cachexia was first reported as a commonly occurring syndrome more than 70 years ago, when an autopsy series of 500 cancer patients documented that the immediate cause of death in cancer patients was secondary to inanition in 114 (22%) of the patients, and that up to two-thirds of this cadre of patients exhibited some degree of cachexia.[7] Since then, the scope of malnutrition in cancer patients has been studied in a wide variety of patient groups. In a series of 3047 patients enrolled in the Eastern Cooperative Oncology Group chemotherapy protocols, who were all assessed for weight loss before initiating chemotherapy, survival was significantly lower in the patients who demonstrated weight loss when compared with those who had not lost any weight before starting chemotherapy.[8,9] In this study group, patients with breast cancer or sarcomas had the lowest frequency of weight loss (31% to 40%), patients with colon cancer had an intermediate frequency of weight loss (48% to 61%), and patients with pancreatic or gastric cancer had the highest frequency of weight loss (83% to 87%), with approximately one-third of these patients having presented initially with greater than 10% weight loss.[8,9] In a prospective study of 280 cancer patients, malnutrition was related predominantly to tumor type and site, with stomach and esophageal cancer patients demonstrating significantly higher degrees of malnutrition compared with the other groups. Moreover, as expected, malnutrition was shown to increase in severity as the disease advanced.[10] In another study of 365 patients with gastrointestinal cancer, almost 50% percent were shown to be malnourished. The incidence of malnutrition was related to the site of the disease, and the stage of the disease was identified as a predictor of weight loss, with more than 50% of stage III patients manifesting malnutrition.[11]

Although nutritional status is usually evaluated by a combination of clinical assessment and anthropometric tests, including body weight, skin-fold thickness, and mid-arm circumference, most clinicians rely on body weight as the major measure of nutritional status, using usual adult body weight as a point of reference.[1] Cachexia should be expected if an involuntary or unexpected weight loss of greater than 5% has occurred within a previous 6-month period, especially when combined with muscle wasting. A weight loss of 10% or more ordinarily indicates severe depletion but can also be used as a starting criterion for the anorexia-cachexia syndrome in obese patients. Body compartment analysis has shown that patients with cachexia lose approximately equal amounts of fat and fat-free mass. Losses of fat-free mass occur primarily from skeletal muscle and reflect decreases both in cellular mass and intracellular potassium concentration.[12] In comparison to patients with stable weight, cancer patients with documented 5% weight loss have a shorter median survival rate, respond more poorly to chemotherapy, and experience increased toxicity to chemotherapy.[1,8,13]

Understanding the multiple nutritional, metabolic, and physiologic changes that can occur provides the basis for evaluating the requirements for nutritional support in various clinical situations and for planning and providing support as indicated. Although a localized tumor may exert various initial systemic and generalized effects in a patient, as the tumor grows and metastasizes, these effects often become even more obvious as a result of the increased tumor burden and its local and distant invasion. Additionally, some malignant tumors can produce effects at a distance from the original tumor or its metastases, further compounding malnutrition.[14] The nutritional problems associated with neoplastic disease that can cause or contribute to the development of cancer cachexia are outlined in **Box 1**.

## METABOLIC PATHOPHYSIOLOGY OF CANCER CACHEXIA

Inability to gain and/or maintain weight despite seemingly adequate nutrient intake could be due to these obvious possibilities: (1) increased metabolic needs generated by the accentuated nutritional demands of the semiautonomous tumor; (2) generalized increased energy expenditure in the cancer patient; and (3) maladaptive metabolism (ie, failure of the cancer patient's host tissues to use the nutrients available efficiently and effectively to satisfy the energy requirements of the body).[3] Although malignant cells do have their own specific nutrient requirements and do expend energy, it has been shown that these does not fully explain the cancer cachexia-anorexia syndrome in human cancer patients.[15] Therefore, it is important to differentiate data reported from animal tumors, which tend to represent a much larger proportion of the total body weight of the organism, from data reported from human tumors, which generally represent a much smaller proportion of the weight of the host.

Many studies of resting energy expenditure (REE) and basal energy expenditure have been performed to establish whether cancer patients are hypermetabolic.[15] These studies have demonstrated that approximately 60% of cancer patients have abnormal REE, of whom approximately 35% are hypometabolic and 25% are hyper-metabolic. A confounding aspect of these studies is that lean body mass, rather than total body mass, correlated with alterations found in measured REE. Thus, cancer patients, who ordinarily have early diminished lean body mass, may be expected to have energy expenditure levels which are low for their total weight and what seems to be hypometabolism may really represent a eumetabolic state. Despite this nonstandard interpretation of REE data in cachectic cancer patients, it seems that although hypermetabolism of the host and/or tumor plays a role in cancer cachexia, hypermetabolism does not suffice as a complete explanation of the cancer-cachexia syndrome.

A summary of the current status of the understanding of the metabolic maladaptation of cancer patients to decreased nutrient intake and increased metabolic caloric needs of both the tumor and the host includes increased hepatic glucose production; failure of uptake of the gluconeogenic glucose by muscle, resulting in proteolysis and production of glycogenic amino acids; uptake and use of glucose by tumor cells with resulting lactate production and occasional lactic acidosis; and increased lipolysis with production of fatty acid and glycerol, ultimately used for energy and further gluconeogenesis (**Box 2**). Thus, the nutritional requirements of the tumor are selectively favored over those of the host by these aberrant metabolic mandates in cancer patients.[3]

## PATHOGENIC MECHANISMS OF ANOREXIA

The intake of energy substrates is significantly reduced in cancer patients who lose weight, and although anorexia is unlikely to be responsible solely for the wasting seen in cancer patients, it may be a substantial contributing factor.[3,16,17] Cancer patients, especially those with gastrointestinal cancer, may frequently suffer from physical obstruction of the alimentary tract, pain, constipation, maldigestion, malabsorption, debility, or the side effects of therapy, including opiates, radiotherapy, or chemotherapy, any of which may lead to decreased food intake.[18,19] Additionally, hypercalcemia associated with cancer is a fairly common condition that can cause nausea, vomiting, and weight loss as well as other untoward side effects. Moreover,

**Box 1**
**Nutritional problems associated with the development of cancer cachexia**

1. Anorexia and early satiety with progressive weight loss and undernutrition

2. Altered taste or dysgeusia causing hypophagia, food aversion, or altered food intake

3. Alterations in protein, carbohydrate, and fat metabolism

4. Increased energy expenditure despite decreased body mass

5. Impaired food intake secondary to

    a. Mechanical obstruction of the gastrointestinal tract at any level

    b. Intestinal dysmotility induced by various tumors

6. Malabsorption secondary to

    a. Deficiency or inactivation of pancreatic digestive enzymes

    b. Deficiency or inactivation of bile salts

    c. Failure of ingested food to mix and interact effectively with digestive enzymes

    d. Intestinal fistulas—internal and/or external

    e. Infiltration of the small bowel wall or lymphatics and mesentery by malignant cells

    f. Blind loop syndrome with associated bacterial overgrowth

    g. Malnutrition-induced villous hypoplasia in the small intestine

7. Protein-losing enteropathy

8. Metabolic abnormalities induced by tumor-derived eutopic hormones or peptides

    a. Hypoglycemia induced by insulin-secreting tumors

    b. Hyperglycemia induced by islet glucagonoma or somatostatinoma

    c. Hypercalcemia and hypophosphatemia with osteomalacia induced by parathyroid hormone–like polypeptides secreted by some tumors

    d. Anemia secondary to chronic blood loss and/or bone marrow suppression

9. Electrolyte and fluid derangements secondary to

    a. Persistent vomiting and intestinal obstruction or intracranial tumors

    b. Intestinal fluid losses through fistulas or diarrhea

    c. Intestinal secretory abnormalities with hormone-secreting tumors, such as

        i. Carcinoid syndrome

        ii. Zollinger-Ellison syndrome (gastrinoma)

        iii. Verner-Morrison syndrome (VIPoma)

        iv. Villous adenoma

        v. Increased calcitonin

    d. Inappropriate antidiuretic hormone secretion associated with specific tumors, such as lung carcinomas

    e. Hyperadrenalism secondary to tumors producing corticotropins or corticosteroids

10. Miscellaneous organ dysfunction with nutritional complications, such as intractable gastric ulcers with gastrinomas, Fanconi syndrome with light chain disease, or coma with brain tumors

11. Tumor products stimulating monocyte production of various interleukins

*Data from* Shils ME. Nutrition and diet in cancer management. In: Shils ME, Olson JA, Shike M, editors. Modern nutrition in health and disease. 8th edition. Philadelphia: Lea & Febiger; 1994. p. 1317–48.

---

**Box 2**
**Abnormalities of carbohydrate, protein, and fat metabolism associated with cancer cachexia**

Carbohydrate Metabolism

    Glucose intolerance

    Insulin resistance

    Abnormal insulin secretion

    Impaired glucose clearance

    Increased glucose production

    Increased glucose turnover

    Increased Cori cycle activity

Protein Metabolism

    Increased whole-body protein turnover

    Increased protein fractional synthesis rates in the liver

    Decreased fractional synthesis rates in muscle

    Increased hepatic protein synthesis

    Recalcitrant muscle protein breakdown

    Decreased plasma levels of branched-chain amino acids

Fat Metabolism

    Excess body fat depletion relative to body protein loss

    Increased lipolysis

    Increased free fatty acids

    Increased glycerol turnover

    Decreased lipogenesis

    Hyperlipidemia

        Failure of glucose to suppress oxidation of free fatty acids.

        Decreased serum lipoprotein lipase activity despite normal insulin availability

*Data from* Shils ME. Nutrition and diet in cancer management. In: Shils ME, Olson JA, Shike M, editors. Modern nutrition in health and disease. 8th edition. Philadelphia: Lea & Febiger; 1994. p. 1317–48.

---

anorexia is an extremely distressing syndrome because appetite and the ability to eat have been reported to be the most important factors in the physical and psychological aspects (especially depression) of a patient's quality of life.[20,21] No clinical cause of reduced food intake is obvious, however, in a large number of patients with cancer and cancer cachexia. The early satiety that accompanies reduced appetite in anorectic cancer patients has been postulated to be caused by the production of tumor cell factors that exert their effects by acting on hypothalamic sensory cells.[22] Possible factors include the satietins, in particular satietin D, which have been purified from human plasma and have been shown to produce a long-lasting anorectic effect when injected into rats, although the role of the satietins in the development of anorexia has not been established. Another possible cause of anorexia is the increased serotonergic activity within the central nervous system of patients with cancer cachexia, attributed to the enhanced availability of tryptophan to the brain. A close relationship between elevated plasma-free tryptophan and anorexia has been observed in patients having cancer and reduced food intake.[23] The fact that uptake of tryptophan into the brain is competitive with uptake of branched-chain amino acids has suggested the use of branched-chain amino acids to decrease the incidence of anorexia.[23] Because weight loss is such a potent stimulus to food intake in healthy human beings, the persistence of anorexia in cancer patients implies a failure of this adaptive feeding response, which is so impressive and effective in normal human beings.[24–27]

A hormone secreted by adipose tissue, leptin, is now known to be an integral component of the mechanism for body weight recognition.[19,28–35] Because weight loss causes leptin levels to fall in proportion to the loss of body fat, it seems that leptin plays an important role in triggering the adaptive response to starvation.[1] The activity of the hypothalamic or orexigenic signals that stimulate feeding and suppress energy expenditure are increased by low leptin levels in the brain, which also increase the activity of anorexigenic signals that suppress appetite and increase energy expenditure.[1,24–27] In experimental animals that are fasted, most of the orexigenic signals are known to be up-regulated, suggesting that these signals play an important role in facilitating the recovery of lost weight. It seems that neuropeptide Y produced in the hypothalamus binds to a receptor (Y-5) in adjacent hypothalamic cells, which in turn increases the response of additional neuropeptide Y and stimulates the neuronal basis of appetite.[3] It has further been shown that leptin also binds to Y-5, inhibiting neuropeptide Y activity and producing satiety.[36] Recently, glucagon-like peptide 1 and urocortin have also been shown to be appetite suppressants.[3,37,38]

The cancer-anorexia syndrome may result from circulating factors produced by the tumor or by the host in response to the tumor, and several cytokines have been proposed as possible mediators of the cachetic process.[19] Elevated serum levels of tumor necrosis factor $\alpha$, interleukin 1, and interleukin 6 have been found in some but not all cancer patients, and the serum levels of these cytokines seem to correlate with the progression of the tumor.[22,39,40] Interferon alpha, interferon gamma, and leukemia inhibitory factor are additional cytokines that have been postulated as playing a role in the etiology of cancer cachexia but have not been proved to be responsible solely for the induction of cachexia.[22] Chronic administration of these cytokines, however, either alone or in combination, is capable of inducing reduced food intake and reproducing the cancer anorexia-cachexia syndrome.[19,22,39–43] These cytokines may produce long-term inhibition of appetite and feeding by stimulating the production and release of leptin and/or by mimicking the hypothalamic effect of excessive negative feedback signaling from leptin, leading to the normal compensatory mechanisms for decreases in food intake and body weight.[1,19,24–27,29,30,32,35,44–47] Thus, the weight loss that occurs in cancer patients differs considerably from that which occurs in simple starvation in otherwise healthy human beings.

Melanocortins, a family of regulatory peptides, which include corticotropin and the melanocyte-stimulating hormones, have recently been reported as potential contributory factors in anorexia and cachexia.[1,48–50] This group of peptides and their receptors are important in memory, behavior, and immunity but also help to regulate appetite and body temperature.[19,31,33,34] In animal studies, the melanocortin system remained active during cancer-induced cachexia, whereas the normal response to marked loss of body weight would have resulted in down-regulation of the anorexigenic melanocortin signaling system to conserve energy stores. Moreover, blockade of the melanocortin receptor reversed the anorexia and cachexia in the animals, suggesting a pathogenetic role for this system.[19,48–50]

The specific role of the various factors in the cancer anorexia-cachexia syndrome and their relative importance remain to be clarified. It is presumed that anorexia is caused by the same mediator or mediators that also produce the metabolic derangements of cancer cachexia itself. Use of antianorectic agents alone may improve quality of life in cancer patients but may not solve the problem of anorexia and its associated morbidity and mortality in cancer patients.[16]

The role of hormones in the cancer anorexia-cachexia syndrome must be considered because of the obvious roles that hormones play in the intermediary metabolism of carbohydrates.[51] Insulin, epinephrine, corticotropin, human growth hormone, and insulin-like growth factor have all been suggested to have a role in the anorexia-cachexia syndrome. During early starvation, decreased insulin levels and increased glucagon and epinephrine result in activation of cyclic adenosine monophosphate and of a protein kinase that activates hormone-sensitive lipase. Failure of this normal mechanism may account for the weight loss in cancer patients, who have increased rates of glycerol and free fatty acid turnover compared with starved healthy patients.[16]

Recent studies have indicated the presence of an acidic peptide in animal tumors, which seems to have lipolytic properties that could lead to some of the characteristics of the cancer-cachexia syndrome.[16,52] This factor seems to be a proteoglycan which has been found in the urine of murine species with tumors as well as in human patients with cancer anorexia-cachexia syndrome involving weight loss of greater than 1.4 kg.[16,52] This proteoglycan has been shown to mobilize free fatty acids from adipose tissue and amino acids from muscle in animals, which prompted the investigators to suggest that the role of these tumor products is to mobilize nutrients for which the tumor has the greatest affinity and which results in further increased tumor growth. Investigations are currently under way to determine whether this proteoglycan is widely present in cachectic human cancer patients and whether its pathophysiologic actions mimic those of the cancer anorexia-cachexia syndrome.[3] A potentially clinically useful feature of this research is the discovery of an antagonist (eicosapentaenoic acid) of this proteoglycan which could have a role in the treatment of the human anorexia-cachexia syndrome.[16,53]

It is highly likely that multiple mediators rather than a single mediator probably account for the metabolic and pathophysiologic abnormalities associated with the anorexia-cachexia syndrome. It is possible, indeed likely, that tumor cells produce multiple active peptides or glycopeptides, that they also stimulate the induction of additional cytokines or lymphokines from host immune cells and that they stimulate abnormal hormonal responses to the metabolic stress induced by the malignancy. Alternatively, it is unlikely that a single factor could account for the hypermetabolism, abnormal glucose metabolism, protein gluconeogenesis, and insulin resistance in addition to the anorexia, anemia and fever that accompany the cancer anorexia-cachexia syndrome.

## NUTRITIONAL SUPPORT WITH CANCER CACHEXIA

Early studies promoted optimism that judicious enteral or parenteral nutritional support might overcome cancer anorexia, and modulate or obviate malnutrition and cancer cachexia.[19,54–56] The failure of aggressive nutritional support to increase lean body mass, however, especially skeletal muscle mass, in patients with cancer cachexia has been disappointing. In a meta-analysis of 28 randomized studies of cancer patients receiving TPN, the use of TPN preoperatively in patients with gastrointestinal cancer helped reduce major surgical complications and operative mortality significantly, but no significant benefit was shown on survival, tolerance of treatment, toxicity, or tumor response in patients receiving chemotherapy and TPN.[57] A survey analyzing results individually for patients receiving radiation therapy and chemotherapy and for patients undergoing major surgery concluded that the routine use of preoperative intravenous feeding should be limited to patients unable to sustain lean body mass by oral or enteral feeding.[58] The investigators stated further that intravenous feeding had not been documented to affect responses either to therapy or survival favorably in patients receiving radiation therapy or chemotherapy. Rhey further stated, however, that selecting patients for support with TPN remains a matter of clinical judgment and that when therapy response rates and malnutritional morbidity are high, intravenous feeding should be instituted until the host can recover from the effects of antitumor therapy.[58] The investigators concluded additionally that there is clear evidence that in individual patients with cancer, intravenous feeding can prevent death from starvation and decrease the morbidity of treatment, but only those patients undergoing surgery for gastrointestinal tract neoplasia have benefited significantly from the addition of adjuvant intravenous feeding.[58] Another subsequent review concluded that chronically malnourished patients given nutritional support often have restoration of a sense of well-being and become more physically functional; however, whether this support results in long-term clinical benefits is difficult to evaluate.[59] The investigators stated also that it seems that routine application of nutritional support to all patients undergoing treatment for malignancy is not justified and that the primary indication for nutritional support is for malnourished patients undergoing a major operation for upper gastrointestinal malignancy and for chemotherapy patients with severe gastrointestinal dysfunction.[59] In another analysis of 18 trials in children with cancer, the investigator acknowledged the clear benefits of nutritional support in patients undergoing bone marrow transplantation; however, he stated that there seems to be little support for routine aggressive nutritional support in nonsurgical oncology patients.[60] Nonetheless, the investigator concluded further that circumstances exist in which aggressive nutritional support by any and all routes should be provided, especially during prolonged inability to eat, when nutrition is secondary to poor intake, when a nutrition support team is available to decrease related complications, and when the tumor present is deemed likely to respond to antineoplastic treatment.[60] Additionally, parenteral nutrition (PN) may facilitate administration of complete chemoradiation therapy dosages in esophageal cancer patients and may have beneficial effects for certain patients with decreased food intake because of mechanical obstruction of the gastrointestinal tract.[61–63] Home PN can also be efficacious and rewarding for such patients.[1] If the gastrointestinal tract can be used for nutritional support, enteral nutrition has the advantage of maintaining the integrity of the enterocytes, the mucosal barrier, and immunologic function as well as the advantage of having lower cost and fewer adverse side effects.[1,61,64] Experience, clinical judgment, and wisdom all are important, although often subjective rather than objective, in making the usually difficult and challenging decisions in the management of these unfortunate patients with their multiple ill-defined, poorly understood, and vexing problems, which have few or no obvious solutions.

The effects of aggressive nutritional support on tumor growth and development have been difficult to delineate in cancer patients and are still being debated.[1,65] A clear benefit of nutritional support, however, may be derived in cancer patients with severe malnutrition who may require surgery or may have an obstructing tumor but one that is potentially responsive to therapy.[1,62,66,67] Experience has also indicated that cancer patients with a severely dysfunctional alimentary tract resulting from radiation, chemotherapy, surgery, or combinations thereof, but who are free of residual malignant disease, are entitled to proper management by oral, enteral, and/or parenteral feeding support, which can lead to a prolonged life of good quality.[14] The best treatment for cancer cachexia, especially that related to cancer of the gastrointestinal tract, is to cure the cancer. Unfortunately, this lofty goal remains an infrequent achievement currently among patients with solid tumors. Because a cure for cancer is still under investigation and forthcoming, the best palliative or therapeutic options available are to stimulate increased nutritional intake and ameliorate or prevent the catabolism of muscle and fat. This can be accomplished to varying degrees with a multitude of pharmacologic agents. A goal as monumental as this, however, would be much easier to achieve if it were possible to identify the exact causes and mechanisms of the cancer cachexia-anorexia syndrome. Currently, only those elements of decreased food intake directly related to the antineoplastic treatment, such as nausea, vomiting, mucositis, and dysfunctional gastrointestinal motility, can be somewhat controlled or modulated clinically. The most realistic and practical options at this time are directed toward minimizing adverse gastrointestinal side effects or complications and increasing appetite and nutritional intake in an effort to improve quality of life. The ability to target the myriad consequences caused by cachexia and its treatment as related to cancer are derived in part from observations made by Cahill[4] in a landmark *New England Journal of Medicine* article that clearly and concisely outlined the physiologic and metabolic derangements and adaptations that occur in fat, carbohydrate, and protein metabolism in the starving human organism.

## THE GENESIS OF MODERN THEORIES ON STARVATION AND MALNUTRITION

Intense interest in studying the effects and management of malnutrition followed World War II, primarily because the scale of the global challenge was so broad and because few scientific data existed on the basic physiologic responses to starvation.[68] Cahill, in his article titled, "Starvation in Man," submitted the proposition that fat and protein are practically the only two fuel repositories in the human body with the caveat that because proteins are metabolically active molecules integral to the daily operation of the human engine, the more expendable fat is the primary and predominant energy cache that is consumed during catabolism, thus conserving the more vital protein for function. His fundamental conclusion was that 3 compensatory mechanisms interact during starvation to spare protein from being used as the fuel for metabolism in the human organism: (1) the exclusion of glucose as a fuel source from the majority of tissues in favor of fatty acids; (2) the adaptation of the Cori cycle to shuttle glucose to the peripheral tissue by breaking down lipid, then returning lactate to the liver, which resynthesizes the lactate into glucose; and (3) the ability of the brain to use keto acids for energy to spare glucose, thus ultimately also preserving protein. He observed further that insulin is the dominant hormone that controls and maintains homeostasis during starvation and that glucagon also has an important role, which at that time was undefined. In addition, he noted that fat and fat-derived fuels are used preferentially and almost exclusively in starvation for energy and demonstrated that during the fasting state, muscle, adipose tissue, the liver, and kidneys all work in conjunction to supply, convert, and conserve fuel for the body.

According to Cahill, the human body in its normal metabolic state incorporates approximately 0.3 kg of glycogen, 10 to 15 kg of triacylglycerol, and 6 kg of mobilizable muscle as potential energy sources. Only skeletal muscle and the liver have enough glycogen stores to provide for the daily needs of the entire body under ordinary circumstances. Liver glycogen is exhausted within 18 to 24 hours of starvation, however, and muscle glycogen is not easily available for use, but it can be converted to glucose through exportation to the liver as pyruvate, lactate (the Cori cycle), and/or alanine. Conversely, liver glycogen is readily available for mobilization and, in the fasting state, is quickly depleted.[69] Hence, as the available glycogen is depleted, gluconeogenesis is required for the production of glucose. Another source of glucose is fat but, unfortunately, most of the energy stored as fat by most organs and tissues is not available completely for general use because it is required to provide this source of glucose primarily to the organ or tissue of origin. In the starved state, other glucose dependent organs, such as the brain, have adapted to the relative glucose deficiency that accompanies starvation by using ketone bodies converted from free fatty acids as their energy source.

The primary goal in caring for nutritionally depleted patients is the preservation of functional protein. Although it was initially thought that supplemental dietary protein would have no effect on lean muscle mass in starvation, studies have now confirmed that high protein intake in energy deficient states does spare and/or restore lean muscle mass.[70–76] This is a most important factor to take into consideration when formulating nutrition support regimens for malnourished critically ill patients regardless of the avenue of nutrient administration.

Despite the scientific progress since Cahill's article, the events leading to, or driving, the metabolic changes in starvation are still incompletely understood. Subtle decreases in plasma glucose concentrations and the subsequent fall in the plasma insulin/glucagon ratio, as well as an increase in plasma epinephrine, has been documented to occur.[77,78] Intuitively, one would think that because these hormones are catabolic, there would be an increase in muscle protein breakdown; however, it is spared. It is postulated that protein preservation is stimulated by the decrease in production of triiodothyronine toward its inactive form, reverse triiodothyronine, which effectively reduces the body's metabolic rate. This may subsequently reduce the rate of overall protein consumption.[79]

Notwithstanding the improved understanding of the biomechanics and physiology of starvation, the rate of malnutrition has not changed significantly in the past 40 years, and malnourishment continues to be documented in up to 50% of hospitalized patients who present with various degrees of protein-calorie malnutrition.[80,81] The degree to which patients are malnourished directly correlates with outcome, in particular, morbidity and mortality. The misunderstanding that patients with a normal serum albumin level cannot be malnourished can lead to inappropriate management. In order to treat these individuals appropriately, it is helpful to categorize them into one of 3 groups: marasmus, kwashiorkor, or mixed malnutrition. The improved understanding of the basic biochemical and physiologic derangements that occur in each of these very different malnourished states has allowed clinicians to focus their attention and management on the fundamental cellular disorder.

Marasmus, or simple starvation, develops insidiously, and it results from the body's attempt to adapt to an insufficient caloric intake. Causative factors include alcoholism, central nervous system insult, old age, and chronic debilitating disease. Cachexia, wasting, and clinical signs of nutritional deficiencies are the clinical hallmarks of marasmic patients. Attempts at aggressive nutritional resuscitation may precipitate development of peripheral edema, which is not otherwise a component of this form of malnutrition.

Experience with kwashiorkor, also known as immunorepressive malnutrition or hypoalbuminemic malnutrition, is drawn predominantly from the third world countries. This form of malnutrition is manifest in patients who have adequate caloric intake but inadequate protein intake.[68] They often have a fatty liver, edema, hypoalbuminemia, hyponatremia, and dermatosis.[82] Although these patients may overtly appear well nourished, they have severe deficits in protein stores and immune function, which have prompted the use of more descriptive, alternative names for kwashiorkor, immunosuppressive malnutrition or hypoalbuminemic malnutrition.[83]

Those patients with mixed malnutrition exhibit a combination of marasmus and immunosuppressive or hypoalbuminemic malnutrition and have a higher morbidity and mortality because of the increased magnitude of the physiologic insult.[82] Patients may initially present with one form of malnutrition secondary to the original physiologic insult that eventually transitions to the other because of advancing metabolic severity. The principal goal of nutritional therapy in these clinical scenarios is to preserve lean muscle mass and function. Clinicians' intuitive response in coping with any of these forms of malnutrition is to re-establish nutritional integrity as quickly and as completely as possible. A pivotal article in 1981 by Weinsier and Krumdieck,[84] who revisited the refeeding syndrome induced by the overenthusiastic application of TPN in starving patients, seemingly paradoxically, cautions against rapid nutritional restoration, especially in chronically cachetic patients who have become well adapted to caloric deprivation.

Their report describes two chronically malnourished patients who were aggressively administered nutritional support with PN and who, in contradistinction to expected results, deteriorated secondary to cardiopulmonary failure and died within 48 hours. Both patients had received approximately twice the recommended load of carbohydrate and protein in their initial PN regimen. Each of these individuals abruptly developed hypophosphatemia, which was postulated to be induced by increased intracellular transport of phosphate for glycolysis in these depleted patients. Because fat catabolism, which is the primary source of energy in the starved state, does not require phosphate, the sudden shift to glucose as a fuel source increased the demand for phospate. Both patients also had clinical and laboratory findings consistent with myocardial ischemia, and their acute cardiac decompensation was thought to be directly related to the rapid onset of hypophosphatemia. They also suffered from other collateral metabolic abnormalities, such as hypomagnesemia, hypocalcemia, hypokalemia, hyperglycemia, and acidosis. The resultant complications from refeeding were all associated with the abrupt shift from the consumption of endogenous fat to the use of exogenously infused glucose as the primary fuel source. After recognition of this problem, it was recommended that total calorie/protein requirements not be provided vigorously in nutritional repletion regimens initially but rather be started cautiously at lower levels and reached gradually over several days, with approximately 20% to 30% of total calories derived from fat.

## THE REFEEDING SYNDROME

Interest in the refeeding syndrome initially arose during World War II when little was known scientifically about human starvation or how to deal with refeeding people who had severe degrees of nutritional deprivation.[85] The question to be answered at that time, and one that remains to be answered completely, is, What is the most effective way of providing nutritional rehabilitation? In 1944, Keys and colleagues[5] designed a human experiment to attempt to answer this question. The results of their studies have prompted researchers to explore the metabolic adaptation of the human body to gain insight into the optimal clinical management of starvation. The main objective of Keys' work was to observe and characterize the physical and mental effects that starvation had on 36 otherwise healthy subjects. The young male volunteers were observed under normal conditions for 3 months while ingesting a 3200-kcal diet. This was followed by a period of 6 months of starvation during which they received an 1800-kcal low-protein diet to simulate the diets of the starved survivors of the ravages of warfare. Subjects then under went a nutritional rehabilitative period for 3 months. Each of 4 groups received different amounts of calories, and within those groups, various subjects received different amounts of protein. Throughout each phase of the study, a detailed record of each patient's physiologic state was maintained, including ECGs, radiographs, laboratory studies, body weight, muscle mass, and the results of endurance tests. During the period of nutritional replenishment, several subjects developed cardiac failure, and Keys' conclusions as to the cause, although rudimentary, were fundamentally the same as those of more recent investigators.[84]

There has been much investigation of the refeeding syndrome since the publication of Weinsier and Krumdieck,[84] and although hypophosphatemia and its associated complications remain the hallmark signs, it is now well documented that patients with refeeding syndrome also develop global electrolyte disorders, dyspnea, hypercapnia, tachycardia, elevated central venous pressure, congestive heart failure, and cardiac arrest, among other clinical manifestations. Refeeding syndrome after the overzealous feeding of malnourished patients via oral, enteral, and/or parenteral routes is well recognized in starved individuals, chronic alcoholics, patients with anorexia nervosa, depleted patients admitted from skilled nursing facilities, morbidly obese patients with recent massive weight loss, and some critically ill postoperative patients.[86–90]

Repleting malnourished patients nutritionally is a complex process and to counteract prolonged starvation effectively, the intricate physiologic and metabolic effects that occur when these depleted individuals are fed again at prestarvation levels must be understood. The effects of depletion, repletion, and compartmental shifts of electrolytes, fluids, and other substrates in response to excessive nutritional resuscitation after prolonged starvation are defined as the refeeding syndrome. This so-called syndrome was originally thought secondary only to hypophosphatemia but is understand to also include hypokalemia, hypomagnesemia, and other derangements in glucose control. The essential features of overly enthusiastic carbohydrate administration in severely undernourished patients include rapid falls in the plasma levels of phosphorus, potassium, and magnesium, coupled with sodium and water retention, leading to fluid overload and altered glucose homeostasis. It must be re-emphasized that aggressive attempts to correct the malnourished state by the well-intended reinstitution of feeding that causes these iatrogenic derangements is not without dire physiologic consequences that can be rather sudden, multiple, diverse, and potentially fatal.

More recent biochemical investigations support earlier work that the overzealous reintroduction of carbohydrate into the system either orally, enterally, or parenterally inhibits fat metabolism and promotes glucose metabolism, causing an increase in the use of phosphate to produce phosphorylated intermediates of glycolysis, adenosine triphosphate (ATP) and 2,3 diphosphoglycerate (2,3 DPG).[91,92] This results in the hypophosphatemia of refeeding. Additionally, the high glucose load induces hyperinsulinemia, which is postulated to be the cause of the increased intracellular water that accompanies refeeding. Although the exact mechanism of this phenomenon is yet to be delineated, it is thought that increased insulin levels may have an antinatriuretic effect.[93] Increased demand for the water-soluble vitamin thiamine also is noted in malnourished patients, and it is difficult to determine if this results from a preexisting deficiency or if it is a result of refeeding. It is known that in malnourished patients, high carbohydrate loads increase the demand for thiamine because it is essential for the metabolism of carbohydrates during glycolysis.[94] Its induced or unmasked deficiency in the refeeding syndrome may be secondary to its increased use when it is already in a scarce state in a malnourished individual.

Clinical manifestations of the refeeding syndrome are related directly to electrolyte and vitamin deficiencies. Hypophosphatemia can lead to critical neurologic, respiratory, and cardiac abnormalities, as can hypokalemia and hypomagnesemia. Vitamin deficiencies can cause severe encephalopathy and lactic acidosis. Sodium retention can contribute to fluid overload, pulmonary edema, and cardiac decompensation[86,95] (**Table 1**). Hence, volume status and electrolyte intake and balance must be closely monitored along with caloric intakes and sources, providing patients with an appropriate mixture of fat and carbohydrate calories.[5,96]

In order to prevent and counteract the deleterious consequences of refeeding, clinicians must understand the homeostatic changes that take place in the starving human organism under a variety of circumstances. The primary step in preventing refeeding syndrome is to identify those individuals at risk before initiating nutritional support. Regardless of the patient, avoiding overfeeding is essential, and, therefore, the feeding regimen should be initiated with a small number of calories and the amount incrementally increased slowly. The first day of nutritional support should comprise approximately 25% of the estimated caloric goal and the quantity increased toward the goal in a graduated manner over 3 to 5 days. Electrolyte abnormalities should be addressed before initiating feedings, and electrolyte supplementation should be provided as needed.[95] Phosphate in particular should be closely monitored since patients with severe malnutrition are likely to have depleted total body concentrations, and, therefore, relatively higher requirements.[97,98] In addition to fluid and sodium intake, body weight should also be closely monitored during the first few days of nutritional repletion to prevent cardiac decompensation in patients with an already compromised cardiovascular system. It is recommended initially that approximately 20 mEq of sodium be given per day, that fluid be restricted to less than 1000 mL per day, and that weight gain be limited to 1 kg per week because any greater accumulation of weight is probably attributable to excessive water retention.[95,99] In critically ill patients, it can also be helpful to monitor central venous pressure and peripheral edema. Multiple vitamins should also be provided in therapeutic doses according to the recommendations of the American Medical Association on a daily basis, and additional supplementation should be given according to a patient's requirements.[100] Clinicians should actively examine patients frequently for the signs and symptoms associated with refeeding syndrome.

If the signs and symptoms of the refeeding syndrome become apparent, the treatment consists of immediate cessation of the nutritional support being administered, the correction of any electrolyte abnormalities, and any other indicated supportive care. Neurologic, cardiac, and pulmonary dysfunction should all be addressed accordingly (ie, intravenous thiamine for mental status changes, supplemental oxygen for respiratory distress, and pressors for hypotension). Once all of these abnormalities have been appropriately managed, nutritional support should be restarted cautiously, preferably at 50% of the rate before symptom development. The volume and rate of nutrient infusion should then be slowly advanced toward goal over several days with close monitoring.[92]

Nutritional care in starved patients is a dynamic process that requires continual monitoring and modification according to the metabolic needs of the patients to maintain stability and to promote nutritional restoration. It is of paramount importance that clinicians understand that cachexia and starvation or malnourishment are separate entities and require an appreciation for the unique complex metabolic abnormalities of each to counteract them most effectively. The development of nutritional support teams has allowed cachectic, starving, and/or malnourished patients to receive coordinated and optimal nutritional care in an effort to correct and reverse the pathophysiologic state in a safe, efficient, and effective manner. These multidisciplinary, expert teams also allow for prevention of the metabolic complications associated with

**Table 1**
Signs and symptoms of refeeding syndrome

| Hypophosphatemia | Hypokalemia | Hypomagnesemia | Vitamin Deficiencies | Sodium Retention |
|---|---|---|---|---|
| Neurologic | Neurologic | Neurologic | Encephalopathy | Fluid overload |
| Paresthesias | Paralysis | Weakness | Lactic acidosis | Pulmonary edema |
| Weakness | Weakness | Tremor | | Cardiac decompensation |
| Delirium | Cardiac | Muscle twitching | | |
| Disorientation | Arrhythmias | Changed mental status | | |
| Encephalopathy | Contraction changes | Tetany | | |
| Areflexic paralysis | Respiratory | Convulsions | | |
| Seizures | Failure | Seizures | | |
| Coma | Gastrointestinal | Coma | | |
| Tetany | Nausea | Cardiac | | |
| Cardiac | Vomiting | Arrhythmias | | |
| Hypotension | Constipation | Gastrointestinal | | |
| Shock | Other | Anorexia | | |
| Deceased stroke volume | Rhabdomyolysis | Nausea | | |
| Deceased mean arterial pressure | Muscle necrosis | Vomiting | | |
| Deceased left ventricular stroke volume | | Diarrhea | | |
| Increased wedge pressure | | | | |
| Pulmonary | | | | |
| Diaphragmatic weakness | | | | |
| Respiratory failure | | | | |
| Dyspnea | | | | |
| Hematologic | | | | |
| Hemolysis | | | | |
| Thrombocytopenia | | | | |
| Leukocyte dysfunction | | | | |

refeeding by identifying those patients at risk, providing proper assessment, coordinating interdisciplinary communication, and delivering timely and effective nutritional intervention. Because of improved understanding of these deranged metabolic states, conscientious, rational, informed, and thoughtful approaches to these patients have decreased the morbidity and mortality associated with attempts to treat them. Now and in the future, all clinicians should be sufficiently knowledgeable, trained, and competent in nutritional support techniques and principles to avoid virtually completely the adverse consequences of uninformed or ill-advised, overly aggressive, nutritional rehabilitation. The paradigm to follow is that the state of starvation of a patient did not occur acutely overnight and, therefore, should not, indeed must not, be corrected acutely in the first few hours or days of treatment. Controversy remains regarding the influence of aggressive nutritional support on the quality of life of patients with advanced cancer, and it is important to consider the risks, benefits, and ethical aspects involved before embarking on such a regimen. Physician attitudes, patient age and prognosis, and family or patient perceptions often play important roles in the decision to administer nutritional support, and these variables will continue as issues during the patient's course.[101]

Finally, the principles, practices, and procedures for safe oral, parenteral, and enteral nutritional repletion of starved patients have been established for oral feeding by Keys and associates more than 50 years ago; for PN by Dudrick and colleagues more than 35 years ago; and for enteral nutrition by the American Society for Parenteral and Enteral Nutrition Guidelines for the Use of Parenteral and Enteral Nutrition in Adult and Pediatric Patients more than 10 years ago.[5,102,103] In accordance with the principles derived from "Goldilocks and the Three Bears" (ie, too large, too small, just right; too hot, too cold, just right; and too high, too low, just right), the ultimate goal is to provide optimal nutritional support to all patients under all conditions at all times in a judicious, rational, and orderly manner. It is incumbent upon all members of the healthcare professions to continue their dedication to teaching excellence, vigilance, prudence, and conscientiousness in efforts to providing nutritional support that is "just right."[104]

## REFERENCES

1. Inui A. Cancer anorexia-cachexia syndrome: current issues in research and management. CA Cancer J Clin 2002;52(2):72–91.
2. Toomey D, Redmond HP, Bouchier-Hayes D. Mechanisms mediating cancer cachexia. Cancer 1995;76(12):2418–26.
3. Puccio M, Nathanson L. The cancer cachexia syndrome. Semin Oncol 1997; 24(3):277–87.
4. Cahill GF Jr. Starvation in man. N Engl J Med 1970;282(12):668–75.
5. Keys A, Austin JB, Henshel A, et al. The biology of human starvation, volumes I–II. Minneapolis (MN): University of Minnisota Press; 1950.
6. DeWys WD. Pathophysiology of cancer cachexia: current understanding and areas for future research. Cancer Res 1982;42(Suppl 2):721s–6s.
7. Warren S. The immediate causes of death and cancer. Am J Med Sci 1932;184: 610–5.
8. DeWys WD, Begg C, Lavin PT, et al. Prognostic effect of weight loss prior to chemotherapy in cancer patients. Eastern cooperative oncology group. Am J Med 1980;69(4):491–7.
9. Harrison L, Fong Y. Enteral nutrition in the cancer patient. In: Rombeau JL, Rolandelli RH, editors. Clinical nutrition enteral and tube feeding. 3rd edition. Philadelphia: WB Saunders; 1997. p. 300–23.

10. Bozzetti F, Migliavacca S, Scotti A, et al. Impact of cancer, type, site, stage and treatment on the nutritional status of patients. Ann Surg 1982;196(2):170–9.
11. Meguid MM, Meguid V. Preoperative identification of the surgical cancer patient in need of postoperative supportive total parenteral nutrition. Cancer 1985; 55(Suppl 1):258–62.
12. Kotler DP. Cachexia. Ann Intern Med 2000;133(8):622–34.
13. Rosenbaum K, Wang J, Pierson RN Jr, et al. Time-dependent variation in weight and body composition in healthy adults. JPEN J Parenter Enteral Nutr 2000; 24(2):52–5.
14. Shils ME. Nutrition and diet in cancer management. In: Shils ME, Olson JA, Shike M, editors. Modern nutrition in health and disease. 8th edition. Philadelphia: Lea & Febiger; 1994. p. 1317–48.
15. Heber D, Tchekmedyian NS. Mechanisms of cancer cachexia. Contemp Oncol 1995;(Special Issue):6–10.
16. Langstein HN, Norton JA. Mechanisms of cancer cachexia. Hematol Oncol Clin North Am 1991;5(1):103–23.
17. Staal-van den Brekel AJ, Schols AM, ten Velde GP, et al. Analysis of the energy balance in lung cancer patients. Cancer Res 1994;54(24):6430–3.
18. Barber MD, Ross JA, Fearon KC. Cancer cachexia. Surg Oncol 1999;8(3): 133–41.
19. Bruera E. ABC of palliative care. Anorexia, cachexia, and nutrition. BMJ 1997; 315(7117):1219–22.
20. Brennan MF. Uncomplicated starvation versus cancer cachexia. Cancer Res 1977;37(7 Pt 2):2359–64.
21. Padilla GV. Psychological aspects of nutrition and cancer. Surg Clin North Am 1986;66(6):1121–35.
22. Tisdale MJ. Biology of cachexia. J Natl Cancer Inst 1997;89(23):1763–73.
23. Cangiano C, Laviano A, Meguid MM, et al. Effects of administration of oral branched-chain amino acids on anorexia and caloric intake in cancer patients. J Natl Cancer Inst 1996;88(8):550–2.
24. Flier JS. Clinical review 94: what's in a name? In search of leptin's physiologic role. J Clin Endocrinol Metab 1998;83(5):1407–13.
25. Inui A. Feeding and body-weight regulation by hypothalamic neuropeptides— mediation of the actions of leptin. Trends Neurosci 1999;22(2):62–7.
26. Schwartz MW, Dallman MF, Woods SC. Hypothalamic response to starvation: implications for the study of wasting disorders. Am J Physiol 1995;269(5 Pt 2): R949–57.
27. Schwartz MW, Seeley RJ. Seminars in medicine of the Beth Israel Deaconess Medical Center. Neuroendocrine responses to starvation and weight loss. N Engl J Med 1997;336(25):1802–11.
28. Bray GA, York DA. The MONA LISA hypothesis in the time of leptin. Recent Prog Horm Res 1998;53:95–117 [discussion: 117–8].
29. Elmquist JK, Maratos-Flier E, Saper CB, et al. Unraveling the central nervous system pathways underlying responses to leptin. Nat Neurosci 1998;1(6): 445–50.
30. Friedman JM, Halaas JL. Leptin and the regulation of body weight in mammals. Nature 1998;395(6704):763–70.
31. Inui A. Transgenic approach to the study of body weight regulation. Pharmacol Rev Mar 2000;52(1):35–61.
32. Inui A. Transgenic study of energy homeostasis equation: implications and confounding influences. FASEB J 2000;14(14):2158–70.

33. Kalra SP, Dube MG, Pu S, et al. Interacting appetite-regulating pathways in the hypothalamic regulation of body weight. Endocr Rev 1999;20(1):68–100.
34. Schwartz MW, Woods SC, Porte D Jr, et al. Central nervous system control of food intake. Nature 2000;404(6778):661–71.
35. Woods SC, Seeley RJ, Porte D Jr, et al. Signals that regulate food intake and energy homeostasis. Science 1998;280(5368):1378–83.
36. Gerald C, Walker MW, Criscione L, et al. A receptor subtype involved in neuropeptide-Y-induced food intake. Nature 1996;382(6587):168–71.
37. Donaldson CJ, Sutton SW, Perrin MH, et al. Cloning and characterization of human urocortin. Endocrinology 1996;137(5):2167–70.
38. Spina M, Merlo-Pich E, Chan RK, et al. Appetite-suppressing effects of urocortin, a CRF-related neuropeptide. Science 1996;273(5281):1561–4.
39. Inui A. Cancer anorexia-cachexia syndrome: are neuropeptides the key? Cancer Res 1999;59(18):4493–501.
40. Moldawer LL, Rogy MA, Lowry SF. The role of cytokines in cancer cachexia. JPEN J Parenter Enteral Nutr 1992;16(Suppl 6):43S–9S.
41. Gelin J, Moldawer LL, Lonnroth C, et al. Role of endogenous tumor necrosis factor alpha and interleukin 1 for experimental tumor growth and the development of cancer cachexia. Cancer Res 1991;51(1):415–21.
42. Matthys P, Billiau A. Cytokines and cachexia. Nutrition 1997;13(9):763–70.
43. Noguchi Y, Yoshikawa T, Matsumoto A, et al. Are cytokines possible mediators of cancer cachexia? Surg Today 1996;26(7):467–75.
44. Haslett PA. Anticytokine approaches to the treatment of anorexia and cachexia. Semin Oncol 1998;25(2 Suppl 6):53–7.
45. Mantovani G, Maccio A, Lai P, et al. Cytokine activity in cancer-related anorexia/cachexia: role of megestrol acetate and medroxyprogesterone acetate. Semin Oncol 1998;25(2 Suppl 6):45–52.
46. Moldawer LL, Copeland EM 3rd. Proinflammatory cytokines, nutritional support, and the cachexia syndrome: interactions and therapeutic options. Cancer 1997;79(9):1828–39.
47. Wigmore SJ, Plester CE, Ross JA, et al. Contribution of anorexia and hypermetabolism to weight loss in anicteric patients with pancreatic cancer. Br J Surg 1997;84(2):196–7.
48. Lechan RM, Tatro JB. Hypothalamic melanocortin signaling in cachexia. Endocrinology 2001;142(8):3288–91.
49. Marks DL, Ling N, Cone RD. Role of the central melanocortin system in cachexia. Cancer Res 2001;61(4):1432–8.
50. Wisse BE, Frayo RS, Schwartz MW, et al. Reversal of cancer anorexia by blockade of central melanocortin receptors in rats. Endocrinology 2001;142(8):3292–301.
51. Bartlett DL, Charland SL, Torosian MH. Reversal of tumor-associated hyperglucagonemia as treatment for cancer cachexia. Surgery 1995;118(1):87–97.
52. Todorov P, Cariuk P, McDevitt T, et al. Characterization of a cancer cachectic factor. Nature 1996;379(6567):739–42.
53. Beck SA, Smith KL, Tisdale MJ. Anticachectic and antitumor effect of eicosapentaenoic acid and its effect on protein turnover. Cancer Res 1991;51(22):6089–93.
54. Copeland EM 3rd, MacFadyen BV Jr, Lanzotti VJ, et al. Intravenous hyperalimentation as an adjunct to cancer chemotherapy. Am J Surg 1975;129(2):167–73.
55. Copeland EM, Souchon EA, MacFadyen BV Jr, et al. Intravenous hyperalimentation as an adjunct to radiation therapy. Cancer 1977;39(2):609–16.

56. Dudrick SJ, MacFadyen BV Jr, Souchon EA, et al. Parenteral nutrition techniques in cancer patients. Cancer Res 1977;37(7 Pt 2):2440–50.

57. Klein S, Simes J, Blackburn GL. Total parenteral nutrition and cancer clinical trials. Cancer 1986;58(6):1378–86.

58. Lowry SF, Brennan MF. Intravenous feeding of the cancer patient. In: Rombeau JL, Caldwell MD, editors. Parenteral nutrition. Philadelphia: WB Saunders; 1986. p. 445–70.

59. Shike M, Brennan MF. Supportive care of the cancer patient. In: DeVita VT, Hellman S, Rosenburg SA, editors. Principles and practice of oncology. 3rd edition. Philadelphia: JB Lippincott; 1989. p. 2029–44.

60. Lipman TO. Clinical trials of nutritional support in cancer. Parenteral and enteral therapy. Hematol Oncol Clin North Am 1991;5(1):91–102.

61. Body JJ. The syndrome of anorexia-cachexia. Curr Opin Oncol 1999;11(4): 255–60.

62. Body JJ. Metabolic sequelae of cancers (excluding bone marrow transplantation). Curr Opin Clin Nutr Metab Care 1999;2(4):339–44.

63. Sikora SS, Ribeiro U, Kane JM 3rd, et al. Role of nutrition support during induction chemoradiation therapy in esophageal cancer. JPEN J Parenter Enteral Nutr 1998;22(1):18–21.

64. Nelson KA, Walsh D, Sheehan FA. The cancer anorexia-cachexia syndrome. J Clin Oncol 1994;12(1):213–25.

65. Miller M. Can reducing caloric intake also help reduce cancer? J Natl Cancer Inst 1998;90(23):1766–7.

66. Nelson KA. The cancer anorexia-cachexia syndrome. Semin Oncol 2000;27(1): 64–8.

67. Nitenberg G, Raynard B. Nutritional support of the cancer patient: issues and dilemmas. Crit Rev Oncol Hematol 2000;34(3):137–68.

68. Golden MH. The development of concepts of malnutrition. J Nutr 2002;132(7): 2117S–22S.

69. Rothman DL, Magnusson I, Katz LD, et al. Quantitation of hepatic glycogenolysis and gluconeogenesis in fasting humans with 13C NMR. Science 1991; 254(5031):573–6.

70. Gelfand RA, Hendler R. Effect of nutrient composition on the metabolic response to very low calorie diets: learning more and more about less and less. Diabetes Metab Rev 1989;5(1):17–30.

71. Calloway DH, Spector H. Nitrogen balance as related to caloric and protein intake in active young men. Am J Clin Nutr 1954;2(6):405–12.

72. Blackburn GL, Flatt JP, Clowes GH Jr, et al. Protein sparing therapy during periods of starvation with sepsis of trauma. Ann Surg 1973;177(5):588–94.

73. Greenberg GR, Jeejeebhoy KN. Intravenous protein-sparing therapy in patients with gastrointestinal disease. JPEN J Parenter Enteral Nutr 1979;3(6):427–32.

74. Hoffer LJ, Bistrian BR, Young VR, et al. Metabolic effects of very low calorie weight reduction diets. J Clin Invest 1984;73(3):750–8.

75. Dickerson RN, Rosato EF, Mullen JL. Net protein anabolism with hypocaloric parenteral nutrition in obese stressed patients. Am J Clin Nutr 1986;44(6):747–55.

76. Choban PS, Burge JC, Scales D, et al. Hypoenergetic nutrition support in hospitalized obese patients: a simplified method for clinical application. Am J Clin Nutr 1997;66(3):546–50.

77. Klein S, Holland OB, Wolfe RR. Importance of blood glucose concentration in regulating lipolysis during fasting in humans. Am J Physiol 1990;258(1 Pt 1): E32–9.

78. Jensen MD, Miles JM, Gerich JE, et al. Preservation of insulin effects on glucose production and proteolysis during fasting. Am J Physiol 1988;254(6 Pt 1): E700–7.

79. Gardner DF, Kaplan MM, Stanley CA, et al. Effect of tri-iodothyronine replacement on the metabolic and pituitary responses to starvation. N Engl J Med 1979;300(11):579–84.

80. Bistrian BR, Blackburn GL, Hallowell E, et al. Protein status of general surgical patients. JAMA 1974;230(6):858–60.

81. Schofield C, Ashworth A. Why have mortality rates for severe malnutrition remained so high? Bull World Health Organ 1996;74(2):223–9.

82. Foxx-Orenstein A, Kirby DF. Understanding malnutrition and reefeeding syndrome. In: Kirby DF, Dudrick SJ, editors. Practical handbook of nutrition in clinical practice. Boca Raton (FL): CRC Press; 1994. p. 19–30.

83. Blackburn GL, Bistrian BR, Maini BS, et al. Nutritional and metabolic assessment of the hospitalized patient. JPEN J Parenter Enteral Nutr 1977;1(1):11–22.

84. Weinsier RL, Krumdieck CL. Death resulting from overzealous total parenteral nutrition: the refeeding syndrome revisited. Am J Clin Nutr 1981;34(3):393–9.

85. Kalm LM, Semba RD. They starved so that others be better fed: remembering Ancel Keys and the Minnesota experiment. J Nutr 2005;135(6):1347–52.

86. Solomon SM, Kirby DF. The refeeding syndrome: a review. JPEN J Parenter Enteral Nutr 1990;14(1):90–7.

87. Hayek ME, Eisenberg PG. Severe hypophosphatemia following the institution of enteral feedings. Arch Surg 1989;124(11):1325–8.

88. Marinella MA. Refeeding syndrome and hypophosphatemia. J Intensive Care Med 2005;20(3):155–9.

89. Mehler PS. Eating disorders: 1. Anorexia nervosa. Hosp Pract (Off Ed) 1996; 31(1):109–13, 117.

90. Cumming AD, Farquhar JR, Bouchier IA. Refeeding hypophosphataemia in anorexia nervosa and alcoholism. Br Med J (Clin Res Ed) 1987;295(6596): 490–1.

91. Travis SF, Sugerman HJ, Ruberg RL, et al. Alterations of red-cell glycolytic intermediates and oxygen transport as a consequence of hypophosphatemia in patients receiving intravenous hyperalimentation. N Engl J Med 1971;285(14): 763–8.

92. Kraft MD, Btaiche IF, Sacks GS. Review of the refeeding syndrome. Nutr Clin Pract 2005;20(6):625–33.

93. DeFronzo RA, Cooke CR, Andres R, et al. The effect of insulin on renal handling of sodium, potassium, calcium, and phosphate in man. J Clin Invest 1975;55(4): 845–55.

94. Van Way CW, Longoria M, Sacks GS. Do surgeons need to worry about vitamin deficiencies? Nutr Clin Pract 2001;16(Suppl):S5–7.

95. Brooks MJ, Melnik G. The refeeding syndrome: an approach to understanding its complications and preventing its occurrence. Pharmacotherapy 1995; 15(6):713–26.

96. Heymsfield SB, Bethel RA, Ansley JD, et al. Cardiac abnormalities in cachectic patients before and during nutritional repletion. Am Heart J 1978;95(5):584–94.

97. Ruberg RL, Allen TR, Goodman MJ, et al. Hypophosphatemia with hypophosphaturia in hyperalimentation. Surg Forum 1971;22:87–8.

98. Hill GL, Guinn EJ, Dudrick SJ. Phosphorus distribution in hyperalimentation induced hypophosphatemia. J Surg Res 1976;20(6):527–31.

99. Apovian CM, McMahon MM, Bistrian BR. Guidelines for refeeding the marasmic patient. Crit Care Med 1990;18(9):1030–3.
100. Multivitamin preparations for parenteral use. A statement by the nutrition advisory group. American medical association department of foods and nutrition, 1975. JPEN J Parenter Enteral Nutr 1979;3(4):258–62.
101. Mercadante S. Parenteral versus enteral nutrition in cancer patients: indications and practice. Support Care Cancer 1998;6(2):85–93.
102. Dudrick SJ, Wilmore DW, Vars HM, et al. Long-term total parenteral nutrition with growth, development, and positive nitrogen balance. Surgery 1968;64(1): 134–42.
103. Wilmore DW, Dudrick SJ. Growth and development of an infant receiving all nutrients exclusively by vein. JAMA 1968;203(10):860–4.
104. Palesty JA, Dudrick SJ. The goldilocks paradigm of starvation and refeeding. Nutr Clin Pract 2006;21(2):147–54.

# Parenteral Nutrition and Nutritional Support of Surgical Patients: Reflections, Controversies, and Challenges

Stanley J. Dudrick, MD[a,b,*], Jose Mario Pimiento, MD[c]

KEYWORDS

• Total parenteral nutrition • Total enteral nutrition
• Surgical patients • Geriatric patients • Nutritional controversies

As with virtually every other innovative advance, proposal, or hypothesis made in the course of the introduction and development of a new or existing area of endeavor or accomplishment in medicine, the development of total parenteral nutrition (TPN) was not only accompanied, but preceded and followed, by controversy throughout the past half century from its inception in the 1960s to the present day. The prevailing dogma among clinicians 50 years ago was that feeding a patient entirely by vein was impossible; even if it were possible, it would be impractical; and even if it were practical, it would be unaffordable.[1] The tedious process by which this disputatious novel technique advanced during the next 2 decades to become the state of the art and science of nutritional support of seriously ill or critically ill patients under a wide variety of clinical circumstances is described in the article by Dudrick and Palesty elsewhere in this issue. Three words that denote discussions involving conflicting points of view are argument, dispute, and controversy. Arising from a discussion in which disagreement is expressed, argument stresses the advancement by each side of facts and reasons buttressing their contentions that are intended to persuade the other

The authors have nothing to disclose.
[a] Department of Surgery, Yale University School of Medicine, 333 Cedar Street, New Haven, CT 06510, USA
[b] Department of Surgery, Saint Mary's Hospital, 56 Franklin Street, Waterbury, CT 06706, USA
[c] Moffitt Cancer Center & Research Institute, Department of Surgery, 12902 Magnolia Drive, Tampa, FL 33612, USA
* Corresponding author. Department of Surgery, Saint Mary's Hospital, 56 Franklin Street, Waterbury, CT 06706.
E-mail address: sdudrick@stmh.org

Surg Clin N Am 91 (2011) 675–692
doi:10.1016/j.suc.2011.04.001
0039-6109/11/$ – see front matter © 2011 Elsevier Inc. All rights reserved.

side. The ensuing debates are usually accompanied by emotions that are seldom swayed by the arguments. Dispute further stresses the division of opinion by its implication of contradictory points of view and often implies animosity, which takes argument to the next level. On the other hand, controversy is especially applicable to major differences of opinion ordinarily involving groups of people rather than individuals. Without the backing of substantive and validating data, arguments and disputes are often based largely on ill-founded opinion and prejudice rather than on data or facts to clarify the search for truth. However, healthy controversy, which, by the acquisition and/or production of legitimate data, experience, and/or information (and based on a measured skepticism that does not destroy creativity), can serve admirably and effectively to augment the scientific method in searching for the truth. It is imperative that principles and practices be applied conscientiously, proficiently, and with precision in every patient at all times and in all situations if optimal outcomes are to be obtained.

In contrast to the intentionally focused and relatively defined areas assigned to the other authors in this issue in acknowledgment of their expertise, the subject of this discussion, as can be gleaned from the title, is potentially broad, deep, and lengthy, in content, space, and time. On the other hand, the magnitude of the parameters is such that a comprehensive account of the reflections, controversies, and challenges of parenteral nutrition and nutritional support cannot possibly be accomplished even if the entire issue were available to the authors. Accordingly, this discussion is essentially an abridged commentary summarizing some of the highlights, thoughts, impressions, opinions, principles, practices, and experiences gained or acquired since the inception of TPN and nutritional support as practical clinical entities. This strategy offers the authors advantages over presenting a formal basic or clinical scientific article by allowing us to express our opinions or impressions with, or without, supporting data; to share relevant personal and professional experiences; to evaluate the work of others; to review and appraise historical teachings and writings; to contribute random thoughts and ideas; to make candid suggestions, additions, modifications, revisions, or corrections regarding current principles, practices, and philosophies; and not to be compelled to reference precisely any or all of our contributions to the commentary/presentation. To complete the connotation of the promise of the title, the other 2 major terms deserve definition. Thus, a challenge implies a demand for explanation or justification or a calling into question, whereas a reflection is a mental concentration, a careful consideration, a thought or an opinion resulting from such consideration, or a looking back.

Nutrition support is an amalgam of art and science, as is essentially the rest of the broad field of medicine. Both had their origins in curiosity; empirical observations; concepts; innovation; experimentation; philosophy; ideals; and the application of newly acquired, accumulated, and evaluated knowledge to practical use. For millennia, this situation had formed the basis for the practice of medicine, and advances had been made arithmetically and tediously for hundreds of years until the late nineteenth century and early twentieth century, when discovery, creativity, science, and technology virtually exploded, and has continued to advance logarithmically to the current time. Moreover, this phenomenal increase in knowledge, technology, and expertise is likely to continue in the foreseeable future and have a significant influence on the application of nutritional support to the practice of medicine, maintenance of health, and achievement of optimal clinical and human performance outcomes. However, it is to be expected that in the future, as throughout the past, every new idea, concept, proposal, or adjunct related to improving the quality of health care in general and nutritional support specifically, will be accompanied by copious amounts of doubt, skepticism, criticism, prejudice, controversy, challenges, and resistance to change. Accordingly, the scientific method must be applied diligently, fairly, dispassionately, honestly, morally, and ethically to allow evaluation of as many aspects of the problem, solution, and situation as possible to achieve optimal evaluation, interpretation, and useful application. In this regard, it is admirable, perhaps even ideal, to follow the example of Benjamin Franklin, America's first scientist, in his lifelong quest to seek, acquire, and share useful knowledge.

It can be said that there are few new or truly unique fundamental ideas regarding nutrition and nutritional support; instead, new data and new technology accumulate that are often related to each other and result from the evolution of ongoing scientific inquiry and endeavor. Thus, the discovery of the circulation of the blood in the body almost 4 centuries ago was an essential prerequisite to the development of TPN, and the idea of using this newly discovered anatomic and physiologic knowledge for the intravenous introduction of nutrient substances and medications into the body followed closely thereafter; however, the accomplishment of providing TPN effectively as the sole support for growth, development, and metabolic maintenance first in animals, and then in adults and infant human beings, required almost three and a half centuries until the early, seminal, original ideas and concepts could be brought to fruition as a result of recently acquired scientific, technological, philosophic, and related, practical advancements in basic science and clinical medicine. Subsequently, many thousands of studies have been conducted by clinicians, scientists, engineers, and many other investigators and empirical observers throughout the world to validate, refine, and advance the art and science of TPN and other forms of nutritional support, as well as to translate and apply new knowledge, technology, data, and expertise to the pursuit of optimal nutrition support and health in the service of society. Inexorably, this process will continue and will repeat itself, each time rising to a higher level, inducing and creating the inevitable and essential changes that will eventually improve the safety, efficacy, efficiency, applicability, and affordability of nutritional support. Ultimately, the risk-benefit, cost-benefit, and outcome data must be accrued, scrutinized, and analyzed to justify the resultant, indicated changes not only to our patients and colleagues but also to the continually enlarging number of stakeholders in our increasingly enormous and expensive health care system. Fortunately for those of us in the health care professions who are interested and involved in maintaining and/or improving the nutritional status of all of our patients, under a wide variety of conditions and a broad spectrum of settings, we have been encouraged, supported, and at times even indulged, thus far, throughout our quest to achieve this lofty goal.

Even after working in this area of endeavor for a short time, one soon becomes aware of, and attracted to, the intricacies, complexities, and precision of the countless and phenomenal biochemical interactions that occur continuously within the body, the result of which we interpret as life. The theoretic possibility of being able to modify these processes to the maximum advantage of the individual is a fascinating and mesmerizing idea to many basic and clinical scientists. In attempting to learn what the optimal substrates might be for the promotion and maintenance not only of optimal molecular and atomic structure (within the limits of genetic control) but also of optimal cellular and systemic function, one soon becomes aware of the differences in those vital relationships among the various age groups, including premature infants, full-term infants, young children, adolescents, young and middle-aged adults, and elderly patients. One also can become enmeshed, fascinated, and challenged by the myriad combinations of disparate factors such as genetics, pathophysiologic processes, nutritional status, indications, operative surgical procedures, trauma, immunocompetence, sepsis, and other comorbidities, which can significantly alter interrelationships among the innumerable individual nutrient substrates and combinations provided. If the idealistic, ambitious, and occasionally overwhelming and frustrating goal of providing optimal nutrition to all patients, under all conditions, at all times, could be achieved, patients would be highly likely to enjoy optimal health and quality of life; and perhaps achieve their maximum potentials for accomplishment, performance, satisfaction, happiness, and productive longevity. On the other hand, the extent to which this goal cannot be achieved, and to which the patients are compromised accordingly in achieving maximum potential of the body cell mass, represents the extent to which the patient is unhealthy, at risk, diseased, disordered, traumatized, or otherwise sick or infirm. What started out as a challenging wonderment to the senior author (SJD) half a century ago, has become a career-long obsession accompanied by periods of elation, creativity, discovery, and successful outcomes, punctuated by the frustrations, disappointments, and despair associated with complications, suboptimal results, and failures. However discouraging this may seem, such is the inherent nature of the medical profession, and if the practice of the broad field of medicine is a true vocation, privilege, and responsibility, in contrast to a job, or a mere means to make a living, one must continue to persevere with resilience, values, and purpose toward achieving excellence, if not perfection, in the provision of nutritional support and all other indicated services to all of our patients, but especially to those whose lives may be dependent on our proficiency in the provision of these services. It is a noble calling; it is not for the fainthearted; and it is not for those who lack courage, dedication, and resilience. Two of the most noteworthy groups of patients for whom these prerequisites are of paramount importance are the small, but critically important numbers of premature infants or full-term infants with catastrophic gastrointestinal tract anomalies, and the large (and increasing daily) group of geriatric individuals in our population. Patients derived from these 2 extremes of the human age spectrum are particularly vulnerable to the vagaries of malnutrition and starvation, more so than any other age groups, and they require special attention, particularly in caring for their nutritional and surgical problems, which can otherwise be inordinately lethal.

## NUTRITIONAL SUPPORT OF THE GERIATRIC PATIENT WITH CANCER

There is more to the nutritional support of the surgical patient, especially the geriatric surgical patient with cancer, than the current standards of the science and clinical practice of medicine and surgery mandate or justify unequivocally.[2] The emotional and psychological support of the patients and their significant others, and the socially important aspects of food or nutrient intake and breaking bread with family and friends cannot be denied. These needs do exist, and they must be addressed and have something active and meaningful done about them rather than being ignored, as all too often occurs in our institutions. For example, after all possibilities of providing reasonable, rational, or justifiable specific antineoplastic and/or nutritional therapy for the patient with an inexorably lethal cancer have been exhausted, it is of utmost importance that neither the patient nor the family are ever abandoned, and that they continue to receive comprehensive support from their health care team to maintain a caring and compassionate human bond with them, relieve their guilt, and above all, reinforce their faith in our humane and core values by being there for them and providing a feeling of comfort and hope that cannot otherwise be accomplished. The frontiers for specialized nutrition support of geriatric patients, especially geriatric patients who have cancer, await the continuing exploration, discovery, and judicious clinical applications not only of all health care professionals but also of all members of humankind.

We must develop and carry out relevant, meticulously controlled study protocols specifically designed for the various cohorts of the geriatric population to provide the data essential to understanding and solving the unique nutritional, functional, and surgical problems of elderly patients. At the same time, we must recognize and allow for the difficulties associated with conducting studies in aged patients with seemingly inevitable multiple comorbidities. Moreover, we must understand that the physiologic changes that accompany the normal aging process, especially those related to nutritional and metabolic needs, can occur at different rates and times among all human beings. The difference between chronologic age and physiologic age in the elderly patients must be determined clinically in as conscientious and scientific a manner as feasible to help guide prudent decision making in their management. Although the adage that the chronologic age of the patient is not an independent risk factor for surgical procedures or actions, the age of elderly patients can become an independent risk factor in some patients in whom a great disparity exists between their chronologic age and their physiologic age. Furthermore, establishing nutrient requirements for a heterogeneous population is not an easy task even when the group is relatively healthy, much less when accompanied by a wide variety of confounding health conditions, comorbidities, disabilities, medications, and variations in fitness and nutritional status, and so forth.

Before the latter part of the twentieth century, people in the 50 to 65 years age range were defined as the geriatric or elderly population, and a reasonable amount of useful clinical data had been accrued to justify various aspects of their health and nutritional recommendations appropriate for their management. However, it has recently become obvious to nutritionists, surgeons, and others that it is not valid to extrapolate information from the data that exist for the 50-year-old to 65-year-old age group upward to the eighth, ninth, and 10th decades of life. This problem ultimately must be solved by the systematic collection of data specifically for the older groups from 65 to 100 years of age (perhaps for each quintile or decile) if they are to receive optimal care based on their scientifically determined requirements, metabolic and performance potentials, and tolerances. The challenges involved are difficult enough in determining nutrient requirements and assessing nutritional and physiologic status, but become increasingly more difficult and complex when evaluating nutritional interventions and appraising the success of other outcomes of implementing ambitious nutritional and/or surgical therapies among the patients in the various deciles of the elderly population. The most difficult group, who are also the most vulnerable from a nutritional standpoint, are elderly patients who are institutionalized, have little or no family support, have multiple health problems, have neurologic challenges, cannot perform the activities of daily living competently, and require assistance not only with feeding but also with total custodial care.

The steady loss of lean body mass (about 8–10% per year) that has been documented to occur in elderly individuals (>50 years of age) is greatest in those who are not able or willing to ambulate or exercise, and who also ingest diets inadequate in protein, thus resulting in a compounding of the usual sarcopenia that results in such patients. Nowhere is the chicken or egg phenomenon more evident than in this group of elderly human beings. In addition to protein deficiencies, energy, macronutrient, micronutrient, and fluid deficiencies are also relatively more common in geriatric patients than in younger adults, although their daily requirements per kilogram body weight are not fundamentally dissimilar. A major problem in elderly patients is the difficulty in convincing them to drink more water and fluids, thus often resulting in dehydration and its untoward consequences. Examples of other nutrient aberrations that occur commonly in elderly patients are calcium and vitamin D deficiencies, which can lead to significant increases in morbidity and mortality; these substances must be provided in larger doses in the diet and/or by supplements. Preventive health measures regarding the recently recommended increased intakes of these important nutrients are likely to result in significant reductions in morbidity, mortality, and health care costs; however, these reductions remain to be confirmed in future studies, and are likely to lead to the usual controversies.

As the current saga regarding health care funding and regulation unfolds, and as the vested interests in the various private and governmental power groups become more transparent, debated, and compromised or modified, it is particularly critical to the welfare of the geriatric population that the highest moral and ethical values be followed, that all age groups receive the respect and quality health care appropriate to their needs, and that the financial burdens be shared equitably among the citizens of this nation not only as a compassionate and caring duty but also as a fulfillment of a humane responsibility to humanity and to society. Of paramount importance is the right of self-determination of elderly individuals and their families or conservators in the provision, modification, and cessation of all aspects of nutritional support, not only from the moral, ethical, and religious points of view but also by legal mandate. A government that guarantees the rights of women to decision making regarding their bodies and fetuses must guarantee the equivalent rights of elderly patients to decision making regarding their nutrition, surgical management, and life support. How we nourish and treat our elderly population during the next decade or two will influence greatly how we define our character individually and as a society, culture, and nation. Nutritional support involves more than merely putting food on the table, putting an enteral feeding tube into the gastrointestinal tract, or putting a parenteral nutrition feeding catheter into a central vein.

## THE PRIMACY OF NUTRITION SUPPORT TEAMS

In the 1980s, a devastating blow was dealt to nutritional support in general, and nutrition support teams specifically, primarily as a result of the establishment and relatively uniform acceptance of diagnosis-related groups, which significantly changed, and had an enormous effect on, the way that medicine is practiced and medical services are reimbursed. Little or no provision was made by the inadequately informed planners of this form of health care for reimbursement of nutritional support. Because of this grievously poor and harmful restriction of medical practice, it is imperative that all members of the health care professions continue their efforts to restore the former prominent role of nutritional support services and qualified, expert nutrition support teams in the provision of optimal nutritional support as essential to comprehensive care for all patients in the future. TPN and other forms of specialized oral, enteral, and parenteral nutritional support have revolutionized the manner in which neonatology and pediatric surgery are practiced today. The members of the American Pediatric Surgical Association (APSA), the Neonatology Society, and the American Academy of Pediatrics are aware of the enormous effect that the judicious early application of parenteral and enteral nutritional support has had on the successful nourishment and management of a large portion of the critically ill, injured, or impaired patients in their specialties. The senior author (SJD) learned at a recent APSA meeting that approximately one-third of all major operative procedures in neonates and infants requiring pediatric surgery would be impossible or would highly likely fail without the successful concomitant application of optimal parenteral and enteral nutritional support. At the 2011 Annual Meeting of the Neonatology Society, the President stated in his introductory remarks that the Society had analyzed data on the management of premature neonates and had derived evidence sufficient to show (conservatively) that the lives of more than 10 million premature neonates have been saved in this country primarily as a result of the successful development and judicious application of parenteral nutrition, and that neonatology as a specialty would not have grown and developed as it has, were it not for the advent of TPN.

## CHALLENGES AND CONTROVERSIES IN NOURISHING PATIENTS WHO HAVE CANCER

When the alimentary tract cannot be used effectively, or at all, when feeding patients who have cancer, parenteral nutrition can be life saving. Moreover, patients who are poor candidates, or noncandidates, for any antineoplastic therapy because of their debility or cachexia, can be converted to reasonable candidates after a course of supplemental or TPN.[3,4] The morbidity and mortality of patients who have cancer can be significantly reduced without stimulating tumor growth when applied conscientiously according to the established principles and techniques, and when integrated with specific antitumor therapy, as discussed by Palesty and Dudrick elsewhere in this issue. The most natural and practical method of nutrient administration is volitional by mouth, and the next most feasible method of nutrient delivery is via nasogastric or nasoduodenal feeding tubes. However, minimally invasive operative insertion of a gastrostomy or jejunostomy tube may be necessary for long-term nutritional maintenance in some patients. Optimal nutritional rehabilitation via the alimentary tract can sometimes require an inordinate amount of time, and specific antineoplastic therapy cannot always be deferred until protein and energy stores have been replenished adequately and in a timely manner by this route alone. A unified cause of the vexing problem of cancer cachexia has yet to be defined, and many questions regarding the cause of the metabolic abnormalities observed in cancer cachexia remain unanswered. Why is it that the metabolism of carbohydrates, fats, and proteins is altered in tumor cells? The metabolic changes seem to place the tumor cells in a position of predominance biochemically and metabolically over the nontumor cells. This is obvious from the inevitable outcomes in untreated patients who have cancer. What is the fundamental difference in the metabolism of malignant cells from that of normal cells? Can it be possibly a mass effect or the result of a large tumor burden? If so, the deranged metabolism should respond to excision or debulking of the tumor, but does it? Certainly, not uniformly or obviously. Additional questions include: why do malignant cells seem inherently to induce the secretion of a large number and variety of host mediators that produce a chronic inflammatory state with adverse effects on nutrient metabolism and appetite?[2] Normal host cells either do not act the same under normal conditions, or do so to a lesser degree. Does the inflammatory response associated with neoplasia indicate that tumor cells are recognized as foreign bodies or invaders? Does the tumor-induced inflammatory response have any measurable beneficial effect in containing, controlling, or destroying the neoplasm? If not, the inflammatory reaction seems to be hysterical or futile. How and why is it that the tumor cells multiply and function apparently autonomously from the rest of the host body cell mass?[2]

The altered metabolism of peripheral hormones that regulate appetite indicates a de facto difference in the processing of the usual nutrients ingested by a patient with cancer from that while the patient host is cancer-free.[5] This finding strongly intimates a different metabolism of normal diet and suggests that special diets specifically tailored from individual nutrient components may help the patient by placing the cancer cell at a relative disadvantage compared with the normal cells, rather than vice versa , which seems to be the rule. Sustained, focused investigations in this critically important area are long overdue. Clinicians and investigators have preferred to attempt to develop magic-bullet surgical operations, radiotherapy, chemotherapy, immunotherapy, and targeted therapy, various combinations of these, and other directed therapies. Preferably, they should also be attempting to identify clearly the differences in the cell biology of the various neoplastic cells from the normal cells from which they originate to take advantage of such differences to treat or help to treat the patient specifically, prudently, rationally, scientifically, and more effectively. The learned food aversions of patients with cancer likely occur as a result of bad experiences with some forms of foods that the patients formerly had enjoyed in their normal diets before development of their cancers. What is it about the foods they avoid that causes the patient to reject them? A study of the most highly avoided foods and the composition of those foods might possibly point the way toward formulating a diet that is not so adverse and that might nourish the body cell mass better than the tumor cell mass is nourished, thus placing the malignant cells at a relative metabolic disadvantage.

Another area that requires more intensive study is the hypermetabolic state that occurs in some, but not all, patients who have cancer.[6] Why is it that only one-fourth of patients who have cancer are hypermetabolic at rest, whereas one-third are hypometabolic, and two-fifths have normal resting energy expenditure? In the opinion of the senior author (SJD) of this article, all too often, the metabolic data reported in patients with cancer have been selected and used to the advantage of the theories of the proponents rather than used or applied to the advantage of the patient. Another enigmatic attitude among a disturbingly large number of clinicians and clinical investigators is that initial weight gain in cachectic patients often may result from increased fluid volume and an increase in fat stores rather than in an early increase in protein mass. Why should this finding surprise them when the body water compartment that comprises 60% of total body weight, and the body fat compartment that comprises 10% to 15% or more of total body weight, are the first areas to be depleted? Restoring body protein mass to normal may be a second or third priority and may take a longer period to restore, but might occur with persistent provision of a high-protein diet and specific tailoring of amino acid formulations of the dietary nitrogen of the protein provided. Contradictions and inconsistencies in the results of studies of carbohydrate metabolism in patients who have cancer may be because many malignant cell types exist, all cancers are not the same, and the extents of all cancers in all patients are not identical. Moreover, the biology of the disease, differing tumor actions, and the variety of antineoplastic agents and techniques used in treating the different malignancies, variations, and collateral factors and comorbidities, and so forth are some of the multiple complicating factors that affect the metabolism of carbohydrates. Thus, it is difficult to standardize carbohydrate metabolism globally in patients who have cancer, and accordingly, it is difficult to obtain definitive, conclusive data. As an analogy, 2 other conditions that are difficult to standardize in studying metabolism are critically ill patients with major trauma and septic patients, because it is virtually impossible to have identical types and extents of trauma and sepsis in nearly identical patients, much less in those also having additional identical collateral factors such as age, gender, and comorbidities. Thus, controversy readily arises and becomes easier to accept and accomplish than the challenging standardization of patient groups in many clinical studies.

The differences in protein metabolism with simple starvation and in patients with cancer imply the relative autonomy of the cancer cells compared with normal cells. The cause of this difference is essential to identify, define, and then to neutralize, diminish, or reverse if success in comprehensively treating the patient with cancer is to be achieved. Certainly, basic cell biologists have not been able to elucidate the answers required. Perhaps research in the area of genomics will be more successful in identifying the cause of the differences in protein metabolism among normal and neoplastic cells. It is well known that the current forms of parenteral nutrition have not been successful in decreasing protein turnover, decreasing muscle protein degradation, or altering hepatic protein synthesis favorably. The therapeutic nihilists among us, therefore, condemn and advise against the use of parenteral nutrition support in the management of patients who have cancer. They do not seem to consider that the current parenteral nutrition formulations were designed to correct malnutrition secondary to periods of starvation rather than for the specific therapy for the special forms of malnutrition and anorexia-cachexia that occur in malignant disorders, severe trauma, sepsis, and other complex pathophysiologies. Successful nutritional rehabilitation, whether it be by the enteral or parenteral route, requires special formulations of the components, tailored specifically to the individual patients, their cancer cell types, the stages of their diseases, and their extents of malnutrition, similar to the manner in which cytotoxic drugs and regimens have been designed for specific cancer types. A new hybrid clinician-scientist must be developed and trained to incorporate the best knowledge, skills, and motivations of basic scientists (including molecular biologists, immunologists, and geneticists) with those of medical oncologists, radiotherapists, pharmacologists, nutritionists, and surgeons, if optimal therapeutic results are to be achieved in the management of patients who have cancer. It is time for the profession to stop seeking the silver bullet or the holy grail and to design collaborative studies that are comprehensive in all aspects of the management of the patient who has cancer. Nutritional support must be an essential component of optimal treatment of the patient who has cancer regardless of the specific other components of the antineoplastic therapy protocol.

Regarding lipid metabolism in patients who have cancer, why is that we know increased lipolysis occurs with virtually all cancers, but we still have not identified, defined, or classified the contributions of the various potential causes of the increased lipolysis? This objective must be accomplished before rational attempts at its prevention, reversal, or correction are attempted. Too much time and effort have been spent on fruitless generalizations and observational investigations rather than directing efforts and resources toward specific answers to specific questions. In their summation of the causes of changes in intake and absorption of patients who have cancer, Russell and Steiger[7] succinctly point out the wide variety of causes for these adverse situations; they essentially mandate that patients who have cancer require the services of a special nutritional support team that can provide specific, individually tailored and formulated nutritional support, comprehensively and integrated with the total antineoplastic care of the patient. We agree that this is key to the successful optimal management of the patient who has cancer. We also agree that it is of utmost importance to attempt to achieve a state of anabolism in patients who have cancer if at all possible before any and all forms of antineoplastic therapy to maximize positive outcomes and to minimize morbidity.

## THE GLYCEMIA CONTROVERSY IN NOURISHING CRITICALLY ILL PATIENTS

Consistently maintaining a euglycemic state in all patients under all conditions during wide variations in their clinical status from that of generally stable and healthy to severely injured, septic and/or otherwise critically ill has been highly desirable and a fundamental goal in the provision of nutritional support, especially by parenteral nutrition. One of the primary early limitations to the successful achievement of adequate delivery of calories to meet the energy needs of surgical patients entirely intravenously was the innate ability of each patient to use and metabolize the infused dextrose caloric load without exceeding the capacity of the body cell mass to incorporate the exogenous energy substrate into its myriad biochemical and physiologic processes. Although some guidelines for maximal use of glucose had been derived from various animal and human studies, the range was broad, and dependent on multiple factors, including age, body mass, activity, health status, and presence or absence of disease, especially diabetes mellitus. Moreover, the technology for measuring plasma insulin levels was not available as a clinical tool when TPN was first studied in the laboratory and then introduced into clinical practice. Therefore, rational and reasonable estimates of the requirements of each patient for calories was made, which was usually 4 to 5 times the caloric ration that the patient had been receiving by routine peripheral intravenous dextrose infusions. The resultant hypertonic dextrose solution was necessarily administered into the superior vena cava to minimize thrombophlebitis; however, it was also obligatory to infuse the solution at a rate at which the body cell mass could assimilate and metabolize the infused dextrose load not only for maximum efficacy and safety but also to maintain the blood sugar concentration within normal limits throughout the infusion. The additional goal was not to exceed the renal threshold for glucose, which could create or aggravate a host of problems related to glycosuria. Therefore, it was mandatory to infuse the calculated quantity of dextrose calories continuously at a constant rate throughout the 24-hour day and to periodically monitor blood and urine glucose concentrations. Essentially, the daily caloric infusions could be thought of as a continuous 24-hour glucose tolerance test. To ensure patient safety as much as possible, TPN was initiated at one-third of the calculated dose for the first 12 to 24 hours and increased to one-half the calculated dose for the next day or so to evaluate the patient's tolerance of, and response to, the dextrose infusion. Using periodic blood sugar concentrations as guidelines, the rate of infusion was advanced to the full calculated dose estimated to fulfill the patient's needs, maintaining the blood sugar level in the normal range. Hypoglycemia was avoided because it was more likely to be accompanied by more serious untoward sequelae than occur with hyperglycemia. Conscientious attention to detail and vigilance in observing and monitoring the patients was essential to the early success of TPN. The early patient candidates for this experimental form of central venous hypertonic dextrose feeding were generally stable, but severely malnourished, patients, who specifically were otherwise not stressed by recent trauma and/or sepsis. In addition, patients with insulin-dependent diabetes mellitus were also not considered in the early experiments as candidates for TPN. Subsequently, the entire spectrum of surgical patients and conditions underwent study and treatment with TPN in the clinical research center and in the surgical units of the Hospital of the University of Pennsylvania. These unprecedented trials and procedures were not accomplished easily or without problems. In the late 1960s, no commercially manufactured pumps were available for clinical infusion of intravenous fluids or medications in the hospitals of this country. All intravenous solutions for the maintenance of body fluids and nutrition were administered by gravity drip, requiring virtually hourly adjustments by the nursing personnel throughout the day. After a few episodes of frightening, but otherwise uneventful, hypoglycemia or hyperglycemia, it became obvious that the infusion of this potent combination of concentrated nutrient substrates must be infused at constant, dependable, predetermined rates if the technique of TPN was to be as safe and efficacious clinically in patients as it had been in the beagle puppies in the laboratory, in which the solutions were all controlled and administered precisely by infusion pumps. Accordingly, a major change in the practice of nursing and medical care was initiated by the introduction of specially designed intravenous pumps for the safe, controlled administration of TPN in surgical patients. Only the most senior practitioners of nursing and surgery today can remember the time in the early 1960s when patients received intravenous fluids without pumps, and when intensive care units (ICUs) were just beginning to be built and developed for the specialized and focused care of critically ill patients.

A flurry of controversy arose when we began to extend the use of TPN to surgical patients with diabetes mellitus. As was the practice at that time, short-acting insulin was administered subcutaneously in doses derived from extrapolation of the usual total dose of insulin, which the patients had been taking to control their blood sugars based on their total caloric oral diets. However, it soon became obvious that the intermittent administration of insulin subcutaneously concomitant with the continuous infusion of dextrose intravenously was problematic for optimal metabolic synchronization. Accordingly, the senior author (SJD) undertook some studies to administer regular insulin intravenously through a burette administration set attached to a side-arm port of the TPN infusion tubing, and to use a second pump to administer the insulin at a controlled constant rate simultaneously with the TPN solution. This strategy allowed more precise control of euglycemia, but added potential complications related to the integrity and safety of the infusion apparatus. Eventually, insulin was added directly to the TPN solution in the pharmacy to simplify and consolidate the process of providing all of the essential nutrients at one time, simultaneously, and in the same infusion system. A great hue and cry arose from many of our colleagues, especially the endocrinologists and internists, who posited that the insulin in the TPN solution would not be so effective as when given subcutaneously, or that the insulin would form bizarre, nonusable biochemical complexes with the nutrient components in the TPN and/or that the insulin would bond to the glass of the intravenous bottles or to the plastic intravenous tubing. This controversy raged for years, during which virtually no serious problems occurred or were detected secondary specifically to the addition of the insulin to the TPN solution. The control of the blood sugar in diabetic patients receiving TPN was greatly improved. Throughout the world, clinical research in this area became active and exciting, with various forms of nutrient infusions given to patients having glucose clamps or insulin clamps together with development of advanced insulin immunoassays, insulin pumps, islet cell and pancreatic transplantation, and so forth. Prototypes are already under investigation, and it will soon be possible to have bedside monitors attached to implanted continuous blood glucose sensors to determine blood glucose levels instantaneously, online, on demand. A servocontrolled, closed-loop, computerized system, including a continuous blood sensor and insulin pump linked to an automated algorithm, will allow precision in the management of blood insulin and blood sugar control heretofore unavailable. However, despite the ingenuity and elegance of current and future technology, nothing will ever replace or approach the excellence of patient care that can be attained by conscientious skilled efforts and care by the members of the nursing and physician health care teams, who strive for perfection.

In the management of a stable, noncomplicated, nondiabetic, nonstressed, significantly malnourished patient, achieving and maintaining euglycemia with the judicious administration and conscientious monitoring of TPN is the objective usually and readily achieved. In such a patient, the sudden or abrupt appearance of hyperglycemia is mostly caused by the development of an occult infection, abscess, or inflammatory process, and this finding should alert the clinician to initiate an immediate and thorough search for the source, including the central venous infusion catheter and skin exit site, the lungs, urine, and wound. It has been our experience that hyperglycemia occurs hours before an increase in the leukocyte count, a shift to the left, or an increase in core body temperature. It is when this early warning signal of potential danger is ignored by the health care team, or treated with a lengthy wait-and-see attitude, that the patient may proceed to increased morbidity, multiple expensive studies, and prolonged ICU and hospital stays. Moreover, such patients are highly likely to continue to require additional and prolonged nutritional support, which may include parenteral nutrition to overcome not only the initial starvation and clinical condition but also to treat the complicating infectious process. Such patients are often subsequently included in a retrospective study which includes patients with similar initiating problems, but without the burden of malnutrition (and thus not requiring specialized nutrition support, especially TPN), and are compared unfavorably by meta-analysis and other forms of pseudoscience initially to condemn the TPN for creating or causing the hyperglycemia, and then blaming the hyperglycemia for the development of the infectious process. Nonetheless, there is clinical evidence of good quality data showing clearly that close attention to glucose control while feeding patients in the ICU is of paramount importance, although more data are required to determine the most appropriate blood glucose target levels in different patient populations under different conditions. It is still unclear which glycemic threshold should be used in many patients as the indication for supplemental insulin initiation, but a reasonable approach in surgical patients receiving an adequate nutrition regimen should be to treat them with sufficient insulin to maintain euglycemia.[8]

Before the turn of this century, interest in the control of the blood glucose concentration in ICUs appeared to be low, although studies of the effects of insulin therapy on infectious complications related to cardiothoracic surgery suggested a benefit of tighter glucose control.[8,9] Bistrian and colleagues[9,10] more recently pointed out that few standardized policies existed regarding this matter, perhaps because stress-related insulin resistance leading to mild hyperglycemia was considered an adaptive phenomenon that might even have benefits for the systemic inflammatory response by providing greater amounts of glucose for anaerobic metabolism to important cells for healing and repair such as macrophages and fibroblasts. Observational data suggested that serum glucose levels greater than 200 mg/dL were associated with increases in infectious complications in hospitalized surgical patients, which led to initiation of subcutaneous insulin therapy only for glucose levels consistently in excess of this threshold.[9,11] However, changes in this ICU policy were implemented abruptly in response to the publication in 2001 of a large, randomized trial showing a mortality benefit from the use of intensive insulin therapy in a mainly surgical critical care unit in Belgium.[12] The experimental group was treated with insulin to maintain true normal glycemia (80–110 mg/dL) with initiation of insulin infusion when the serum glucose value rose to more than 110 mg/dL. The control group was not given insulin unless hyperglycemia was shown by a serum glucose level greater than 215 mg/dL. A major strength of this study was its large size of 1548 patients and complete follow-up.[9] However, 70% of those studied were cardiothoracic surgical patients and only 20% had medical conditions. In a follow-up study by this same group in 2006 in medical ICU patients, 1200 patients were randomized, and no overall significant difference in mortality was reported.[13] However, the incidence of infectious complications and kidney injury was reduced in the tight glucose control group. To muddy the waters further and to add fuel to the controversy, a recent randomized trial in 2009[14] (NICE-Sugar) comparing tight glucose control (80–108 mg/dL) with regular glucose control (<180 mg/dL) in 6000 patients showed an increase in mortality together with an increased incidence of hypoglycemic episodes in the tight glucose control group. An even more recent Brazilian study[15] randomized 109 patients undergoing cardiac surgery to intensive versus regular glucose control and showed no differences in morbidity or mortality among the groups. This is such an important topic that many other trials of tight and less stringent glycemic control are currently under way, with the goal being to define a threshold for glucose levels above which the complications of hyperglycemia become evident.[9] Until that time, for surgical patients receiving 200 to 300 g/d of dextrose, an attempt to maintain values as close to normal glycemia as can safely be achieved within the limits of the institution is prudent.[9] The pendulum has swung from the old criterion of attempting to maintain glucose levels less than 200 mg/dL to a more recent short period of tight glucose control less than 110 mg/dL, and now is swinging back to maintaining a blood glucose level less than 180 mg/dL. The ideal goal of achieving and maintaining nutritional and metabolic homeostasis remains noncontroversial. However, the means by which this lofty goal is achieved is likely to remain controversial until science overtakes the art in the practice of nutritional support and parenteral nutrition.

In a recent, concise, definitive review of the subject, Bistrian and McCowen[9] discussed the importance of the route of feeding in patients in the ICU, stating that the traditional ICU doctrine is that enteral is always better than parenteral nutrition. Early studies of TPN in ICUs showed high rates of infection, usually related to hyperglycemia because the ease with which TPN can be administered allows the delivery of large quantities of dextrose with consequent hyperglycemia in critically ill, insulin-resistant patients unless insulin therapy is judiciously added to the regimen.[16] Because of this finding, in part, many of the studies in which enteral and parenteral nutrition have been compared are seriously flawed in that the quantities of nutrients delivered were not equivalent; overfeeding occurred more frequently in patients receiving TPN, in all likelihood because of poor control of the TPN infusion, and different rates and degrees of hyperglycemia presumably contributed to the differences in the incidence of infectious complications.[9] Moreover, a plethora of flawed meta-analyses that failed to show any benefit of TPN over enteral feeding, coupled with animal data showing that enteral nutrition is associated with lower rates of bacterial translocation, have stimulated subsequent ICU nutrition support guidelines stressing the use of enteral nutrition whenever possible in preference to parenteral nutrition.[9] However, a more recent meta-analysis of studies comparing TPN with enteral nutrition (which excluded poor quality studies with pseudorandomization and high dropout rates), showed a significant mortality benefit for TPN over total enteral nutrition (TEN), with little evidence of heterogeneity among the 9 randomized trials in the study that provided intention-to-treat results.[17] However, a higher rate of infectious complications in critically ill patients fed with TPN prevails overall. As discussed earlier, in this era when the deleterious effects of even small increases in plasma glucose concentrations have been established, the conscientious efforts, especially in patients in the ICU, to attain and maintain normal glycemia with precision, may allow the potential for other benefits of TPN to be fully appreciated.[9] In nutritionally depleted patients, it has been easier to achieve goal-feeding with TPN earlier than with enteral nutrition. Mortality advantages of TPN were found primarily compared with late enteral feeding; however, this advantage for TPN disappeared when compared with early parenteral feeding, suggesting at least for patients at high nutritional risk that the ability to feed earlier in the illness is of paramount importance, and that any way adequate feeding can be accomplished is appropriate.[18] Delayed feeding in the ICU is associated with poorer outcomes, and meta-analyses of early versus delayed enteral nutrition have generally shown better results, including fewer infectious complications and shorter lengths of hospital stay from early feeding, with no effects on noninfectious complications or mortality. Accordingly, evidence-based protocols have been designed with a focus on early enteral nutrition whenever possible.[19–22] Early enteral feeding and/or parental feeding are likely to benefit patients in the ICU if the nutritional support regimen can be accomplished without inducing hyperglycemia, and aggressive approaches of feeding in the ICU are warranted from recent studies.[23–27] We agree with Bistrian's assessment that the content of the nutritional support in critically ill patients in the ICU has not yet been satisfactorily resolved, but that nutrient requirements should be provided as comprehensively and as judiciously as possible, and as early as possible, by whatever means possible, in patients in the ICU.[9] Both the parenteral and enteral techniques are complementary, have clear indications, and can be used individually, together, or sequentially, as appropriate and as needed to meet nutrient requirements. Most problems arise when the indications are not followed, when the enteral route is not initiated as soon as possible, or when parenteral nutrition is not used to supplement early enteral feeding that cannot meet the requirements.[28–30] A study by Hasenberg and colleagues[31] in 2006 randomized 82 patients with late-stage colorectal cancer receiving chemotherapy either to enteral supplementation alone or to enteral supplementation and parenteral nutrition together, and showed weight stabilization, improved quality of life, and fewer chemotherapy-related complications in the group receiving the parenteral nutrition, underscoring the benefits of using both techniques in a complementary manner in specific clinical situations for achievement of optimal outcomes.

## REFLECTIONS ON THE TPN VERSUS TEN CONTROVERSY

On a personal note, the senior author (SJD) would like to express a continuing major disappointment during a 4-decade to 5-decade career in complex general surgery, reoperative surgery, surgical critical care, and surgical nutritional support.[1] This disappointment arises from the somewhat immature and irresponsible arguments and disputes (rather than potentially constructive controversy), engendered by the postures and attitudes associated with TPN versus TEN or parenteral nutrition versus enteral nutrition, especially among many in the health care professions who should know better. Anyone interested and competent in providing optimal nutrition support to their patients knows that it is essential that knowledge, judgment, proficiency, and competency must prevail in choosing the best nutrient constituents of a feeding regimen and in deciding how these formulations might best be provided for the benefit of the patient under virtually any condition or with any adverse situation. Not to know, use, or have proficiency with every tool in our clinical toolbox detracts from our education and training; our trust, competence, and professionalism; and our morals and ethics. The practice of optimal nutritional support should not be adversely influenced by ambition, self-interest, prejudice, financial gain, and so forth. Health care practitioners who always treat their patients with enteral nutrition, and those who always treat their patients with parenteral nutrition, are both likely to be practicing less than optimal nutritional support. The judicious use of the most appropriate nutritional support modality in every conceivable situation requires broad versatility, experience, judgment, proficiency, wisdom, and equanimity. An example analogous to situations commonly witnessed in our hospitals and outpatient settings today *vis-à-vis* comprehensive nutritional support is that it is possible, although awkward and inefficient, to insert a screw with a pair of pliers, but it is more appropriate, suitable, and efficacious to use a screwdriver for this purpose; similarly, it is possible to pound a nail into a board with a wrench, but it is better, more effective, and more precise to use an appropriately designed hammer. It bodes well for practitioners of nutritional support to appraise a given clinical situation comprehensively, to identify and define the goals of nutritional support, and to choose and use the most appropriate nutritional support tools proficiently in the overall comprehensive management of the patient. It would be a noble endeavor for the members of the health care professions to direct our efforts, talents, and limited resources to perfecting nutritional support to the point that we all could nourish our patients by the most efficacious methods and techniques possible to provide substrates sufficient in quantity and quality to allow the maximum number of cells in the body cell mass to perform optimally the functions for which they were designed. We owe it to our patients to do so.

## REFLECTIONS ON GERIATRIC NUTRITIONAL SUPPORT

The following discussion summarizes our thoughts on the status of geriatric nutritional support. Comprehensive geriatric health care should include the maintenance of normal nutrition status in those who are in good health and provision of adequate nutrition for sick and infirm patients. Elderly patients may be at risk for development of malnutrition because of a variety of physiologic and socioeconomic factors. Hospitalized patients are a heterogeneous population, but they are at significant risk for presenting to the hospital with, or developing afterward, protein-energy, electrolyte, divalent mineral, and micronutrient deficiencies. Accordingly, nutritional assessment should be routine on admission and at regular intervals thereafter. In elderly patients requiring nutritional support, parenteral nutrition is indicated when the early establishment of effective enteral nutrition is not reliable or possible, and it should be initiated early in the hospital course. Peripheral parenteral nutrition can be a valuable interim solution in the clinical course when volitional or enteral intakes are uncertain or potentially unsafe. Dietary counseling and nutritional support are just 2 of the interventions required for the optimal care of this important, vulnerable, and rapidly increasing segment of our society. Further research in basic and clinical areas is necessary to define more clearly the many nutritional events that occur with aging and to define optimal management of these changes to provide the best possible nutrition to all patients, under all conditions, at all times.

## REFLECTIONS ON LEGACIES OF TPN

In reflecting on the past 45 years of a passionate pursuit of providing optimal nutritional support to all patients, the senior author (SJD) has compiled a lengthy list of perceived significant contributions of the development and successful clinical application of TPN to the overall fund of useful medical knowledge. They include the following:

1. The first demonstration that all nutrients required for normal growth and development in any animal species (initially in beagle puppies and later in other species) could be provided long-term entirely intravenously
2. The first demonstration subsequently that all nutrients required for normal growth and development in human beings (initially in a term newborn infant and later in premature infants and older infants and children) could be provided long-term entirely intravenously for the first time
3. The demonstration that positive nitrogen balance, weight gain, wound healing, reduced morbidity and mortality, and many other desirable clinical outcomes, could be accomplished in critically ill patients nourished entirely intravenously for as long as required
4. The development of a wide variety of parenteral macronutrient and micronutrient substrates for standard and special nutritional and metabolic support of seriously ill patients of all ages
5. The development of safe, effective, percutaneous central venous catheterization techniques

6. The development of safe, long-term intravenous infusion principles and techniques for nutritional support, resuscitation, and pharmacotherapy

7. The stimulation of a technological revolution in the development, advancement, and use of infusion pumps, together with alarms, safety features, servomechanisms, miniaturization, portability, precision, dependability, and so forth

8. The stimulation of the development of intravenous fluid bags, reservoirs, infusion tubing, administration apparatus, and so forth, tailored to specific individual patient requirements, infusates, and situations

9. The development of a variety of central venous catheters, antimicrobial solutions and ointments, reservoir injection ports, cuffed implanted catheters, inline filters, infusion tubing, administration apparatus, and so forth

10. The stimulation of a technological revolution and transformation of pharmacy practice, including automated, computerized preparation and admixture apparatus, filtered laminar airflow areas, cold sterilization by filtration, nutrient-nutrient and nutrient-medication interactions and compatibilities

11. The stimulation of the advancement of the specialty of clinical pharmacology and nutrition support among pharmacists and the origin of solution preparation technicians in the pharmacy profession

12. The demonstration of the multidisciplinary scope of clinical nutrition and the initiation and organization of nutrition support teams

13. The subsequent inspiration for, and stimulation of, the establishment of scores of multidisciplinary professional, educational, scientific, and clinical societies for the advancement of nutritional support worldwide (eg, American Society of Parenteral and Enteral Nutrition, ESPN, PENSA, POLSPEN)

14. The demonstration of the usefulness of inducing a period of bowel rest together with TPN in the management of selected conditions or disorders of the gastrointestinal tract

15. The establishment, beyond a doubt, of the relevance of adequate nutritional support in achieving optimal results, minimizing morbidity and mortality, and improving outcomes in the adjunctive or primary therapy for critically ill patients

16. The stimulation of the subsequent accentuated interest and advancement in enteral nutritional support as an adjunctive, additional, or alternative technique of nutritional support of patients with an adequately functioning alimentary tract

17. The stimulation of the study and analysis of cost-benefit, risk-benefit, outcomes, policies and procedures, standards, regulatory legislation and oversight, credentialing, reimbursement, medical-legal, and ethical issues, and so forth of nutritional support

18. The stimulation of the development of nutrient solutions for specific metabolic needs, such as renal failure, hepatic failure with encephalopathy, pulmonary insufficiency, and immunomodulation

19. The stimulation of the concept of nutrients, either individually, or in various combinations, as medical foods for use in the therapeutic management of a medical disorder, disease or condition (eg, nutriceuticals and prescription foods)

20. The development and advancement of the concept that the practice of clinical nutrition support is not merely the provision of foodstuffs but also involves the integration and/or modulation of cellular biochemistry, molecular biology, immunology, genetics, and function

21. The development of the concepts, apparatus, expertise, and systems of ambulatory home nutritional support, leading to the virtually explosive growth in the home care industry and outpatient therapy

22. The evolution and advancement of the concept, management, and biology of intestinal failure, and the development of expertise and services in this vital area of sophisticated nutritional support and complex gastrointestinal management
23. The stimulation of rehabilitation support for patients requiring long-term parenteral and/or enteral nutrition, including psychological, emotional, spiritual, social, economic, legal, custodial, occupational, educational, and physical therapy support
24. The development of standards of care, principles and practices, adjunctive medications, assessments, and other guidelines related to the safe, efficacious, and competent provision of optimal nutrition to virtually all patients under all conditions
25. The demonstration of the essentiality for fundamental, integrated, and continuing nutritional education in the curricula of medical professional schools, postgraduate training programs, and for lifelong learning.

## REFERENCES

1. Dudrick SJ. A 45 year obsession and passionate pursuit of optimal nutritional support: puppies, pediatrics, surgery, geriatrics, home TPN, ASPEN, et cetera. JPEN J Parenter Enteral Nutr 2005;29(4):272–87.
2. Dudrick SJ, Palesty JA. Commentary: specialized nutritional support for cancer patients. Chapter 3. In: Silberman H, Silberman AW, editors. Principles and practice of surgical oncology. Multidisciplinary approach to difficult problems. Baltimore (MD): Wolters Kluwer/Lippincott Williams & Wilkins; 2009. p. 59–66.
3. Dudrick SJ, Palesty JA. What we have learned about cachexia and gastrointestinal cancer. Dig Dis 2003;21:198–213.
4. Palesty JA, Dudrick SJ. The goldilocks paradigm of starvation and refeeding. Nutr Clin Pract 2006;21(2):147–54.
5. Laviano A, Meguid MM, Inui A, et al. Therapy insight: cancer anorexia-cachexia syndrome–when all you can eat is yourself. Nat Clin Pract Oncol 2005;2:158–65.
6. Dempsey DT, Feurer ID, Knox LS, et al. Energy expenditure in malnourished gastrointestinal cancer patients. Cancer 1984;53:1265–73.
7. Russell MK, Steiger E. Specialized nutritional support for cancer patients. Chapter 3. In: Silberman H, Silberman AW, editors. Principles and practice of surgical oncology. Multidisciplinary approach to difficult problems. Baltimore (MD): Wolters Kluwer/Lippincott Williams & Wilkins; 2009. p. 51–9.
8. Furnay AP, Kerr KJ, Grunkemeier GL, et al. Continuous intravenous insulin infusion reduces the incidence of deep sternal wound infection in diabetic patients after cardiac surgical procedures. Ann Thorac Surg 1999;67:352–60.
9. Bistrian BR, McCowen KC. Nutritional and metabolic support in the adult intensive care unit: key controversies. Crit Care Med 2006;34(5):1525–31.
10. McCowen KC, Malhotra A, Bistrian BR. Stress-induced hyperglycemia. Crit Care Med 2001;17:107–24.
11. Pomposelli JJ, Baxter JK 3rd, Babineau TJ, et al. Early postoperative glucose control predicts nosocomial infection rate in diabetic patients. JPEN J Parenter Enteral Nutr 1998;22:77–81.
12. Van den Berghe G, Wouters P, Weekers F, et al. Intensive insulin therapy in the surgical intensive care unit. N Engl J Med 2001;345:1359–67.
13. Van den Berghe G, Wilmer A, Hermans G, et al. Intensive insulin therapy in the medical ICU. N Engl J Med 2006;354:449–61.

14. Finfer S, Chittock DR, Su SY, et al. Intensive versus conventional glucose control in critically ill patients. N Engl J Med 2009;360:1283–97.

15. Chan RP, Galas FR, Hajjar LA, et al. Intensive perioperative glucose control does not improve outcomes of patients submitted to open-heart surgery: a randomized controlled trial. Clinics (Sao Paulo) 2009;64:51–60.

16. Simpson F, Doig GS. Parenteral vs enteral nutrition in the critically ill patient: a metabolic analysis of trials using the intention to treat principle. Intensive Care Med 2005;31:12–23.

17. Peter JV, Moran JL, Phillips-Hughes J. A metaanalysis of treatment outcomes of early enteral versus early parenteral nutrition in hospitalized patients. Crit Care Med 2005;33:213–20.

18. Marik PE, Zaloga GP. Early enteral nutrition in acutely ill patients: a systematic review. Crit Care Med 2001;29:2264–70.

19. Martin CM, Doig GS, Heyland DK, et al. Multicentre, cluster randomized clinical trial of algorithms for critical-care enteral and parenteral therapy (ACCEPT). CMAJ 2004;170:197–204.

20. Barr J, Hecht M, Flavin KE, et al. Outcomes in critically ill patients before and after the implementation of an evidence-based nutritional management protocol. Chest 2004;125:1446–57.

21. Mackenzie SL, Zygun DA, Whitmore BL, et al. Implementation of a nutrition support protocol increases the proportion of mechanically ventilated patients reaching enteral nutrition targets in the adult intensive care unit. JPEN J Parenter Enteral Nutr 2005;29:74–80.

22. Heyland DK, Dhaliwal R, Day A, et al. Validation of the Canadian practice guidelines for nutrition support in mechanically ventilated critically ill patients: results of a prospective observational study. Crit Care Med 2004;32:2260–6.

23. Caparros T, Lopez J, Grau T. Early enteral nutrition in critically ill patients with a high-protein diet enriched with arginine, fiber, and antioxidants compared with a standard high-protein diet: the effect on nosocomial infections and outcomes. JPEN J Parenter Enteral Nutr 2001;25:299–308.

24. Hall JC, Dobb G, Hall J, et al. A prospective randomized trial of enteral glutamine in critical illness. Intensive Care Med 2003;29:1710–6.

25. Woodcock NP, Zeigler D, Palmer MD, et al. Enteral versus parenteral nutrition: a pragmatic study. Nutrition 2001;17:1–12.

26. Maykel JA, Pazirandeh S, Bistrian BR. Is there a benefit to postpyloric feeding? Crit Care Med 2002;30:1654–6.

27. Maykel JA, Bistrian BR. Is enteral feeding for everyone? Crit Care Med 2002;30:714–6.

28. McClave SA, Martindale RG, Vanek VA, et al. Guidelines for the provision and assessment of nutrition support therapy in the adult critically ill patient: Society of Critical Care Medicine (SCCM) and American Society of Parenteral and Enteral Nutrition (ASPEN). JPEN J Parenter Enteral Nutr 2009;33:277–316.

29. De Jonghe B, Appere-De-Vechi C, Fournier M, et al. A prospective survey of nutritional support practices in intensive care unit patients: what is prescribed? What is delivered? Crit Care Med 2001;29:8–12.

30. Peterson SJ, Tsai AA, Scala CM, et al. Adequacy of oral intake in critically ill patients 1 week after extubation. J Am Diet Assoc 2010;110:427–33.

31. Hasenberg T, Essenbreis M, Herold A, et al. Early supplementation of parenteral nutrition is capable of improving quality of life, chemotherapy-related toxicity and body composition in patients with advanced colorectal carcinoma undergoing palliative treatment. Results from a prospective, randomized clinical trial. Colorectal Dis 2010;12:e190–9.

# Historical Highlights of the Development of Total Parenteral Nutrition

Stanley J. Dudrick, MD[a,b,*], J. Alexander Palesty, MD[b,c]

**KEYWORDS**

- Total parenteral nutrition • TPN history • Development of TPN
- Philosophy of TPN

The hypothetical concept of nourishing patients using means other than the alimentary tract, by injecting nutrient substances or fluids subcutaneously, or infusing them directly intravenously, was advocated and attempted for many decades before its successful achievement. The fulfillment of this seemingly fanciful dream required centuries of fundamental research and discovery, coupled with myriad technological developments and judicious applications dating back to the early 17th century. The prerequisites to rational, fruitful clinical studies in this challenging but vital area included knowledge of the anatomy and physiology of the circulatory system; knowledge of the biochemical nature of nutrient substrates; the interrelationships of these active and potent substrates with microbiology, immunology, asepsis, and antisepsis; and some knowledge of the complex interactions of food substances with metabolism, multiple pharmacologic agents, and the spectrum of pathophysiologic processes.[1–11] Although complete or Total Parenteral Nutrition (TPN) has been available as a practical, effective, and useful clinical adjunct for almost 50 years, the relatively modern development of this mode of therapy was initiated in the fourth decade (1930s) of the last century and crystallized by the focused investigations of Elman in the late 1940s.[12,13] However, the practical clinical application and effective use of TPN did not emerge until the 1960s. Elman[14] performed a series of orderly and logical original experiments, and was instrumental in developing protein substrates

The authors have nothing to disclose.

[a] Department of Surgery, Yale University School of Medicine, 333 Cedar Street, New Haven, CT 06510, USA

[b] Department of Surgery, Saint Mary's Hospital, 56 Franklin Street, Waterbury, CT 06706, USA

[c] Department of Surgery, University of Connecticut School of Medicine, 263 Farmington Avenue, Farmington, CT 06030, USA

* Corresponding author. Department of Surgery, Saint Mary's Hospital, 56 Franklin Street, Waterbury, CT 06706.

E-mail address: sdudrick@stmh.org

Surg Clin N Am 91 (2011) 693–717

doi:10.1016/j.suc.2011.02.009

0039-6109/11/$ – see front matter © 2011 Elsevier Inc. All rights reserved.

in the form of protein hydrolysates and crystalline amino acids, which presumably would have led him inevitably to the development of an efficacious and reliable technique of TPN. However, his work was unfortunately interrupted in large part by the events related to World War II, in which national priorities were shifted dramatically and abruptly away from basic scientific medical efforts to military and humanitarian endeavors. Following the end of the war, Elman[15] compiled his studies in a classic tome entitled, *Parenteral Alimentation in Surgery with Special Reference to Proteins and Amino Acids*, published by Hoeber, Inc in 1947. This is a classic treatise, which should be read by all those interested in metabolic and nutritional support, especially for surgical and other seriously ill patients. Although Elman resumed his basic research and clinical investigative efforts in the late 1940s, his health failed, and he never regained the momentum he had achieved earlier in his career. We teach our students that there are not very many entirely unique new ideas, but rather new techniques, technology, and data that primarily allow the full definition and validation of ideas that have often been expressed previously. Evidence for this premise is manifested by the fact that the recorded history of this field of endeavor dates back almost 400 years. The axiom that we "make progress by standing on the shoulders of our predecessors" is obvious from the number of important scientific contributions that have been essential to the eventual development and advancement of TPN and that are outlined in **Table 1**.

It seems fair and appropriate to state that the seminal discovery that enabled the development of intravenous infusion and parenteral nutrition was the discovery and demonstration by Harvey[16] of the circulation of the blood in 1616, which he subsequently published in 1628. Consequently, it became reasonable to assume that whatever matter entered the bloodstream would circulate throughout the body, and that the nutrients provided in ingested food would eventually be processed to molecular substances that could be transported to all of the tissues in the body. Before the 17th century, scientists and physicians did not understand fully the anatomy and physiology of blood vessels and body fluids until Harvey introduced them to the concepts of experimentation and biologic research. A physician and investigator, he first described the circulatory system in 1616 after conducting studies and experiments with deer carcasses. Afterward, in research on vivisected animals, he discovered that the heart propels the blood throughout the body, acting as both a muscle and a pump and producing a continuous circulation of the blood. Until that time, it was believed that, although arteries and veins both contained blood, the blood flowed back and forth like "human breath." Indeed, until Harvey[16] eventually identified the capillary network, the liver was regarded as the center of the circulatory system. Well into the 19th century, many physicians believed that a "useless abundance of blood" was a principal cause of all disease, and accordingly, blood was commonly removed by practitioners with lancets, cupping, and leeches to treat a variety of disorders. Moreover, 200 years after Harvey's discovery of blood circulation, medical students were still instructed to treat hemorrhage by bleeding patients to the point of syncope, and venesection was considered a useful treatment to encourage coagulation and to arrest hemorrhage.[17]

About a generation later, in 1658, Wren[18] first injected ale, wine, and opium into the veins of dogs, using a goose quill attached to a pig's bladder as his infusion apparatus. In 1665, Lower first successfully transfused blood from one live dog to another, and 2 years later, in 1667, both Lower and Denis, working independently, reported the "successful" transfusion of blood from a sheep to a man, presumably inferring that their patients survived.[19–21] Meanwhile, Escholtz,[22] in 1665, published the first description of techniques and illustrations of intravenous access and infusion equipment, including metal cannulas connected to sections of excised animal veins as flexible tubing in *Clysmatica Nova*. Other investigators had injected and infused a variety of salts, medications, nutrients, blood, and other substances into the vasculature before this classic publication, but their sophistication increased afterward (see **Table 1**). Subsequently, in 1678, Courten[23] infused vinegar, salts, and urine into veins of dogs without untoward results, but found that the animals infused with olive oil died of severe respiratory distress, leading him to conclude that oil or fat would require special preparation or modification before successful tolerance of intravenous infusion of these substances.

Medical experimentation and discovery were quite limited in the 18th century, but progress began to occur more rapidly in the 19th century, when knowledge was increasingly gained regarding human physiology.[17] Early in the 19th century, Blundell[24] was the first physician to transfuse blood successfully from one human being to another in 1818, and in 1831, Latta[25] infused intravenous solutions into patients successfully in the treatment of cholera. His work, and that of O'Shaughnessy,[26] demonstrated that the large amounts of water and salts lost in diarrhea by cholera victims must be replaced by copious infusions of water and salts into the bloodstream. Their work ultimately revolutionized the understanding both of the cause of death in patients with cholera and its alleviation by the judicious restoration of circulating blood volume.

The following year, in 1832, Latta was credited with saving 8 of 25 victims of cholera, whom he treated by injecting intravenous saline using a small silver tube attached to a syringe containing a hypotonic solution of sodium, chloride, and bicarbonate.[27,28] However, the medical profession was prolific in its criticism of the infusion work of Latta and did not readily adopt the use of saline injections because it was thought that this would hasten death, probably because it was used only in patients about to die.[17] In view of the insufficient knowledge of physiologic chemistry and microbiology in the 1800s, the concepts and work of O'Shaughnessy and Latta were well ahead of their time.[17] When one thinks of the mind-sets among members of the medical profession, which exist even today regarding resistance to change and to acceptance of new ideas, techniques, and technology, it appears that attitudes, responses, and reactions fundamentally have not changed much throughout the centuries.[29] Certainly, the presentations of new techniques and technologies related to vascular access, such as percutaneous subclavian vein catheterization, and to intravenous nutritional support, such as TPN, did not escape severe criticism and skepticism in the early stages of their development and clinical application by Dudrick[30] and others; and controversies continue to abound relevant to indications, techniques, complications, risks, costs, outcomes, etc, of virtually all aspects of nutritional support, as evidenced in this issue.

In 1843, Bernard infused various sugar solutions into animals, primarily rabbits, and over the next 2 decades, infused egg whites, milk, and other nutrients into animals with various degrees of success.[31] His work introduced and popularized the concept of *Le Milieu Interior* and, in 1859, he demonstrated the essentiality and primacy of glucose as an energy source in maintaining normal metabolism.[32] During the middle of the 19th century, many investigators attempted to provide nutrients by subcutaneous injection. Menzel and Perco injected fat, milk, and camphor subcutaneously in dogs in 1869; in 1875, Krug injected oil and protein extract into a patient with anorexia nervosa; and in 1876, Whittaker attempted to feed a woman who was unable to eat, by injecting milk, beef extract, and cod liver oil subcutaneously.[31,33,34] Later, in 1904, Friedrich[35] carried the subcutaneous studies further by injecting peptone, fat,

**Table 1**
**Early historical highlights in the development of total parenteral nutrition**

| Year | Accomplishment | Investigator |
|------|----------------|--------------|
| 1616 | Discovery of the circulation of blood | Harvey |
| 1628 | First published report of circulation of blood | Harvey |
| 1658 | First intravenous injection in animals (ale, wine, and opium) | Wren |
| 1665 | Transfusion of blood from one live animal to another (dogs) | Lower |
| 1665 | Techniques of intravenous entry and infusion first described and illustrated (*Clysmatica Nova*) | Escholtz |
| 1667 | Transfusion of blood from an animal (sheep) to a man | Lower/Denis |
| 1678 | Intravenous infusion of olive oil, vinegar, salts, and urine into a dog | Courten |
| 1818 | Transfusion of blood from human to human | Blundell |
| 1831 | Intravenous infusion of water and saline in humans for successful treatment of cholera | Latta |
| 1843 | Intravenous infusion of sugar in animals | Bernard |
| 1859 | Intravenous infusion of egg white, milk, and other foods in animals (rabbits) | Bernard |
| 1869 | Subcutaneous injection of fat in animals (dogs) | Menzel/Perco |
| 1870 | Aseptic and antiseptic techniques for surgery in humans | Lister |
| 1873 | Intravenous infusion of milk in humans for treatment of cholera (2 of 3 patients survived) | Hodder |
| 1876 | Subcutaneous injection of milk in humans for nutrition | Whittaker |
| 1877 | Discovery of microbes and the microbial relationship to infection | Pasteur |
| 1887 | Intravenous infusion of sucrose in humans for treatment of shock | Landerer |
| 1891 | Intravenous infusion of saline solution in humans for treatment of shock | Matas |
| 1895 | Discovery of colloid osmotic functions of plasma proteins | Starling |
| 1896 | Intravenous infusion of glucose in humans | Biedl/Kraus |
| 1901 | Discovery of first 3 of the 4 human blood groups | Landsteiner |
| 1904 | Subcutaneous injection of peptone, fat, glucose, and electrolytes in humans for parenteral nutrition | Friedrich |
| 1905 | Development of methods for analysis of urea, creatinine, and other nitrogenous fractions useful for nutritional assessment | Folin |
| 1907 | Discovery of fourth blood group and classification of 4 blood groups | Jansky |
| 1911 | Intravenous infusion of glucose postoperatively in humans for nutrition | Kausch |
| 1912 | Discovery of vitamins (vital amines) as essential nutrients | Funk |
| 1913 | Intramuscular injection of thiamine (yeast extract) for treatment of polyneuritis in pigeons | Funk |
| 1913 | Intravenous infusion of hydrolyzed proteins in animals (goat) with demonstration of use for nutrition | Henriques/Andersen |

(continued on next page)

**Table 1**
*(continued)*

| Year | Accomplishment | Investigator |
|------|----------------|--------------|
| 1913 | Intravenous infusion of hydrolyzed proteins in animals (dogs) with demonstration of use for nutrition | VanSlyke/Meyer |
| 1915 | Intravenous infusion of fat in animals with demonstration of use for nutrition | Murlin/Riche |
| 1915 | Demonstration of rate of use of intravenous glucose in humans (0.85 g of glucose/kg/h) | Woodyatt/Sansum/Wilder |
| 1918 | Intravenous infusion of orange juice in man for treatment of scurvy | Hess/Unger |
| 1920 | Intravenous infusion of emulsified fat in humans | Yamakawa |
| 1923 | Discovery of cause of pyrogens in sterile water | Seibert |
| 1924 | First continuous intravenous drip infusion of glucose in humans | Matas |
| 1932 | Transfusion of human serum in humans | Kunz |
| 1932 | Description of increased nitrogen losses in urine resulting from catabolic response to major limb trauma in animals and humans | Cuthbertson |
| 1934 | Intravenous infusion of plasma proteins in dogs and humans with demonstration of metabolic use | Holman/Mahoney/Whipple |
| 1934 | Identification of the essential amino acids for growth in rats | Rose |
| 1935 | First intravenous infusion of cottonseed oil emulsions in humans | Holt |
| 1938 | Identification of the essential amino acids and their requirements in humans | Rose |
| 1939 | Demonstration of use of amino acids in hydrolyzed casein infused intravenously in humans | Elman/Weiner |
| 1940 | Demonstration of use of crystalline amino acids infused intravenously in humans | Shohl/Blackfan/Dennis |
| 1944 | Infusion of hypertonic dextrose, insulin, and plasma protein by peripheral vein in high-risk surgical patients | Dennis |
| 1944 | First complete intravenous feeding (water, saline, fat, carbohydrate, amino acids) for 5 days in a 5-month old infant with Hirschsprung's disease | Helfrick/Abelson |
| 1945 | Intravenous infusion of fat emulsions, dextrose, and protein hydrolysate by peripheral vein in humans | McKibbin/Hegsted/Stare |
| 1945 | Development of first polyethylene catheters for intravenous infusions in humans | Zimmermann |
| 1946 | Intravenous infusion of plasma proteins in humans with demonstration of positive nitrogen balance | Albright/Forbes/Reifenstein |
| 1947 | First intravenous protein hydrolysate available commercially in Europe | Wretlind |
| 1948 | Intravenous infusion of cottonseed oil emulsions in dogs | Meng/Freeman |
| 1949 | Development of first continuous delivery technique for long-term intravenous infusion of nutrients in dogs | Rhoads/Parkins/Vars |

glucose, and electrolytes, but reported unequivocally that the subcutaneous injections of these nutrients were too painful to be practical clinically, and accordingly, these attempts at feeding were abandoned.

In 1873, Hodder[36] infused fat in the form of fresh cow's milk intravenously for fluid replacement, and *not* for nutritional purposes, into 3 cholera patients. Two of the patients survived, but the third patient died, adding credence to Courten's earlier observations that unmodified fats could not be given safely and effectively by vein.[23,36]

The discovery by Pasteur of the association of microorganisms with infection, and the introduction by Lister of the concepts of asepsis and antisepsis, together with the early development of anesthesia in the late 19th century, paved the way for safe and effective performance of surgical procedures in the 20th century.[37–39] Because major surgery required attention to maintaining fluid and electrolyte balance, intravenous fluid administration gradually was incorporated into the treatment regimen of the preoperative, operative, and postoperative patient.[17]

In 1895, Starling[40] made the important discovery of the colloid osmotic functions of plasma proteins, which continue to confound us today in the nutritional management of protein-depleted, septic patients, especially those in intensive care units with multiple systems failure. The following year, in 1896, Biedl and Kraus were the first to infuse glucose intravenously into human beings, but it was not until 15 years later, in 1911, that Kausch first infused glucose intravenously for nutritional purposes in to a surgical patient postoperatively.[41,42] In 1915, while using a pump to ensure constant infusion, Woodyatt and his coworkers[43] were the first to establish a dose-response relationship for intravenous glucose by varying the infusion rate while monitoring urinary glucose excretion. This classic human study demonstrated that up to 0.85 g of glucose per kilogram per hour, could be infused without causing glycosuria, thus establishing that providing intravenous glucose for nutrition was feasible clinically, and paving the way for experimentation with intravenous amino acids, polypeptides, lipids, and so forth.

At the turn of the 20th century, physicians and basic scientists were performing landmark research in several areas of importance to the optimal clinical management of patients including, but not limited to, the discovery of the 4 human blood groups; the development of dependable, accurate methods for analysis of urea, ammonia, creatinine, and other nitrogenous fractions of body fluids, useful for nutritional assessment; the discovery of vitamins as essential nutrients; the demonstration of use for nutritional therapy of intravenously infused hydrolyzed protein, plasma proteins, human serum, and emulsified fats; and the identification of the essential amino acids and their requirements for humans.[44–51]

By 1890, the medical literature had stressed the importance of sterilizing syringes and parenteral solutions, but febrile reactions accompanying infusions were common.[17,30] In 1923, Seibert[52] discovered that sterilized and stored metabolic products of microorganisms, called pyrogens, caused febrile reactions if the sterilized water had not been also properly distilled. Following this landmark discovery, the development and commercial production of intravenous solutions became possible, profitable, and practical, and began to flourish. The next year, in 1924, Matas,[53] a surgeon in New Orleans, was the first to use a continuous drip infusion of glucose in humans.

In the 1930s, another major milestone was reached by Cuthbertson's[54] persistent, elegant investigations and findings of the obligatorily increased urinary excretion of nitrogen, sulfur, phosphorus, and potassium (apparently secondary to muscle breakdown), particularly following major accidental injury such as fracture of one or more of the long lower limb bones, major burns, and multiple injuries. Increased urinary excretion of zinc and 3-methyl histidine and creatinine were also found in these patients who concomitantly exhibited associated increases in oxygen consumption and body core temperature with fever. This "catabolic response to injury" had occasionally been observed and noted before in patients following battle injuries, major operations, or major blood loss, but special attention to the unexpected, seemingly inordinate increase in urinary losses of nitrogen and the potential significance of this phenomenon had not been realized previously. Cuthbertson's observations and work redefined the understanding of, and revolutionized the approaches to, management of these patients to this day.[55,56]

In 1935, when a patient received an "IV feeding," as it was commonly called, the solution was poured into an open glass flask and capped with a plug of gauze until used. At the time of infusion, the neck of the flask was attached to a rubber stopper through which a glass tube, with one end in the fluid in the flask, was connected at the outside end to rubber intravenous (IV) tubing, and the flow rate was controlled with a metal screw clamp. Infusions took a few hours and then were discontinued. The glass flasks containing blood or fluids were often wrapped in hot water bottles "to prevent shock" to the patient, and while a patient received IV fluids, a nurse usually stayed at the bedside constantly.[17] Twenty-five years later, when the senior author (Stanly J. Dudrick) was a medical student at The Hospital of the University of Pennsylvania, more than 90% of IV solutions were manufactured in the hospital pharmacy and continued to be administered in this manner. Enormous progress has been made in parenteral fluid therapy in the past 50 years since then!

Another major contributor to the nutritional field during this time was Whipple, a pathologist and Nobel Laureate, who demonstrated the adverse effect of infection and nonbacterial injury on nitrogen catabolism.[31] He made the distinction between the *labile* protein (later known as visceral protein) reserves, which broke down easily and quickly in response to injury and appeared in the urine as urea, and the *stable* or fixed protein (later known as somatic or skeletal protein) reserves, which did not break down as early or easily. These studies complemented the earlier work of Folin,[57] who made the distinction between exogenous (dietary) and endogenous (body) protein metabolism based on the urinary output of creatinine, which was constant and represented endogenous protein metabolism versus urea, which fluctuated as a result of nitrogen intake and represented exogenous protein metabolism. Whipple showed further that if the labile protein reserves were depleted by a protein-deficient diet or by previous injury, the body lost its ability to respond to subsequent surgical or traumatic injury with the usual rapid and extensive protein catabolism and mobilization of protein moieties for recovery, repair, and healing. He also demonstrated in dogs that various proteins had different effects on restoring plasma proteins; for example, 10 grams of hemoglobin in the oral diet was required to produce 1 gram of plasma protein in a depleted dog, in contrast to 3 grams of plasma protein required orally to accomplish the same result (which led to the identification and designation of the biologic value of food proteins). He demonstrated that a dog could be maintained in nitrogen equilibrium when given intravenous plasma as the sole source of protein, provided that protein-sparing dosages of carbohydrate and fat were given simultaneously by mouth.[58] Later, in the 1950s, Allen and colleagues[59] repeated these experiments in immature, young dogs showing that the animals would grow when given intravenous plasma as the sole source of their protein requirements, provided that they received all other nonprotein requirements by mouth. These studies actually served as an encouraging intermediate step toward the TPN experiments performed in Beagle puppies a decade later by Dudrick.[31] Another important contribution by Allen[60] was his observation that storage of human plasma for 6 months at temperatures of 70° to 80°F inactivated any contaminating hepatitis virus. After confirmation by others, these findings led to major changes in blood-banking procedures, especially for plasma storage and transport.

In 1946, Albright and colleagues[61] studied the metabolic fate of human plasma protein infused intravenously into human beings who were not acutely ill and concluded that the 3 potentialities for intravenously infused plasma protein were (1) to be consumed or catabolized, which could be measured by increased nitrogen excretion; (2) to be converted into protoplasm, which could be measured by the decreased excretion of phosphorus and/or potassium; or (3) to remain in the recipient unchanged in form. However, their data did not provide direct evidence for, or against, the Whipple hypothesis that infused plasma protein is incorporated into protoplasm without first being broken down into amino acids and resynthesized. Despite the exhaustive work of Whipple, Albright, Allen, and others, considerable skepticism still exists among many investigators and clinicians to this day regarding the conclusiveness of the evidence for the precise metabolic use of intravenously infused plasma proteins.[62] At or about the same time, in the early 1940s, Cohn and colleagues,[63] stimulated by the involvement of the United States in World War II, performed successful fractionation of the proteins in human plasma. Their isolation of intact human serum albumin represents a most important accomplishment, especially for parenteral nutritional therapy.[62] The following excerpt from Levenson and colleagues[62] states the case for intravenous infusion of plasma proteins, especially albumin: *"Current practice varies among different physicians regarding the use of I.V. plasma proteins (principally albumin) as part of complete (or total) parenteral alimentation of patients. Our view is as follows: We would not use infusions of plasma proteins (principally albumin) as the only or chief parenteral source of amino acids, peptides and protein, but using them judiciously in conjunction with the infusion of amino acids when physiologically and clinically significant hypoalbuminemia is present seems eminently sensible. Hepatitis is not a risk with the commercially available albumin and plasma protein preparations, albumin generally making up about 85% of the total protein in the latter preparations. The ability to safely infuse albumin and thereby correct physiologically and clinically significant hypoalbuminemia without depending on hepatic albumin synthesis, which may be depressed in seriously ill and injured patients, is important. We are aware that the rate of albumin catabolism may be accelerated in seriously ill and injured patients; this is so for endogenously synthesized albumin as well as exogenously infused albumin, although catabolism of the latter may be faster if denaturation of the albumin has occurred during its processing."*[62(pp1391–406)]

The foregoing statement clearly and concisely also represents our philosophy for the use of albumin intravenously in malnourished critically ill patients, but with the added important caveat that albumin should not be infused intravenously into patients who are febrile or septic or for other reasons have lost normal structural capillary integrity. The infused albumin under those circumstances will likely leak through the porous vascular endothelium into the interstitial space, greatly increasing the risk of acute respiratory distress syndrome or shock lung syndrome and thereby increasing, rather than decreasing, morbidity and mortality. However, nonalbumin-containing TPN regimens can be given judiciously to such patients until sepsis and/or multiple systems failure are controlled, and afterward, albumin can be added safely to the nutritional regimen and increased cautiously as indicated, desired, or tolerated.

Major progress was made in the field of protein metabolism by the classic studies of Rose[64] in the 1930s, who determined the essential amino acids first in rats and then in humans, and subsequently proposed the ideal mixture and dosages of amino acids that might support protein synthesis in healthy adult human beings. As referred to earlier, one of his students was Elman,[14] a surgeon who published the first successful studies evaluating the intravenous infusion of amino acids in humans in the form of protein hydrolysates. Elman's work represents an important landmark in the development of TPN, which established unequivocally the importance of these nutrients in the nutritional support of seriously ill and injured patients. He greatly emphasized the importance of preventing nutritional deteriorization in surgical patients and the primacy of treating malnutrition if it were already present. He stated that *"the eventual behavior of amino acids after they leave the blood stream is not known in detail, although it would seem that basically it differs very little from the metabolism of amino acids absorbed into the portal circulation… that relatively little is lost as urine and that protein synthesis actually occurs is shown by the fact that the injection of adequate amino acid mixtures leads to the achievement of positive nitrogen balance, and to increase in serum albumin even when no other form of protein nourishment is given."*[13(pp437–40)] In the laboratory, Elman[13] showed further that serum proteins were regenerated faster in dogs that were proteins depleted by repeated hemorrhage, when a solution of 5% amino acids and 5% dextrose was infused than when 10% dextrose was infused alone. He began an intensive clinical investigation during the next several years, initially with acid hydrolysates of casein fortified with added tryptophan, and later with an enzymatic hydrolysate of casein with no added amino acid fortification.[65] Stimulated by Elman's studies, a large number of studies were performed by multiple other investigators using enzymatic protein hydrolysates, crystalline amino acids, or acid hydrolysates of casein with added tryptophan.[62] The first intravenous protein hydrolysate solution in Europe was developed by Wretlind[66] in 1944. In contrast to the acid hydrolysis preparations of Elman, Wretlind[66] hydrolyzed casein with pancreatic enzymes and dialyzed the resultant mixture to remove the larger polypeptides from the solution.

In part, related to the technological revolution associated with World War II, previously unprecedented basic and clinical scientific investigations throughout the world produced data and advances in technology at a higher rate than ever before, laying the groundwork for the enormous progress made in advancing nutritional support during the past half century. In the basic science laboratory of Rhode and colleagues,[67] the first continuous delivery technique for long-term IV infusion of nutrients was developed in dogs in 1949. In 1951, Yuilie and colleagues[68] infused isotopically labeled plasma proteins into dogs and found that after the IV injection of the carbon-labeled plasma, there was a rapid drop in plasma protein radioactivity, followed by a slow gradual decline, so that as much as 30% of the initial dose was still present in the circulation 1 week later. These findings contrasted markedly with those in animals in which the labeled plasma protein was fed orally. Yuilie and colleagues[68] interpreted their data as showing a rapid, complete breakdown of plasma protein to amino acids when it was given orally, but not when it was infused by vein. This observation was also somewhat in conflict with the Whipple hypothesis that intravenous plasma proteins could be incorporated into tissue protoplasm without first being broken down completely into amino acids.[62] This controversy remains unresolved and serves as a challenge to nutritional scientists for future clarification (**Table 2**).

Clinically, Aubaniac[69] published the first description of percutaneous subclavian venipuncture for the achievement of rapid blood transfusion in severely injured war victims in 1952. Another important and practical access advance was made in 1945 by Zimmermann,[70] who developed the first polyethylene catheters for IV infusions in humans. In 1959, Moore[6] demonstrated that the optimal nonprotein calorie:nitrogen ratio was 150:1 in humans. Although hundreds of fat emulsions of varying composition were studied throughout the world between 1920 and 1960, the cottonseed oil fat

**Table 2**
**Modern historical highlights in the development of total parenteral nutrition**

| Year | Accomplishment | Investigator |
|------|----------------|--------------|
| 1952 | First description of subclavian percutaneous venipuncture to achieve rapid transfusion in severely injured war victims | Aubaniac |
| 1956 | Demonstration that intravenous infusion of plasma protein in dogs fed a protein-free diet could support growth | Allen/Stemmer/Head |
| 1959 | Demonstration of optimal nonprotein calorie:nitrogen ratio as 150:1 in humans | Moore |
| 1961 | Development of first safe, standardized, and stable intravenous fat emulsion (soybean oil stabilized by egg phosphatides) | Schuberth/Wretlind |
| 1962 | Diuretics as an adjuvant in disposing of extra water used as a vehicle in parenteral nutrition | Rhoads |
| 1965 | Achievement of positive nitrogen balance by infusing high-volume nutrient solutions and diuretics by peripheral vein in humans | Rhoads et al |
| 1966 | Demonstration of long-term normal growth and development in Beagle puppies receiving total parenteral nutrition by central vein | Dudrick/Vars/Rhoads |
| 1967 | Infraclavicular subclavian percutaneous catheterization for central venous pressure monitoring in humans | Mogil/DeLaurentis/Rosemond |
| 1968 | Normal growth and development in an infant nourished entirely by central venous total parenteral nutrition; first use of in-line intravenous filter | Dudrick/Wilmore |
| 1968 | First comprehensive technique for long-term total parenteral nutrition in humans | Dudrick/Wilmore/Vars/Rhoads |
| 1968 | First patient supported entirely by total parenteral nutrition at home for 6 months | Dudrick/Steiger |

emulsion that emerged for commercial production and clinical investigation in the United States was associated with multiple serious adverse effects, including chills, fever, nausea, vomiting, dyspna, hypoxia, tachycardia, and hypotension, as well as hemolytic anemia, thrombocytopenia, hepatomegaly, splenomegaly, hyperbilirubinemia, and nondescript abdominal, flank, and back pain, and was withdrawn from the market.[71] These discouraging experiences occurred in the middle of the Dudrick puppy experiments and required modification of the originally used complete parenteral nutrition mixture, which included the cottonseed oil emulsion, to a formula that did not contain any fat as an energy source, both in the laboratory animals, and also subsequently clinically in the United States from 1964 until 1978.[55,72,73] The first nontoxic readily available fat emulsion was developed by Schuberth and Wretlind[74] in 1961. Initially, it seemed impossible to them to find any fat emulsions that did not cause adverse reactions in experimental animals. After several years, however, they found that an IV emulsion prepared from "natural food products" consisting of soybean oil with egg yolk phospholipids as an emulsifying agent, was nontoxic and without adverse effects when tested in animals for 28 days, even when given in amounts up to 9 g of fat per kilogram body weight per day.[75] Hallberg and colleagues[75] subsequently tested the new IV fat emulsion in surgical patients in 1963 and found that they tolerated the preparation very well. Subsequently, in 1966, Hallberg and colleagues[75] alleged that the fat particles in the soybean oil emulsion were eliminated from the bloodstream in the same way and at the same rate as natural chylomicrons. This declaration has subsequently been found to be incorrect, and it is now well known that the emulsified soybean oil particles are not metabolized like chylomicrons, but are actually ingested in a similar manner to foreign bodies or bacteria by macrophages and other cells in the reticuloendothelial system. Subsequently, the 1-$\mu$m oil droplets are broken down intracellularly in the leukocytes and released through their cell membranes back into the blood as fatty acids for distribution to the body cell mass by the circulation.[76] This represents a fruitful area for future basic and clinical investigation. On the positive side, IV fat emulsion not only serves as a high-density caloric source that can be infused into peripheral as well as central veins, but also provides essential fatty acids (for which the requirements are increased in seriously ill and injured patients) and choline (as part of the egg phosphatide stabilizer).[62] Despite years of investigation, controversies persist regarding the relative protein-sparing effects of intravenous glucose and/or intravenous fat emulsion in critically ill and injured patients who are hypermetabolic; and the likelihood of impairment of pulmonary and/or reticuloendothelial cell function and the secondarily decreased resistance to infection after infusions of IV fat emulsions.[77] Increasing evidence to date suggests that IV emulsions of medium-chain triglycerides may be better used by severely injured patients than IV long-chain triglycerides, although the requirement for some long-chain fatty acids will still exist.[62]

Another area of controversy related to the infusion of the currently available fat emulsions is the biochemically and biophysically unsound admixture of the fat emulsions with the crystalloid components of complete parenteral nutrition mixtures, despite the currently popular introduction of the "all-in-one" system, in which all nutrients of the parenteral nutritional regimen, consisting of water, carbohydrates, fat, amino acids, vitamins, and trace elements, are mixed in one bag shortly before infusion, primarily to simplify and reduce the costs of the formulations.[71,78] Additionally, it is believed that the steatosis and cholestasis, especially of newborn infants requiring long-term TPN, but also in some adults, is most likely caused by the currently nonphysiologic fat emulsions, and several studies appear to substantiate this hypothesis.[78,79] The need for the development of truly physiologic fat emulsions for the maximal safety and efficacy of all patients requiring TPN in the future is obvious—another opportunity for future research and development. This important area of endeavor is presented and discussed extensively in the article by the Puder group elsewhere in this issue.

It is interesting that other than blood, the first substance infused intravenously to achieve potential beneficial effects more than 350 years ago was alcohol.[18] In 1891, Atwater and Benedict[80] showed that oral ethyl alcohol was used efficiently as a caloric and protein-sparing nutrient in human beings, providing 7 calories per gram. More than 60 years later, Rice and Stricker,[81] in 1952, showed comparable use when ethyl alcohol was infused intravenously. They showed further that the intoxicating level of blood alcohol is about 0.15 g per deciliter, that sedation occurs at a blood alcohol level of about 0.06 to 0.08 g per deciliter, and that ethyl alcohol could be infused slowly and continuously in amounts to provide a maximum of 700 calories per day in human subjects while maintaining the blood level below the intoxicating level. Subsequently, a commercial preparation became available in the United States for intravenous infusion, containing casein hydrolysate, dextrose, and ethyl alcohol.[62] It was used sparingly for a number of years without obvious and adverse effects, but intravenous ethyl alcohol is used extremely rarely today as a caloric source following the demonstration by Lieber[82] that ethyl alcohol can be hepatotoxic even when the nutrient intake is otherwise adequate.

Although most clinicians in the 1950s were aware of the negative impact of malnutrition on morbidity, mortality, and outcomes, only a relatively small percentage of practicing physicians and surgeons understood the necessity for providing optimal nutritional support for their malnourished patients if optimal clinical results were to be obtained. However, the prevailing dogma in the 1960s was that feeding entirely by vein was impossible; if it were possible, it would be impractical; and even if it were practical, it would be unaffordable. TPN was considered a "Holy Grail" or "Gordian Knot" pursuit by most physicians and surgeons of that time. This negative attitude formed the wall of ignorance, prejudice, and indifference that had to be penetrated by, first, developing all of the substrates in a compatible form that could be delivered to a seriously ill patient intravenously to provide adequate nourishment. Second, demonstrating in the experimental laboratory that such a solution, together with an appropriate safe, and effective delivery system, could provide all essential nutrients in quality and quantity sufficient to support animals for long periods of time. And third, if the animal experiments were successful, applying the techniques and technology, and the knowledge gained in the basic laboratories to safe, effective clinical use in human beings.[83,84]

The initial fundamental hindrances to the development of TPN in the 1960s were (1) insistence on use of a peripheral vein as the infusion route for nutrient fluids; (2) the inherent limitation of the volume of water that could be tolerated per day by the average adult patient (2500–3500 mL); (3) the inadequacy of the number, type, form, and compatibility of nutrient substrates available commercially for parenteral use; and (4) inadequate facilities and resources for solution formulation, modification, storage, and distribution in most hospitals.[83]

The standard of care at that time was to infuse isotonic or near-isotonic solutions into the peripheral veins of the upper extremity after inserting metal needles of various sizes into the lumens of the limited number of accessible veins in the arms and hands. Indwelling plastic catheters were not yet available for routine clinical indwelling use, and the sharp needles inserted directly into the veins for infusion often penetrated the back or side walls of the veins with subsequent infiltration of the infusate into surrounding tissues and even back-bleeding into the tissues. Phlebitis and thrombosis were frequently encountered despite changing the site of venipuncture virtually daily. Armboards or other devices that were used to stabilize the venipuncture site limited the motion and use of the extremity, contributing to patient dissatisfaction and discomfort, and compromising patient ambulation. During the course of a prolonged hospitalization, the accessibility of available upper extremity veins was usually exhausted within a few days. Despite a reluctance to use lower extremity veins because of the attendant increased incidence of associated phlebitis, thrombosis, pulmonary embolism, and infection, saphenous vein cut-downs were used at times for life-saving infusions, especially in dire emergency situations, and were usually removed in 3 to 4 days. The only medical-grade plastic tubing available for use in these situations was polyethylene, which was nonstandardized, often stiff, and had a tendency to kink or fragment in addition to causing inflammatory, thrombotic, and/or toxic reactions in some patients.

Another hindrance to providing adequate nutrient substrates by peripheral veins was the requirement that solutions be isosmotic with the body fluids (290–300 mOsm/L) to minimize physical and chemical trauma to the intima of the blood vessels and to the formed elements of the blood. Because of the limited volume of water that could be infused safely in the average adult patient (25–35 mL/kg/d or 2000–3000 mL/d), especially in seriously ill malnourished patients, excessive water retention and large increases in total body water accompanied attempts to increase the volume of intravenous isotonic nutrient solutions, often precipitating pulmonary edema, congestive heart failure, atelectasis, pneumonia, pleural effusions, and ileus. No safe, effective intravenous diuretics were available clinically at that time, and the responsiveness to the standard mercurial intramuscular diuretics was poor or unreliable, and often accompanied by metabolic derangements.[83]

The inherent caloric value of the basic individual nutrients, ie, 3.5 to 4.0 kcal per gram of carbohydrate, 4.0 to 4.25 kcal per gram of protein or amino acids, 9.0 to 9.1 kcal per gram of fat, and 7.0 kcal per gram of ethanol, were immutable metabolic restrictions, just as they are today. Moreover, the maximum effective metabolic rate of use of these and the other nutrients (vitamins, minerals, and trace elements) had to be determined and calculated individually, and in combinations, to avoid potentially untoward effects of administering these biochemically active substrates injudiciously. The nutrient products available commercially for safe and effective long-term total or complete parenteral nutrition were inadequate at their worst, and suboptimal at their best. No intravenous formulations of amino acids were available clinically, and the only source of protein moieties available for clinical intravenous infusions were unstable, nonstandardized, incompletely hydrolyzed fibrin and casein hydrolysates. The only source of intravenous lipid was an experimental cottonseed oil emulsion that was unstable, nonstandardized, incompletely emulsified, and accompanied by a sufficiently high rate and severity of complications that it was withdrawn even from investigational availability in the mid-1960s.[56,83] The divalent cations that were available for IV therapeutic infusion (calcium, magnesium) were not intended for use as admixtures for nutritional purposes and were incompatible when combined together. Moreover, none of the other divalent cations essential for TPN were available commercially in IV form, nor were IV solutions of iron or phosphorus. No commercial sources of intravenous trace elements were available either individually or as mixtures. There were no commercially available complete IV vitamin mixtures, no complete IV water-soluble vitamin mixtures, no complete fat-soluble vitamin mixtures, and no specific combinations of IV vitamins formulated specifically to meet pediatric or adult maintenance or therapeutic requirements. Thus, the impediments to the development of TPN were quite formidable and frustrating for those who sought to provide adequate nutritional support parenterally 4 to 5 decades ago.[85]

The general prerequisites that had to be met for developing safe and effective TPN included (1) formulate complete parenteral nutrient solutions; (2) concentrate the subsequent nutrient substrate components to 5 to 6 times isotonicity without adverse interactions or precipitation to meet tolerable fluid restrictions; (3) demonstrate the utility and safety of central venous catheterization access; (4) demonstrate the practicality, efficacy, and safety of long-term continuous central venous infusion of hypertonic nutrient solutions; (5) maintain asepsis and antisepsis throughout the entire continuum of solution preparation, admixture, and infusion; and (6) anticipate, avoid, and correct nutritional and metabolic imbalances or derangements. Additionally, the requirements for nutrients given intravenously to achieve TPN had to be determined or estimated from existing oral nutritional data because precise comprehensive parenteral nutrient requirements or recommendations were not available. The compatibility of the individual components of the intravenous nutrient regimen had to be determined, ensured, and maintained under a number of variable situations, including ambient temperature changes, exposure to light, time from formulation to infusion, transportation, shelf life, and so forth. The risk of infection had to be eliminated or minimized to an acceptable level. As the former was probably impossible, in view of the fact that a foreign body (catheter) had to be passed through the skin into the bloodstream and remain in place for prolonged periods of time, the latter was essential. Pharmaceutical and medical technology companies had to be convinced to develop, produce, and market the nutrient components and apparatus for administration of TPN within a reasonably affordable cost. Procedures and tests had to be established to assess and monitor the safety and efficacy of a TPN program. Continuous infusion of the solution at a constant rate throughout each 24-hour period had to be maintained to ensure the administration of the maximal metabolizable or utilizable dosages of each of the nutrients in the mixture. This concept was quite different from the usual infusion practices at that time. Physical, fiscal, and personnel resources had to be appraised to determine the feasibility of an undertaking of this magnitude. Furthermore, it was essential to overcome decades of written and verbal expressions by prominent physicians and scientists that long-term TPN was either impossible, improbable, impractical, or folly. Plausible fundamental evidence to the contrary had to be generated if skepticism and prejudices were to be neutralized or overcome, and if widespread clinical acceptance was eventually to occur. Accordingly, efforts were directed toward designing experiments in the laboratory to explore and verify the efficacy and safety of TPN with the ultimate goal of applying clinically to patients the basic knowledge, skills, and techniques that had been acquired, developed, and mastered in animals.[83]

The decision to abandon peripheral venous infusion in favor of central venous infusion as the preferred route for providing all required nutrients entirely by vein was a key factor leading to the successful development and clinical application of TPN. The quantity of high-quality nutrients required to achieve and maintain positive nitrogen balance and its associated clinical benefits in a critically ill patient had to be concentrated in a volume of water that could be tolerated without untoward "overload" complications. The resulting hypertonic nutrient solutions exceeded the normal osmolarity of the circulating blood approximately sixfold (1800 mOsm/L) or more. The infusion of hypertonic solutions of this order of magnitude into peripheral veins caused an intolerable degree of pain, together with an inevitable and unjustifiable inflammation of the intima of the vein and damage to the formed elements of the blood, resulting in inordinate phlebitis and thrombophlebitis, and associated adverse secondary consequences and complications. However, it was discovered and demonstrated in the animal laboratory, and subsequently confirmed in human subjects and patients, that hypertonic solutions, when infused at a constant rate over the 24 hours of each day through a catheter with its tip in a large central vein, such as the superior vena cava, were rapidly diluted virtually to iso-osmolarity by the high blood flow in this major vein. By titrating the nutrient and water administration precisely to the metabolic needs and tolerances of each patient, the nutrients and the water were removed or extracted from the circulation at approximately the rate of infusion, thus avoiding problems of hyperosmolarity, overhydration, exceeding renal excretion thresholds for the nutrients, and/or nutrient losses in the urine. Accordingly, the successful development of TPN was eventually possible in large part because of the associated technical advances leading to safe, long-term, central venous access.[83]

The fundamental principles of the Total Parenteral Nutrition Project were to (1) calculate the calories, amino acids, and all micronutrients required for the achievement of positive nitrogen balance, weight gain, tissue synthesis and repair, and/or normal growth and development; (2) concentrate the nutrient substrates in the volume of water that the patient can tolerate and metabolize safely and efficaciously; (3) infuse the resultant nutrient formulation continuously at the rate of optimal use, preferably by a pump, into a large central vein wherein the high blood flow (about 50% of cardiac output) can instantly dilute the relatively small incremental volume of the hypertonic infusate to near isotonicity; (4) maintain aseptic and antiseptic conditions during all phases of preparation, modification, and infusion of the formulation, and throughout the achievement and long-term maintenance of central venous access; during handling, transport and management of all components of the infusion and administration apparatus; and in all other aspects of the comprehensive care of the patient to minimize the ever-present threat of infection and sepsis. Before these principles could be applied morally, ethically, and practically to human subjects or patients, they required testing and validation in the basic experimental laboratories of the Harrison Department of Surgical Research.

After an extensive survey of the available literature, a plan evolved to concentrate the nutrients required for growth and development of Beagle puppies into the quantity of water the animals could tolerate per day and infuse the resultant 30% hypertonic solution (1800–2400 mOsm/L) into a large-diameter, high blood flow central vein where it could be diluted instantly to isotonicity.[14,59,86,87] Continuous infusion of the nutrient formulation at the maximum rates of use and tolerance, without exceeding renal threshold for the individual nutrients, was an additional goal of the protocol. An effective practical apparatus that was counterbalanced and used a specially designed swivel to permit maximum mobility of the animal in the cage was engineered, crafted, and tailored over a period of several months specifically for continuous intravenous infusions into active, unrestrained puppies.[67,72,88–90]

An intravenous dietary regimen was formulated that most closely approximated that of the known oral dietary requirements for growth and development of Beagle puppies. Although attempts were initially made to grow newborn puppies, the technical, biochemical, and immunologic difficulties encountered in this endeavor were so overwhelming at that time that this ambitious, idealistic goal was temporarily abandoned. Therefore, the next logical hallmark of growth and development at which to initiate total parenteral feeding experiments was at 8 weeks of age when puppies are normally weaned from the breast.[83]

Although the recommended daily allowance of protein for an 8-week-old Beagle puppy is 8.8 g per kilogram body weight per day, only 4 grams of protein per day in the form of fibrin hydrolysate could be infused without inducing toxicity reactions in the puppies, manifested by lethargy, vomiting, and periorbital and perioral swelling and redness. Accordingly, in addition to infusing the daily recommended carbohydrate dose, 4 additional grams of carbohydrate per kilogram as dextrose was given to spare the administered nitrogen maximally and to maintain the recommended daily total caloric ration. Because the experimental cottonseed oil emulsion was still available at that time, it was possible to provide the exact recommended ration of fat intravenously in this form. Over a period of approximately 2 to 4 hours per day, 2.6 g of fat per kilogram body weight were infused into the puppies during the initial experiments. However, when the cottonseed oil emulsion was withdrawn abruptly from the market, the IV diet was modified in the second group of experimental animals so that the daily dosage of fat was calculated to provide only the minimal requirements for linoleic acid (0.6 g fat emulsion per kilogram body weight per day). In the third set of animals, fat was necessarily eliminated completely from the IV regimen because the supply of the lipid emulsion had been exhausted. As the fat in the IV diet was decreased, carbohydrate calories in the form of dextrose were increased equivalently to maintain an isocaloric ration of 130 calories per kilogram body weight per day.[83]

To provide all electrolyte requirements in one solution, it was necessary to bind the calcium and phosphate ions organically individually to prevent precipitation as calcium phosphate. Calcium was added in the form of calcium gluconate and/or calcium heptonate, and phosphate was supplied as sodium or potassium glycerophosphate. Several months of tedious trial and error experiments were required to formulate the electrolyte and trace element solutions in which all of the components were mutually soluble and compatible. During the course of the experiments, a trace element solution evolved that contained cobalt, copper, iodine, manganese, molybdenum, and zinc. The remaining essential electrolytes in the solutions were necessarily added individually.[83]

Providing the recommended vitamins for growth in Beagle puppies was problematic. First of all, no vitamin preparation containing all of the vitamins required for growth in Beagle puppies in parenteral form was available commercially. Moreover, vitamin C, essential for human beings, is not required by dogs; biotin and choline, which at that time were considered conditionally essential for human beings, are required for dogs; and para-amino-benzoic acid (PABA) is a vitamin in dogs, but not in human beings. Biotin, choline, and PABA were obtained in crystalline form, dissolved in water, sterilized, and added to the solution individually. Commercial mixtures of the B-complex vitamins, vitamin A, vitamin D, and vitamin K were added separately. When an experimental multivitamin infusion became available several months after the puppy experiments began, the ease of providing most of the water-soluble and fat-soluble vitamins for dogs, including vitamin E, was enhanced greatly. Vitamin $B_{12}$, folic acid, and vitamin K, however, had to be added individually to the solution immediately before infusion because they were not in the original multiple vitamin infusion mixture.

The superior vena cava was chosen as the best venous route for delivery of the hypertonic nutrient mixtures. To confirm that adequate mixing of the continuously infused solution occurred within a reasonable distance from the tip of the catheter, preliminary studies were performed as follows. Two catheters were inserted into the superior vena cava, one via a jugular vein and the other via an iliac vein, and advanced so that the tips of the catheters were virtually touching each other. As the hypertonic solution was infused at the appropriate rate through the cephalad catheter, the caudad catheter was withdrawn 1 centimeter at a time sequentially, and blood samples were obtained carefully at each level to avoid a streaming effect through the caudad catheter for determination of osmolarity and glucose concentration. In this way, it was shown consistently that the blood in the superior vena cava had normal osmolarity and normal glucose concentration within 1.5 to 2.5 cm from the tip of the infusion catheter while the nutrient solutions were administered at appropriate rates.[83]

Every commercially available infusion catheter known to exist at the time was tested for tissue tolerance and toxicity, by initially implanting them in subcutaneous tissue and subsequently in peripheral veins in adult dogs and observing the relative tissue reactivity to the various plastic products. Subsequently, the least reactive catheters were inserted into an external jugular vein of various mongrel dogs, advanced into the superior vena cava distally until the tip of the catheter was situated just above the right atrium of the heart, secured with sutures, and tunneled proximally subcutaneously from the base of the neck to emerge through the skin at a point midway between the scapulae under meticulous aseptic and antiseptic operating room conditions. A custom-made soft canvas harness was attached to an aluminum or stainless steel support apparatus, which secured the catheter to the animal at its exit site while providing a point of attachment to the infusion administration apparatus. Polyethylene catheters were found to be the most reactive, most thrombogenic, and least durable, and were associated with the highest incidence of kinking, spontaneous rupture, and other mechanical difficulties. Polytetrafluoroethylene (Teflon) catheters were too rigid in the forms available at that time and were associated with untoward perforation of the venous system. Silicone rubber (Silastic) catheters were the least reactive, but were the most difficult to insert and advance into the proper position, the most difficult to maintain secured in place, and the most likely to rupture spontaneously. Moreover, they were not radiologically opaque at that time. Polyvinyl chloride catheters had the best overall properties and characteristics and were, therefore, chosen for use in the Beagle puppy study. Parenthetically, the original polyvinyl tubing used was not medical grade, but was designed for use as insulation for electrical wire. One such catheter remained in situ safely and usefully for 170 days before it polymerized and fractured. It was successfully replaced by another identical catheter, which survived and functioned well for the 12 subsequent weeks in that experimental animal.[83]

To minimize the introduction of microorganisms around the catheter exit site, a 2-inch-square area of skin surrounding the site was kept shaved, and was prepared with a 2% tincture of iodine followed by application of 1 gram of triple antibiotic ointment daily at the exit site. The solutions were admixed in a relatively clean area of the laboratory, with strict adherence to the usual aseptic and antiseptic principles and precautions during addition of the components to the reservoir bottle, but about 18 individual manipulations were required to complete the preparation of each unit of the nutrient solution. The high risk of contamination during preparation was obvious and ever present. Formulation was eventually performed in a laminar-flow, filtered air environment, which reduced solution contamination to 1% to 3%. To reduce further the risk of delivery of microorganisms to the puppies via the infusate, a 1-inch-diameter membrane filter (Millipore) having an average pore size of 0.22 $\mu$m, was incorporated into the delivery system as a "final filter" to prevent the infusion of any microorganisms that might have been introduced into the solution inadvertently during preparation. The reduction in the incidence of sepsis in the pilot series of animals following this innovation was dramatic and significant and allowed progression of the experimental protocol to the next stage with reasonable expectations of success.[83]

The original aim of the study was to support growth and development in the puppies for 10 weeks. During the academic year 1965–1966, 6 male pedigreed Beagle puppies were fed entirely by central venous infusion for 72 to 256 days and compared with their littermates fed orally.[72] After weaning at 8 weeks of age, the puppies were paired according to their size and weight since birth, housed individually in metal cages, and fed a standard oral diet for 4 weeks to determine their indigenous growth rates. At 12 weeks of age, a polyvinyl catheter was inserted into an external jugular vein and advanced into the mid-superior vena cava of one of the puppies in each pair. The proximal end of the catheter was directed subcutaneously with a trocar and brought out through a puncture wound in the skin between the scapulae. A blunt needle was inserted into the catheter and secured to the back of the animal by a specially designed stainless steel support apparatus and an adjustable, tailored canvas harness. A counterbalanced, swiveled infusion assembly was connected internally to delivery tubing attached to the catheter by a Luer fitting and externally from the swivel to the support apparatus on the animal's back by a modified speedometer cable, which protected the vinyl delivery tubing. A peristaltic pump anchored to the top of the cage propelled the solution dependably to the animal below at the desired rate through a 0.22-$\mu$m membrane filter attached to the swivel assembly.[91] This specifically engineered apparatus allowed the animal freedom of movement within the cage. During the continuous infusion daily over a 21-hour to 23-hour period, the animals received the dosages of dextrose, protein hydrolysate, and all of the vitamins and minerals recommended for growth. In the dietary regimens, which included intravenous lipid, the emulsion was infused separately over a 2 to 3 hours. The puppies were disconnected from the infusion apparatus for the remaining 0.5 to 1.0 hour daily for exercise and recreation. The 6 puppies fed entirely intravenously outstripped their control orally fed littermates in weight gain and matched them in skeletal growth, development, and activity for the study periods of 72 days, 100 days (3 puppies), 235 days, and 256 days. Moreover, no significant differences could be discerned among the puppies receiving the 3 experimental diets, which differed primarily in fat content.[83]

The 2 longest-term animals, which were fed for 235 and 256 days, more than tripled their body weights and developed comparably to their control littermates. In both groups, the deciduous teeth were shed and replaced with permanent teeth at the same time. The intravenously fed animals were just as energetic as the controls and demonstrated no obvious abnormalities of their skin, coats, or bony development. Having thus demonstrated beyond a doubt that it was possible and practical to feed animals entirely by vein for prolonged periods of time without excessive risks, or compromises of growth and development potential, attention was directed toward applying what had been learned in the laboratory to the treatment of surgical patients.[83]

Accordingly, 6 severely malnourished patients with chronic complicated gastrointestinal problems were nourished for 15 to 48 days entirely by vein with a modified puppy formula.[72] The human adult parenteral solution, consisting of 20% dextrose, 5% fibrin hydrolysate, electrolytes, trace minerals, and vitamins, was infused continuously through an indwelling catheter inserted percutaneously into the external jugular vein and advanced into the mid-superior vena cava. Strict aseptic and antiseptic surgical technique was observed during the insertion and long-term maintenance of the central venous catheter.[92] To minimize contamination with microorganisms, the skin around the catheterization site was cleansed every 3 days with an iodine solution, antibiotic ointment was applied, and the sterile gauze occlusive dressing was replaced. Infusion catheters were maintained in place safely and effectively sepsis-free for several weeks.[93,94]

The basic nutrient solution, composed of 1000 calories (1 kcal/mL) and 6 grams of nitrogen per liter, was formulated and membrane sterilized daily by the manufacturing pharmacist at The Hospital of the University of Pennsylvania.[95] Each morning after biochemical and hematologic indices had been determined, appropriate electrolytes, trace elements, and vitamins were added to the base solution. Starting in each patient at established levels of fluid metabolism and carbohydrate use (about 2400 mL), the intravenous nutrient infusion was gradually increased to maximum levels of tolerance (up to 4500 mL). For optimal efficiency of use, the solution was administered as constantly as possible over 24 hours daily by gravity drip because intravenous pumps and apparatus were not then available clinically. Daily weight measurements; fluid balance and urine sugar determinations every 4 hours; and regular serum concentrations of electrolytes, glucose, urea nitrogen, and creatinine served as fundamental guides for monitoring the administration of the embryonic TPN solution.[96–98]

Positive nitrogen balance was achieved in all of the first 6 patients, together with weight gain, normal wound healing, and increased strength, activity, and sense of well-being in a variety of generally catabolic clinical situations. All were discharged from the hospital in good condition despite the originally grave prognoses related to their severely malnourished state.[72,73]

Although these seriously malnourished adults were studied initially, the opportunity and challenge to adapt and apply the puppy experience to a human infant arose within a few months after the laboratory successes with intravenously fed puppies.[99] In July 1967, at the Children's Hospital of Philadelphia, a newborn female infant underwent operation for near-total small bowel atresia.[100] Following massive intestinal resection, her duodenum had been anastomosed to the terminal 3 cm of ileum; her weight had declined from 5.5 pounds at birth to 4.0 pounds at 19 days of age; she appeared catabolic, hypometabolic, and moribund; she had no jejunum; and had only 1% to 2% of her ileum; and it was obvious that she was dying of starvation.

Accordingly, a polyvinyl catheter was inserted via cut-down into her right external jugular vein, advanced into her superior vena cava, and the other end passed subcutaneously behind her right ear to emerge through the parietal scalp. It was anticipated theoretically, and based on the puppy experience, that the skin tunnel would reduce the chances of introducing microorganisms into the circulatory system. The infant was initially infused cautiously with a basic nutrient mixture containing hypertonic dextrose, fibrin hydrolysate, electrolytes, and vitamins. Each day or so, another nutrient was added to the mixture so that if the infant experienced an adverse reaction related to the formula change, the probable cause would likely be more apparent. The infusion was delivered continuously by a Harvard peristatic pump though a closed intravenous administration system containing an in-line 0.22-μm membrane filter.[91] Prevention of infection was foremost in this model because it was anticipated that the infection rate associated with an indwelling central venous foreign body inserted percutaneously would be 100% if left in place indefinitely.

The baby weighed 5.1 pounds at birth and 4.0 pounds when the catheter was inserted. Forty-five days later, she had gained 3.5 pounds in weight and had increased 5.5 cm in length. Her head circumference increased by 6.5 cm, and she manifested normal activity and development for her age.[100] She was fed for 22 months primarily by vein and achieved a maximum weight of 18.5 pounds. She had undergone central venous catheterization via her jugular veins 6 times, her saphenous vein once, her cephalic vein once, and her subclavian veins 8 times. Although she eventually died, clinicians gained a tremendous experience metabolically and technologically during her management, and her legacy to pediatric parenteral nutrition is unparalleled.[101–103]

In the first few adult patients to whom the technique of central venous feeding was applied via the superior vena cava, the catheters were inserted through an external jugular vein by cut-down or percutaneously. However, because of troublesome problems either in advancing the catheter to the desired position or maintaining it free of infection, a more proximal and less mobile site of insertion was desirable. Thus, percutaneous subclavian vein catheterization, which had been used infrequently clinically, since its inception in 1952, for monitoring central venous pressure, was explored as an access route for continuous long-term hypertonic central venous feeding.[69,104,105] The principles and techniques of asepsis and antisepsis, and the advances both in catheter and insertion technology that developed during subsequent clinical trials, have minimized the risks of infection and, with appropriate care and management, have allowed long-term feeding catheters to remain in place safely and effectively for months or years.[106,107] The components of TPN solutions have improved over the years and are likely to continue to undergo modification, testing, and application as more knowledge and experience are gained in this vital area of clinical biochemistry and nutritional support.[108–111]

Although currently available knowledge, components, and techniques of parenteral nutritional support have been shown to be utilitarian and life-saving in a wide variety of clinical conditions, TPN support today is still not ideal.[112–122] Much basic and clinical investigation remains to be accomplished and must be stimulated, encouraged, and supported if this technique is to be perfected to achieve the ultimate goal of providing optimal nutrition to all patients, under all conditions, at all times.[123] In the words of the eminent biochemist and nutritionist, Sir David Cuthbertson,[55(pp1–11)] *"Lest we forget, I would remind you that we all owe our foetal life till parturition to the passage of the nutrients we require from the blood vessels of our mothers into our blood vessels as they traverse the chorionic villi in close relation."* It is important for us to recall that we all began our lives as human beings in utero, receiving our nourishment entirely by vein, and we must continue our quest to attempt to emulate that ideal model of intravenous feeding for the support of those who might require a period of TPN for sustaining postnatal life.

Long-term TPN was inaugurated successfully as a safe and efficacious basic and clinical feeding technique more than 40 years ago. It has been credited for having been instrumental in saving countless lives, and has clearly demonstrated the relevance of adequate nutrition to the achievement of optimal clinical results in surgical patients of all ages, leading to the enormous increase in the use of enteral feeding in all varieties of patients whose oral intakes are inadequate to support normal nutritional status and metabolic function. Furthermore, the subsequently obvious need for special ambulatory and home parenteral and enteral feeding capabilities has stimulated the unbridled development of home health care not only in the United States, but throughout the world. Innovative development and maturation of the technology and techniques that are likely to occur in this field in the future are most promising, almost incomprehensible, and virtually unlimited.

## REFERENCES

1. Dudrick SJ. Foreword. In: Langas A, Goulet O, Quigley EM, et al, editors. Intestinal failure—diagnosis, management and transplantation. Malden (MA): Blackwell Publishing Co; 2008. p. xiii, xv.
2. Beal JM, Payne MA, Gilder H, et al. Experience with administration of an intravenous fat emulsion to surgical patients. Metabolism 1957;6(6 Pt 2):673–81.
3. Dennis C. Ileostomy and colectomy in chronic ulcerative colitis. Surgery 1945; 18:435–40.
4. Dudrick SJ, Lehr HB, Senior JR, et al. Nutritional care of the surgical patient. Med Clin North Am 1964;48:1253–69.
5. Holden WD, Krieger H, Levey S, et al. The effect of nutrition on nitrogen metabolism in the surgical patient. Ann Surg 1957;146(4):563–77 [discussion 577–9].
6. Moore FD. Metabolic care of the surgical patient. Philadelphia: W.B. Saunders Company; 1959.
7. Ravdin IS, McNamee HG, Kamholz JH, et al. The effect of hypoproteinemia on susceptibility to shock resulting from hemorrhage. Arch Surg 1944;48:491–7.
8. Rhoads JE, Alexander CE. Nutritional problems of surgical patients. Ann N Y Acad Sci 1955;63(2):268–75.
9. Rhoads JE, Kasinskas W. The influence of hypoproteinemia on the formation of callus and experimental fracture. Surgery 1942;11:38–43.
10. Thompson WB, Ravdin IS, Frank IL. Effects of hypoproteinemia on wound disruption. Arch Surg 1938;35:500–3.
11. Mecray MC, Barden RP, Ravdin IS. Nutritional edema: its effects on gastric emptying time before and after gastric operations. Surgery 1937;1:53–5.
12. Elman R, Weiner DO. Intravenous alimentation with special reference to protein (amino acid) metabolism. J Am Med Assoc 1939;112:796–802.
13. Elman R. Amino acid content of the blood following amino acid injection of hydrolyzed casein. Proc Soc Exp Biol Med 1937;37:437–40.
14. Elman R. Parenteral replacement of protein with the amino-acids of hydrolyzed casein. Ann Surg 1940;112(4):594–602.
15. Elman R. Parenteral alimentation in surgery with special reference to proteins and amino acids. New York: Hoeber Inc; 1947.

16. Harvey W. Exercitatio Anatomica de Motu Cordis et Sanguinis in Animalibus. Francofurti (Italy): Sumptibus F. Fitzeri; 1628.
17. Millam D. The history of intravenous therapy. J Intraven Nurs 1996;19(1):5–14.
18. Wren C. An account of the method of conveying liquors immediately into mass of blood. As reported by Henry Oldenburn. Philos Trans R Soc Lond 1665.
19. Denis JB. A letter concerning a new way of curing diseases by the transfusion of blood. Philos Trans R Soc Lond 1667;2:489–504.
20. Lower R. The method observed in transfusing blood out of one live animal into another. Philos Trans R Soc Lond 1666;1666(1):353–8.
21. Lower R. An account of the experiment of transfusion, practiced upon a man in London. Philos Trans R Soc Lond 1667;2:557–64.
22. Escholtz J. Clysmatica Nova. Sive Ratio qua in Venam Sectam Medicamenta Immitti Possint. Amsterdam: Berloni; 1665.
23. Courten W. Experiments and observations of the effects of several sorts of poisons upon animals made at Montpellier in the years 1678 and 1679 by the late William Courten. Philos Trans R Soc Lond 1712;27:485–500.
24. Blundell J. Successful case of transfusion. Lancet 1829;431–2.
25. Latta T. Relative to the treatment of cholera by the copius injections of aqueous and saline fluids into the veins. Lancet 1831;2:274–7.
26. O'Shaghnessy WB. Proposal of the new method of treating the blue epidemic cholera by the injection of highly oxygenated salts into the venous system. Lancet 1831–1832;1:366–71.
27. Latta T. Malignant cholera. Lancet 1831–1832;2:274–7.
28. Latta T. Injections in cholera. Lond Med Gazz 1832;379–82.
29. Nuland SB. The Doctors' plague: germs, childbed fever, and the strange story of Ignac Semmelweis (Great discoveries). New York: W.W. Norton; 2003.
30. Dudrick SJ. History of vascular access. JPEN J Parenter Enteral Nutr 2006; 30(Suppl 1):S47–56.
31. Rhoads JE, Dudrick SJ. History of intravenous nutrition. In: Rombeau JL, Caldwell MD, editors. Clinical nutrition-parenteral nutrition. Philadelphia: W.B. Saunders Company; 1993. p. 1–10.
32. Bernard C. Lecons sur les Proprietes Physiologiques et les Alterations Pathologiques de Liquides de l' Organsisme. Paris: J B Balliere 1859;2. p.459.
33. Whittaker JT. Hypodermic alimentation. The Clinic 1876;10:37.
34. Menzel A, Perco H. Ueber die resorption von, Nahrungs Mitteln Vom Unterhautzellgewebe Aus. Wien Med Wochenschr 1869;19:517.
35. Friedrich PL. Die kunstliche subkutane ernahrung in der praktischen chirurgie. Chir Arch klin Chir 1904;73:507–16.
36. Hodder E. Transfusion of milk in cholera. Practitioner 1873;10:14–6.
37. Bigelow HJ. Insensibility during surgical operations produced by inhalation. Boston Med Surg J 1846;35:309–17.
38. Lister J. On the effects of the antiseptic system of treatment upon the salubrity of a surgical hospital. Lancet 1870;1:4–6, 40–2.
39. Pasteur L, Joubert JV. Charbon et septicemie compte V Hebd Seave. Acad Sci Paris 1870;85:101–15.
40. Starling EH. On the absorption of fluids from the connective tissue spaces. J Physiol 1895;19:312–26.
41. Kausch W. Ueber intravenose und subkutane emahrung mit traubenzucker. Dtsch Med Wochenschr 1911;37:8.
42. Biedl A, Kraus R. Uber intavenose traubenzucker infusionen an menschen. Wien Med Wochenschr 1896;9:55–8.

43. Woodyatt RT, Sansum WD, Wilder RM. Prolonged and accurately timed intravenous injections of sugar. JAMA 1915;65:2067–70.

44. Folin O. Laws governing the chemical composition of urine. Am J Physiol 1905; 13:66–115.

45. Funk C. The etiology of the deficiency disease. J State Med 1912;20:341–68.

46. Rose WC. Nutritional significance of amino acids. Physiol Rev 1938;18:109–36.

47. Schmidt JE. Medical discoveries: who and when. Springfield (IL): Bannerstine House; 1959.

48. Murlin JR, Riche JA. Blood fat in relation to depth of narcosis. Proc Soc Exp Biol Med 1915;13:7–8.

49. VanSlyke DD, Meyer GM. The fate of protein digestion products in the body III. the absorption of amino-acids from the blood by the tissues. J Biol Chem 1913; 16:197–212.

50. Henriques V, Andersen AC. Uber parenterale ernahrung durch intravenose injecktion. Hoppe Seylers Z Physiol Chem 1913;88:357–69.

51. Lansdsteiner K. Uber intravenose traubenzucker infusionen an menschen. Wien Med Wochenschr 1901;9:55–8.

52. Seibert FD. Fever producing substance found in some distilled waters. Am J Physiol 1923;67:90–104.

53. Matas RM. The continued intravenous "drip". Ann Surg 1924;79:643–61.

54. Cuthbertson DP. Observation on the disturbance of metabolism produced by injury to the limbs. Q J Med 1932;25:233–46.

55. Cuthbertson D. Historical background to parenteral nutrition. Acta Chir Scand Suppl 1980;498:1–11.

56. Cuthbertson DP. Second Annual Jonathan E. Rhoads Lecture. The metabolic response to injury and its nutritional implications: retrospect and prospect. JPEN J Parenter Enteral Nutr 1979;3(3):108–29.

57. Folin O. The American Journal of Physiology volume XIII: 117–138, 1905. A theory of protein metabolism. Nutr Rev 1975;33(5):141–3.

58. Terry R, Sandrock WE, Nye RE, et al. Parenteral plasma protein maintains nitrogen equilibrium over long periods. J Exp Med 1948;87:547–59.

59. Allen JG, Head LR, Stemmer E. Similar growth rates of litter mate puppies maintained on oral protein with those on the same quantity of protein as daily intravenous plasma for 99 days as only protein source. Ann Surg 1956;144(3): 349–55.

60. Allen JG. The epidemiology of post-transfusion hepatitis. Basic blood and plasma tabulations. Stanford (CA): J. Garrott Allen; 1972.

61. Albright F, Forbes AP, Reifenstein EC. The fate of plasma proteins administered intravenously. Trans Assoc Am Physicians 1946;59:221–34.

62. Levenson SM, Hopkins BS, Waldron M, et al. Early history of parenteral nutrition. Fed Proc 1984;43(5):1391–406.

63. Cohn EJ, Oncley JL, Strong LE, et al. Chemical, clinical and immunological studies on the products of human plasma fractionation. 1. The characterization of the protein fraction of human plasma. J Clin Invest 1944;23:417–32.

64. Rose WC. The significance of amino acids in nutrition. Harvey Lect 1934;30: 45–65.

65. Cox M, Mueller AJ. Nitrogen retention on casein digestions. Proc Soc Exp Biol Med 1939;42:658–63.

66. Wretlind A. Free amino acids in a dialyzed casein digest. Acta Physiol Scand 1947;13:45–54.

67. Rhode CM, Parkins W, Vars HM. Method for continuous intravenous administration of nutritive solutions suitable for prolonged metabolic studies in dogs. Am J Physiol 1949;159(3):409–14.
68. Yuilie CL, Lamson BG, Miller LL, et al. Conversion of plasma protein to tissue protein without evidence of protein breakdown. Results of giving plasma proteins labelled with carbon 14 parenterally to dogs. J Exp Med 1951;95: 539–57.
69. Aubaniac R. Subclavian intravenous injection; advantages and technic. Presse Med 1952;60(68):1456 [in Undetermined Language].
70. Zimmermann B. Intravenous tubing for parenteral therapy. Science 1945; 101(2631):567–8.
71. Vinnars E, Wilmore D. Jonathan Rhoads symposium papers. History of parenteral nutrition. JPEN J Parenter Enteral Nutr 2003;27(3):225–31.
72. Dudrick SJ, Wilmore DW, Vars HM, et al. Long-term total parenteral nutrition with growth, development, and positive nitrogen balance. Surgery 1968;64(1): 134–42.
73. Dudrick SJ, Wilmore DW, Vars HM, et al. Can intravenous feeding as the sole means of nutrition support growth in the child and restore weight loss in an adult? An affirmative answer. Ann Surg 1969;169(6):974–84.
74. Schuberth O, Wretlind A. Intravenous infusion of fat emulsions, phosphatides and emulsifying agents. Acta Chir Scand Suppl 1961;278:1–21.
75. Hallberg D, Schuberth O, Wretlind A. Experimental and clinical studies with fat emulsion for intravenous nutrition. Nutr Dieta Eur Rev Nutr Diet 1966;8(3): 245–81.
76. Seidner DL, Mascioli EA, Istfan NW, et al. Effects of long-chain triglyceride emulsions on reticuloendothelial system function in humans. JPEN J Parenter Enteral Nutr 1989;13(6):614–9.
77. Abbott WC, Grakauskas AM, Bistrian BR, et al. Metabolic and respiratory effects of continuous and discontinuous lipid infusions. Occurrence in excess of resting energy expenditure. Arch Surg 1984;119(12):1367–71.
78. Clayton PT, Bowron A, Mills KA, et al. Phytosterolemia in children with parenteral nutrition-associated cholestatic liver disease. Gastroenterology 1993;105(6): 1806–13.
79. Iyer KR, Spitz L, Clayton P. BAPS prize lecture: new insight into mechanisms of parenteral nutrition-associated cholestasis: role of plant sterols. British Association of Paediatric Surgeons. J Pediatr Surg 1998;33(1):1–6.
80. Atwater WO, Benedict FC. An experimental inquiry regarding the nutritive value of alcohol. Mem Natl Acad Sci 1897;8:235.
81. Rice CO, Stricker JL. Parenteral nutrition in elderly surgical patients. Geriatrics 1952;7:232–40.
82. Lieber CS. Hepatic and metabolic effects of alcohol. Gastroenterology 1966; 50(1):119–33.
83. Dudrick SJ. Early developments and clinical applications of total parenteral nutrition. JPEN J Parenter Enteral Nutr 2003;27(4):291–9.
84. Dudrick SJ. Rhoads lecture: a 45-year obsession and passionate pursuit of optimal nutrition support: puppies, pediatrics, surgery, geriatrics, home TPN, A.S.P.E.N., et cetera. JPEN J Parenter Enteral Nutr 2005;29(4):272–87.
85. Geyer RP. Parenteral nutrition. Physiol Rev 1960;40:150–86.
86. Clark DE, Brunschwig A. Intravenous nourishment with protein, carbohydrate and fat in man. Proc Soc Exp Biol Med 1942;49:329–32.

87. Helfrick FW, Abelson NM. Intravenous feeding of a complete diet in a child: report of a case. J Pediatr 1944;25:400–3.

88. Dudrick SJ, Steiger E, Wilmore DW, et al. Continuous long-term intravenous infusion in unrestrained animals. Lab Anim Care 1970;20(3):521–9.

89. Dudrick SJ. Total intravenous feeding and growth in puppies. Fed Proc 1966; 1966(25):481.

90. Dudrick SJ, Vars HM, Rhoads JE. Growth of puppies receiving all nutritional requirements by vein. Fortschr Parenteral Ernahrung 1967;1:1–4.

91. Wilmore DW, Dudrick SJ. An in-line filter for intravenous solutions. Arch Surg 1969;99(4):462–3.

92. Wilmore DW, Dudrick SJ. Cannula sepsis. N Engl J Med 1967;277(8):433–4.

93. Dudrick SJ, Wilmore DW. Long-term parenteral feeding. Hosp Pract 1968;3: 65–78.

94. Wilmore DW, Dudrick SJ. Safe long-term venous catheterization. Arch Surg 1969;98(2):256–8.

95. Serlick SE, Dudrick SJ, Flack HL. Nutritional intravenous feeding. Bull Parenter Drug Assoc 1969;23(4):166–73.

96. Travis SF, Sugerman HJ, Ruberg RL, et al. Alterations of red-cell glycolytic intermediates and oxygen transport as a consequence of hypophosphatemia in patients receiving intravenous hyperalimentation. N Engl J Med 1971;285(14):763–8.

97. Allen TR, Ruberg RL, Dudrick SJ. Hypophosphatemia occurring in patients receiving total parenteral hyperalimentation. Fed Proc 1971;30:580.

98. Sugerman H, Travis SF, Pollock T. Alterations in oxygen transport and red cell metabolism as a consequence of hypophosphatemia in intravenous hyperalimentation. Clin Res 1971;19:487.

99. Steiger E, Dudrick SJ, Daly JM. Growth and development of puppies nourished intravenously with crystalline amino acids as the sole source of dietary nitrogen. Fed Proc 1970;29:364.

100. Wilmore DW, Dudrick SJ. Growth and development of an infant receiving all nutrients exclusively by vein. JAMA 1968;203(10):860–4.

101. Dudrick SJ, Groff DB, Wilmore DW. Long-term venous catheterization in infants. Surg Gynecol Obstet 1969;129(4):805–8.

102. Wilmore DW, Dudrick SJ. Effects of nutrition on intestinal adaptation following massive small bowel resection. Surg Forum 1969;20:398–400.

103. Wilmore DW, Groff DB, Bishop HC, et al. Total parenteral nutrition in infants with catastrophic gastrointestinal anomalies. J Pediatr Surg 1969;4(2):181–9.

104. Dudrick SJ, Rhoads JE. Total intravenous feeding. Sci Am 1972;226(5):73–80.

105. Mogil RA, DeLaurentis DA, Rosemond GP. The infraclavicular venipuncture. Value in various clinical situations including central venous pressure monitoring. Arch Surg 1967;95(2):320–4.

106. Dudrick SJ, Ruberg RL. Principles and practice of parenteral nutrition. Gastroenterology 1971;61(6):901–10.

107. Dudrick SJ, Long JM, Steiger E. Intravenous hyperalimentation. Med Clin North Am 1970;54:577–89.

108. Daly JM, Dudrick SJ, Vars HM, et al. The effects of protein depletion on colonic wound healing in rats. Fed Proc 1971;30:298.

109. Daly JM, Vars HM, Dudrick SJ. Correlation of protein depletion with colonic anastomotic strength in rats. Surg Forum 1970;21:77–8.

110. Ruberg RL, Dudrick SJ, Long JM, et al. Pre- and postoperative nutrition using crystalline amino acid as the sole source of nitrogen. Fed Proc 1971;30:300.

111. Steiger E, Dudrick SJ, Daly JM, et al. Effects of postoperative intravenous nutrition on serum proteins, body weight and liver morphology in protein depleted rats. Fed Proc 1971;30:580.
112. Dudrick SJ. Intravenous feeding as an aid to nutrition in disease. CA Cancer J Clin 1970;20:198–211.
113. Dudrick SJ, Steiger E, Long JM, et al. Role of parenteral hyperalimentation in management of multiple catastrophic complications. Surg Clin North Am 1970;50:1031–8.
114. Dudrick SJ, Wilmore DW, Steiger E, et al. Reversal of uremia and body wasting with intravenous essential amino acids. Fed Proc 1969;28:808.
115. Dudrick SJ, Wilmore DW, Steiger E, et al. Intravenous essential amino acids and hypertonic glucose in the treatment of renal failure. Medizin und Ernährung 1970;11:111–7.
116. Dudrick SJ, Wilmore DW, Steiger E, et al. Spontaneous closure of traumatic pancreatoduodenal fistulas with total intravenous nutrition. J Trauma 1970;10: 542–53.
117. Wilmore D, Dudrick SJ. Treatment of acute renal failure with intravenous essential L-amino acids. Arch Surg 1969;99:669–73.
118. Wilmore D, Dudrick SJ, Samuels GSA, et al. The role of nutrition in small bowel adaptation following massive intestinal resection. Fed Proc 1969;28:305.
119. Dudrick SJ, Rhoads JE. New horizons for intravenous feedings. JAMA 1971; 215:939–49.
120. Dudrick SJ, Steiger E, Long JM. Renal failure in surgical patients: treatment with intravenous essential amino acids and hypertonic glucose. Surgery 1970;68(1): 180–5.
121. Long JM, Steiger E, Dudrick SJ, et al. Total parenteral nutrition in the management of esophagocutaneous fistulas. Fed Proc 1971;30:30.
122. Steiger E, Wilmore DW, Dudrick SJ, et al. Total intravenous nutrition in the management of inflammatory disease of the intestinal tract. Fed Proc 1969; 28:808.
123. Dudrick SJ. Presidential address: the common denominator and the bottom line. JPEN J Parenter Enteral Nutr 1978;2(1):13–21.

# Index

Note: Page numbers of article titles are in **boldface** type.

Surg Clin N Am 91 (2011) 719–726
doi:10.1016/S0039-6109(11)00056-9
0039-6109/11/$ – see front matter © 2011 Elsevier Inc. All rights reserved.

surgical.theclinics.com

# Moving?

## Make sure your subscription moves with you!

To notify us of your new address, find your **Clinics Account Number** (located on your mailing label above your name), and contact customer service at:

**Email: journalscustomerservice-usa@elsevier.com**

**800-654-2452** (subscribers in the U.S. & Canada)
**314-447-8871** (subscribers outside of the U.S. & Canada)

**Fax number: 314-447-8029**

**Elsevier Health Sciences Division**
**Subscription Customer Service**
**3251 Riverport Lane**
**Maryland Heights, MO 63043**

*To ensure uninterrupted delivery of your subscription, please notify us at least 4 weeks in advance of move.